MACROBIOTIC PREGNANCY
and Care of the Newborn

By the same Authors:

MICHIO KUSHI: *The Book of Macrobiotics: The Universal Way of Health and Happiness*

————— : *The Book of Do-In: Exercise for Physical and Spiritual Development*

————— : *Natural Healing Through Macrobiotics*

————— : *How to See Your Health: The Book of Oriental Diagnosis*

————— : *Cancer and Heart Disease: The Macrobiotic Approach to Degenerative Disorders*

AVELINE KUSHI: *How to Cook with Miso*

MACROBIOTIC PREGNANCY
and Care of the Newborn

by Michio and Aveline Kushi

edited by Edward and Wendy Esko

foreword by Christiane Northrup, M.D.

Japan Publications, Inc.

Note to the reader: It is advisable to seek the guidance of a qualified
health professional and macrobiotic counselor before implementing the
dietary and other suggestions for specific conditions presented in this
book. It is essential that any reader who has any reason to suspect
serious illness in themselves or their family members seek appropriate
advice promptly. Neither this or any other book should be used as a
substitute for qualified care or treatment.

Published by JAPAN PUBLICATIONS, INC., Tokyo

Distributors:
UNITED STATES: *Kodansha International/USA, Ltd., through Harper & Row,
Publishers, Inc., 10 East 53rd Street, New York, New York 10022.* SOUTH
AMERICA: *Harper & Row, Publishers, Inc., International Department.*
CANADA: *Fitzhenry & Whiteside Ltd., 150 Lesmill Road, Don Mills,
Ontario M3B 2T6.* MEXICO AND CENTRAL AMERICA: *HARLA S. A. de C. V.,
Apartado 30–546, Mexico 4, D. F.* BRITISH ISLES: *International Book
Distributors Ltd., 66 Wood Lane End, Hemel Hempstead, Herts HP2 4RG.*
EUROPEAN CONTINENT: *Boxerbooks, Inc., Limmatstrasse 111, 8031 Zurich.*
AUSTRALIA AND NEW ZEALAND: *Book Wise (Australia) Pty. Ltd., 101 Argus
Street, Cheltenham Victoria 3192.* THE FAR EAST AND JAPAN: *Japan Publica-
tions Trading Co., Ltd., 1–2–1, Sarugaku-cho, Chiyoda-ku, Tokyo 101.*

First edition: January 1984

ISBN 0–87040–531–4

Foreword

So often during my medical training I've been struck by how much time we spend treating chronic degenerative diseases that might have been prevented in the first place. Renowned epidemiologist, Denis Burkitt, M.D., has likened the problem to a sink overflowing with water. Despite hours of mopping and even the creation of chief moppers, subspecialty moppers, improved mops, and even institutions devoted to mopping skills, the water keeps overflowing unless someone turns off the tap.

The information contained in this book is a very good way to start turning off those taps. One of the main reasons I went into obstetrics is because I can't think of a better place to enhance health and prevent illness than before one is born, and, in my practice, more and more couples are seeking preconception advice as well as prenatal care.

As the working mother of two small children, one of whom is still nursing, I know well the stress of raising children in our current society. There never seem to be enough hours in the day to do all the tasks required, let alone to exercise, meditate, and engage in other health-enhancing activities. This is precisely why macrobiotics is so practical and fulfilling, because, no matter what else happens during the day, you know that the meals you've prepared will enhance your family's health, and not a day goes by in which one doesn't eat. Cooking this way is sort of a daily meditation, and as my pregnant sister-in-law said after a recent meal with us, "Eating this way makes me happy."

It's very important, though, particularly with children, not to get too rigid about diet. Children must not be made to feel socially isolated by their food. Healthy children will want to try all types of food no matter what their quality may be. If a child's constitution is basically strong, she or he will be able to process almost anything without much of a problem. That is why it's so important to eat well prior to and during pregnancy as well as during lactation because then, by virtue of a strong constitution, you'll be giving your child the gift of freedom to experience the world relatively free of illness. Remember, though, that our daily thoughts are also part of our daily nourishment, and, for that reason, constant worry and concern over what goes into our mouths, especially when pregnant, can potentially have a negative effect on our unborn child. In fact, Thomas Verney's book, *The Secret Life of the Unborn Child*, documents the far-reaching effects of a mother's thoughts on her unborn child!

So, as in all things, we must strive to make balance between our physical and mental nourishment.

This book should be used as a guideline for your childbearing and childrearing experience but not as a rigid set of rules.

Remember that each individual is different and each woman brings to her pregnancy her own set of values, beliefs, and state of health. So, for some, for example, a cesarean delivery done in a large medical center with a good nursery may be a more holistic and fulfilling setting than a birthing center just as for some women the benefits of anesthesia during delivery far outweigh the disadvantages. In general, though, in most deliveries, the less intervention the better.

In my current practice, straddling the fence between traditional Western allopathic medicine and more alternative modalities such as macrobiotics, I am reminded daily of how much each has to offer. The best of both worlds would be to combine them into one all-encompassing, nonjudgmental approach. Although it seems that all too often our scientific left-brained training precludes this, more and more physicians are awakening to this need.

For those of you just getting started with macrobiotics and wanting to do what is best for your families, let me leave you with the following thoughts:

- Don't feel guilty if you didn't know about macrobiotics when you were pregnant and, therefore, think you might have been responsible for some problem a child has. Remember that all the cells in our body are replaced every seven years and that the human body is amazingly adaptable. So, it's never too late to start. I am constantly amazed by how quickly positive results can be achieved through changes in diet.

- You needn't be concerned about the adequacy of the diet. With study, care, and planning, the macrobiotic diet for pregnancy and childrearing can contain all the nutrients needed for optimal growth and development without all the pesticide residues and saturated fats of the standard American diet. In fact, recent studies point out that without consuming whole grains and legumes, the average American cannot obtain enough nutrients from his or her daily food without supplements.

- In my three years of involvement with macrobiotic people I've found that regardless of what their parents look like, macrobiotic children are consistently beautiful. A grain-based diet returns to us the facial features we were meant to inherit.

- Macrobiotics, in my opinion, is second only to love in its power to heal and make balance, and because so much love and caring goes into good cooking, you can give your children both at the same time.

- Finally, remember that you and I are pioneers in this new (though ancient) way of life. It's not yet a comfortable position to occupy, but with a sense of humor, it can be exhilarating.

CHRISTIANE NORTHRUP, M.D.
Fellow of the American College of
Obstetricians and Gynecologists
Portland, Maine
July, 1983

❀ | Preface

Our civilized world is facing a great crisis of human existence on this planet Earth, especially as we approach the 21st century. This crisis has two aspects: 1) possible nuclear warfare which may instantaneously annihilate a majority of the world's population in industrialized societies, and 2) rapid biological degeneration of human life which may result in the physical, psychological, and social deterioration of the species.

These two issues, however, are closely related and the second—biological degeneration of human life—is actually the basis for the first crisis.

The problem we all are confronted with today is to discover how to maintain and improve the quality of human life, not through theory, idealism, or other conceptual means, but by the practical method of recovering our health and developing our judgment.

To prevent and relieve degenerative disorders such as heart disease, cancer, arthritis, allergies, sexually transmitted disease, mental disorders, and wild, anti-social behavior is, of course, a paramount issue to be solved as soon as possible. However, for the future of human society, the physical and psychological health of coming generations, our children, grandchildren, and their offspring, is a more essential task.

This book deals with securing the health and well-being of the coming generation, especially in the all-important beginning stage of pregnancy and birth and discusses how to avoid possible defects and disorders that are increasingly affecting the newborn. The purpose of this book, although it appears to be on the subject of health, is to offer a possible entrance to a new world of peace and happiness which will be built by parents and children who have recovered their vitality and understanding. The solution presented in this book is simple. It involves the correction of environmental conditions and dietary habits as well as the reorientation of modern life toward more simple, clear, and natural ways of living. Unlike conventional medical texts and complicated technologies, this book suggests more common, intuitive approaches to solve complex problems.

Macrobiotic education began more than sixty years ago. It started in America and Europe thirty-five years ago, and has since spread throughout the world. It revolutionized the food patterns of modern society by starting the natural foods movement and it has contributed simple and revolutionary solutions for all contemporary health issues, especially physical and psychological disorders. As the number of families following this approach grows, macrobiotic education will also provide the foundation for the recovery of family happiness and community health. Macrobiotics further offers a solution for complex world issues, including social, economic, and political difficulties and even a solution for the prevention of nuclear war. As it spreads internationally, the macrobiotic way of life will create better health at all levels, elevate the human spirit, and eventually lead to the realization of our common dream of one peaceful world.

The contents of this book have been gathered, reviewed, revised, and edited from lectures and seminars which we have presented in various countries for the past thirty years and from ongoing classes at the Kushi Institute, the East West Foundation, East West Centers, and other macrobiotic educational institutions. We are especially grateful to Edward and Wendy Esko, who have been long time associates in our educational activities and who are both qualified macrobiotic teachers and counselors, for compiling and editing these materials. We are also grateful to Christiane Northrup, M.D. of Portland, Maine, who is a pioneer in the field of a natural and macrobiotic approach to pregnancy, childbirth, and women's health issues, for reviewing the manuscript and contributing valuable insights based on her experience as an obstetrician. We also extend our gratitude to Alex Jack of Brookline, Massachusetts who has studied with us for more than ten years and to Phillip Jannetta, now living in Tokyo, who has also studied with us for more than seven years, for reviewing the text and making many helpful suggestions. We further wish to thank Florence Nakamura, Diane Coffey, and Phoebe Hackett for their efforts in typing and preparing the manuscript in correct form, and also extend appreciation to Pamela Snyder, Judith Waxman, Carol Smith, Tonia Gagne, and Carolyne Cesari for contributing personal accounts of pregnancy and giving birth. We also wish to mention the special participation of Peter Harris and Melissa Sweet, who contributed the charts, diagrams, and illustrations. The publisher, Japan Publications, Inc. of Tokyo, and their representatives, Mr. Iwao Yoshizaki and Mr. Yoshiro Fujiwara, have been a constant source of encouragement in making this information available to you and your family.

We sincerely hope this book will contribute to the health and well-being of mothers, fathers, babies, and children, now and in the future. With endless prayer for the betterment of humanity, let us join together to realize one peaceful world on this wonderful planet.

MICHIO KUSHI
Brookline, Massachusetts
July, 1983

There are two events in our life that are inevitable. These two events are birth and death. All other happenings—travel plans, career plans, family plans, study, and others—are changeable.

In simple words, we can compare our life to that of an arrow which has been shot by an archer. The way in which the arrow proceeds to its target depends on the archer and how well he or she has mastered the bow. The best archer can make the arrow go swiftly, strongly, and directly to its target. So it is with our life. We can compare the pregnant mother to the archer and the unborn child to the arrow. The target is a long, healthy, and happy life, ending in a peaceful death. A very strong start with a natural pregnancy and birth will guide or direct us through an easy, happy, and healthy life. This strong-quality force or power to direct our lives is a tremendous gift from our parents, which we, in turn, pass on to our children. It is truly more valuable than material possessions.

I come from a family with nine brothers and sisters. I am the third eldest. My mother actually had a total of twelve pregnancies. During my mother's last pregnancy, the doctor felt that she was too weak to carry the baby for the entire nine-month period. He recommended that she have an abortion. I was twenty-two years old at the time and I accompanied my mother to the hospital. The pregnancy was terminated. I remained at the hospital with my mother for a couple of days. The next to the last baby was very big at birth. The doctor had to use forceps to remove it, and the baby was injured. It lived only a very short time afterwards. Between my mother's seventh and eighth child there was a very healthy boy baby, but when he was two-and-a-half years old he drowned in a nearby pond. I remember my mother crying every night after my brother's death for three years until the birth of her next baby. Nine of us grew up without any particular difficulties or sickness. The second child, a daughter, was married to a border police guard who was stationed in Manchuria toward the end of World War II. During this time the Soviet Union attacked Manchuria. After the war somebody told us that my sister, her husband, and their son had committed suicide rather than be captured. The remaining eight children now have families and are happy without any serious problems.

As a child I can remember listening to conversations between my parents and our family doctor. He was a very traditional physician and in addition to his regular practice was also in charge of 600 children at school. According to his experience a child would have a healthy, strong constitution and live a long life if the parents, which at that time meant especially the husband, did not indulge in drinking *sake* or other alcoholic beverages. Many cultures around the world have had the same view. Today we are now being warned of alcoholic substances as well as drugs, coffee, and other stimulants. This is important not only for the wife but also for the husband, as you will see by reading this book. Of course, when I was a child, over a half century ago, there was less danger because we did not have chemicalized foods, drugs, or other dangerous substances, especially in the countryside of Japan. My father, after the age of twenty-one, never drank *sake* or smoked cigarettes and, of course, my mother never did so during her whole life.

My parents were very honest people and pioneers of the Christian movement. They were the first couple in my village to be married in a Christian service instead of the traditional ceremony. My father was drafted into military training around this time and always carried a Bible with him. He was put into military prison for carrying his Bible but was such an excellent soldier that he was soon released and permitted to carry his scriptures.

Reflecting back on this time, I can now see just how much my parents have given me, through their discipline and dedication. They gave my brothers and sisters and me a strong power of perseverance and endurance which is so important to sustain us through life. Because of them I was able to put my whole life's effort into preventing future wars and to furthering peace. Shortly after World War II I discovered macrobiotics and found that it was a tool to help accomplish this goal. Because of my parents I could pursue my life's goal with stamina and clarity. I deeply appreciate my parents' life and all that they have given to me and my family.

My husband and I have five children, one daughter and four sons, and three grandchildren. When we came to this country, few macrobiotic or high quality natural foods were available as they are now. Breast-feeding was not so popular at that time, but I would not have raised my children in any other way. From the beginning we ate very simple macrobiotic meals. Each child was so different, and I often asked myself what food did I take with each pregnancy to accoun tfor the change. I can now recall how each of their conditions and personalities was shaped and influenced by my activity, eating, lifestyle, and environment.

As we have mentioned in the book, the nine-month period during pregnancy is a very important time to create a happy, strong, and healthy baby. The unborn child is influenced physically, mentally, and spiritually by the mother's way of eating, thinking, activity, and behavior. If during this period you can care well for your unborn child, it makes a great difference. Ideally, it is best to prepare for pregnancy before conception arises. This can be done by living the macrobiotic way of life and eating a macrobiotic diet.

I have had the good fortune to have met Miss Gloria Swanson, to become her friend, and to know her personality and life story. She was truly a remarkable person. In fact, I can honestly say that she was one of the greatest women I have met in my lifetime. There are many things which I clearly remember having learned from her. She was kind enough to write the introduction to my first book —How to Cook with Miso— and I would like to share a part of that introduction with you here because I feel that her words perfectly express our feelings concerning the importance of pregnancy. Miss Swanson is writing about a dinner Michio and I had at her home and she says:

> "My wife is much more strict about what she eats than I am," he (Micho) explained. Mrs. Kushi blushed faintly, lifting her hand to her face. "But I must be," she smiled. "I have five children. I never know when I may be pregnant again. By the time I discover I am pregnant, three, four or six weeks might have passed. The first weeks are so important. I must be careful never to eat anything not right for this new life inside me."

An increasing number of children are brought into existence each year deformed and retarded. We may be approaching the point where healthy children are becoming a minority group. Government or medical science cannot save us.

We can only save ourselves if women can liberate themselves and can accept personal responsibility for the future of their children, as Mrs. Kushi has shown us where it begins. Let us be grateful for this opportunity to learn from her.

There are many things in our lives which we forget or allow to pass by unnoticed, but Gloria Swanson very carefully watched her friends and nature as you can see from her remarks. I feel embarrassed by her compliments and am grateful to have known such a woman.

I hope this book will be helpful for you and that you share its message with your relatives and friends. Let us work together to create one peaceful world for our children, who are the future of humanity.

AVELINE KUSHI
Brookline, Massachusetts
June 23, 1983

❀ |Editors' Note

We stand at the crossroads of time. Like the grains of a cereal plant, we are both the fruit of an endless past and the seed of an infinite future. The influence that we receive from parents and ancestors is therefore incalculable, as is that which we pass on to our children and their descendants. A story from our family illustrates this well.

About a year ago, Edward's parents visited Brookline together with his mother's mother, who is now close to eighty. They brought a stack of books that had been in his grandmother's attic for many years. They were dusty and yellow with age and had titles like *Nature Cure*, *Food Is Your Best Medicine*, and *Be Happier, Be Healthier*. We were delighted to learn that she had long ago become interested in natural foods and healing and at one time had practiced a natural diet with plenty of whole grains and fresh local vegetables.

Edward's paternal grandmother had a similar interest in good food as a result of her experiences in early life. About ten years ago, before we were married, we visited her at her small country store outside of Philadelphia. She was in her eighties and listened approvingly as we described our macrobiotic diet. When we happened to mention *kasha*, or whole buckwheat, her eyes lit up and she began to reminisce, saying, "When I was a girl, growing up on a farm in the old country, *kasha* was our meat." She then told us about her diet during childhood which consisted mainly of whole grains, including *kasha* and dark wheat and rye breads, and fresh local vegetables. She was especially fond of cabbage which was often fermented and eaten as sauerkraut. She told us that meat and other animal products were eaten rarely; much less so than at present.

As Michio has often said, our dream of life is inherited from our parents and ancestors. We now know that our macrobiotic way of life, and the dream of a healthy and peaceful world, is simply the outcome of the diet, way of life, and vision of the future which these and other ancestors cherished.

It is with great joy that we offer this book, *Macrobiotic Pregnancy and Care of the Newborn*, to you. After a long gestation period—more than a year and a half— it has been delivered naturally, at home, and without complications, and is ready to begin an independent life in the world. We hope that you find as much joy in reading and using it as we have had in conceiving and delivering it.

As we mention throughout the book, a positive attitude based on faith in God or the infinite order of the universe is a very important factor in a healthy pregnancy. We would like to offer you a short poem which we feel symbolizes this spirit. We have set it to a universally known melody, the *Ode to Joy* chorus from Beethoven's *Ninth Symphony*. Please feel free to make it your own and to sing it throuhout pregnancy together with your friends and family members.

The poem is as follows:

Macrobiotica
The way of health and happiness.
Yin, yang in harmony
With life and nature guiding us.
Self-reflection
And transformation
Living with an endless dream.
One grain, ten thousand grains
With gratitude eternally.

EDWARD and WENDY ESKO
Brookline, Massachusetts
July, 1983

❃ | Contents

8 | Recipe Guide, 213

9 | Pregnancy and Birth Experiences, 231

1 | Reproducing Ourselves

All things in the universe can be divided into two: day and night, birth and death, spring and fall, man and woman, sperm and egg. One category is created and influenced more by centrifugality, or expansion. This tendency is referred to as yin and is often represented by an inverted triangle ($\triangledown$). The other, complementary category is created more by the force of centripetality, or contraction. This tendency is referred to as yang and is often represented by an upright triangle ($\triangle$). The terms yin and yang were coined many thousands of years ago and are still used throughout the Orient. Although the terminology may be different, a similar view of nature and the universe is common to all great cultures in both East and West and North and South.

Yin and yang do not represent certain phenomena, however, nor are they pronouns for certain things. Rather, they show relative tendencies, compared dynamically. The comparative classifications on the next page show practical examples of the antagonistic, complementary nature of yin and yang.

On this planet the tendencies of yin and yang appear as the forces of heaven and earth. Spiralling in from infinite space towards the center of the earth, heaven's force—including cosmic rays, electromagnetic and light radiation, solar energy and air pressure—moves in a counterclockwise motion. This is the same direction as the rotation of the earth. In the Orient, this more yang force is called *Ten-no-Ki*, meaning the energy of heaven.

Earth's force is generated outward from the center towards infinite space, by the rotation of the planet. It moves in a clockwise spiral. (These directions are the opposite in the Southern Hemisphere.) This more yin force is called *Chi-no-Ki*, or the energy of the earth. Between these two antagonistic yet complementary motions, all things on the earth and in the relative, ever changing world, are created, sustained, destroyed and are eventually reborn in the eternal cycle of life.

Nothing can exist by one force alone. For instance, if something were dominated totally by heaven's force, it would immediately contract to an infinitesimal point and disappear. If something manifested earth's force alone, it would expand to an infinitely large size and would also no longer exist. Both forces act in every phenomenon.

Men receive heaven's counterclockwise force through the spiral at the back of the head. Heaven's force enters the head and, passing downward, charges the midbrain. This central region, deep within the brain, is the center of the nervous system and consciousness. All nervous impulses and stimulation gather here and are then distributed to the left and right hemispheres of the brain and to the entire body.

Passing downward, heaven's force creates the *uvula*, the fleshy lobe that hangs down at the entrance to the throat. From here, it is transmitted to the root of the tongue and, passing further downward, charges the heart and makes it beat.

Examples of Yin and Yang

General	YIN ▽ * Centrifugal force	YANG △ * Centripetal force
Tendency	Expansion	Contraction
Function	Diffusion	Fusion
	Dispersion	Assimilation
	Separation	Gathering
	Decomposition	Organization
Movement	More inactive and slower	More active and faster
Vibration	Shorter wave and high frequency	Longer wave and low frequency
Direction	Ascent and vertical	Descent and horizontal
Position	More outward and periphery	More inward and central
Weight	Lighter	Heavier
Temperature	Colder	Hotter
Light	Darker	Brighter
Humidity	More wet	More dry
Density	Thinner	Thicker
Size	Longer	Smaller
Shape	More expansive and fragile	More contractive and harder
Form	Longer	Shorter
Texture	Softer	Harder
Atomic particle	Electron	Proton
Elements	N, O, K, P, Ca, etc.	H, C, Na, As, Mg, etc.
Environment	Vibration . . . Air . . . Water . . . Earth	
Climatic effects	Tropical climate	Colder climate
Biological	More vegetable quality	More animal quality
Sex	Female	Male
Organ structure	More hollow and expansive	More compacted and condensed
Nerves	More peripheral, orthosympathetic	More central, parasympathetic
Attitude	More gentle, negative	More active, positive
Work	More psychological and mental	More physical and social
Dimension	Space	Time

* For convenience, the symbols ▽ for Yin, and △ for Yang are used.

It also produces the rhythm of breathing. Going further, it charges the stomach and generates energy in the liver, spleen, pancreas, and kidneys. Heaven's charge then passes down to the center of the intestines, charging the region, known in Oriental countries as the *Hara, Tan-Den,* or, the abdominal energy center. Here it produces the rhythmic expansion and contraction of the intestines, bladder, and kidneys.

Heaven's force then proceeds to the lower region of the body where it creates another organ, similar to the uvula, known as the penis. When heaven's force creates the uvula, two glands, known as the adenoids, differentiate on either side of the upper throat. Similarly, heaven's force differentiates in the genital region into a pair of glands known as the testes.

A woman's orientation is complementary. In her case, the upward and expanding force of the earth is predominant.* For example, men are generally taller than women, meaning that their bodies extend further in a downward direction as a result of the greater influence of heaven's descending force. A woman's long, flowing hair is created primarily by the upward, expanding force of the earth, while a man's facial and body hair grows in a more downward direction under the influence of heaven's force.

Of course, just as men also receive earth's force, women receive heaven's force, which creates the hair spiral and uvula and vitalizes the charge of energy within the brain. The differences between men and women are most apparent in the sex organs. Because heaven's force is more downward, the male sex organs develop in an outward and downward manner. Conversely, earth's more expansive energy causes the female reproductive organs to develop a more upward and inward structure. Since the influence of heaven's force is less, women do not develop an extended "uvula" in the genital region. A smaller version, known as the clitoris, develops instead.

As earth's force passes upward through the body, it meets the force of heaven which flows in the opposite direction. When these forces collide deep within the female body in the intestinal region, they create a pair of spirals which later develop into the uterine tubes and ovaries. When a collision occurs in the region of the heart, the resulting spirals eventually take the form of the mammary glands and breasts. The collision of the two forces also creates a pair of spirals in men which later become nipples. However, because earth's energy is much weaker in men, these spirals do not normally develop into more yin, or expanded breasts.

As earth's force proceeds upward, it produces the tongue. The tongue is similar, both structurally and in terms of its energy quality, to the womb. Both are created primarily by earth's expanding force. Just as the womb is surrounded on either side by the ovaries, the tongue is surrounded by a pair of glands, the tonsils, which are similar to the ovaries in structure. Because of this relationship, when we have the tonsils removed, there is a weakening of sexual vitality. A weakening of vitality also occurs when the adenoids are removed, since these glands are closely related to the testes. These operations may therefore contribute to the widespread sexual unhappiness that many people now experience.

Heaven and earth's forces run along an invisible channel located deep within the body. The centrally charged regions along this primary energy channel were known in ancient cultures as the "seven *chakras*" or "energy centers." The intensive charge of energy produced in these regions is distributed throughout the body, charging and vitalizing all of its functions. The life energy produced in the heart *chakra*, or energy center, for example, is distributed throughout the upper chest, down to the arms and out to the tips of the fingers. The energy of the heart *chakra* produces the movement and life activity of the arms, chest, and hands. Similarly, the energy produced by the small intestine *chakra* creates the movement and life activity of the legs, lower abdomen, and feet.

---

* The complementary flow of heaven and earth's forces can be seen when a pendulum, such as a nail clipper attached to a string, is held above the head spiral. In men, the pendulum will begin to rotate in a counterclockwise direction; in women, it will begin to rotate clockwise. These directions are reversed in the Southern Hemisphere.

Sex is the act of connecting a man's positively charged magnetic pole and a woman's negatively charged magnetic pole in order to make these energies one. Heaven and earth's forces always seek one another in order to become one. As they connect their channels, a charge starts to build and both feel more harmonized.

Heaven and earth's forces become more unified during sex. Like an alternating current with a plus and minus attraction, these forces pass through the human body during intercourse. Conductivity begins as soon as a couple touches, at which time they start to exchange a very subtle charge of energy.

The flow of energy between heaven and earth does not take place in a smooth, constant manner, but alternates, first heaven, then earth, then heaven, etc. To coordinate with this, a couple will instinctively begin a rhythmic motion as the sexual act progresses, further harmonizing their respective charges with each other and with the environment.

As the charge intensifies, motion automatically becomes more rapid, causing the charge to intensify even further. Higher temperatures are produced and energy deep within the organism is generated and distributed throughout the body, charging the *chakras*, arms, and legs. The midbrain becomes especially charged, and so most people lose control over their thinking during sex.

The generation of heat, energy, and vibration continues to intensify until it reaches a peak as a spark, like thunder and lightning, that passes through the primary channel of both partners. We refer to this spark as orgasm. Then, the man's excessive accumulation of heaven's force and the woman's excessive accumulation of earth's force cancel each other out. Both partners then enter into balance with the surrounding environment.

The Female Reproductive System

Earth's more yin, expansive energy, produces many of the qualities associated with the female sex. The female reproductive organs are created and nourished more by this force and the female hormones, especially the *estrogens*, carry this more yin quality. The female reproductive organs include:

External Sex Organs (Vulva): The external sex organs include: 1) the *labia majora* and *labia minor* (outer and inner lips)—the two folds of soft skin which surround and protect the vagina; and 2) the *clitoris*, the small erectile organ which becomes filled with blood during sexual activity.

Internal Sex Organs: These include: 1) the *vagina*, a muscular tube which extends upward and backward from the vulva; 2) the *cervix*, or narrow neck of the womb (the lowest portion of the uterus that extends down into the vagina); 3) the *uterus*, a hollow, pear-shaped organ that lies in the center of the lower abdomen; 4) the *oviducts*, or *Fallopian tubes*, which are paired tubes about five inches long, extending from the top of the uterus to the ovaries; and 5) the *ovaries*, the primary organs of reproduction, located on either side of the uterus.

The ovaries produce mature egg cells and hormones which create feminine bodily and sexual characteristics. The ovarian hormones also play a primary role in the changes that comprise the monthly menstrual cycle, which involves the following:

Ovarian Changes: The almond-shaped ovaries are about 1½ inches long and an inch wide. At birth their outer layer, or *cortex*, contains up to 400,000 immature *primary ovarian follicles* in each ovary. Each follicle is a spirallically formed mass of cells at the center of which lies an *ovum*, or egg cell.

At the beginning of the first menstrual cycle, and during every cycle that follows, several follicles begin to mature. Normally, only one reaches maturity in each cycle, while the others degenerate. The menstrual cycle is normally repeated once every month throughout a woman's reproductive years, beginning at the time of *menarche*, or the onset of menstruation (ages twelve to fourteen) and continuing until *menopause*, or the cessation of menstruation (ages forty-five to fifty-five).

As a follicle matures, it accumulates fluid and increases in size until it occupies as much as one-fourth of the ovary. At maturity, the follicle, now known as a *Graffian follicle*, will bulge from the surface of the ovary. About ten days after it begins to develop (or about ten days after the last menstrual period), the mature follicle bursts and releases its ovum. The ovum then enters the finger-like, or fimbriated, end of the Fallopian tube. The discharge of the ovum is known as *ovulation* and occurs about once every twenty-eight days.

Once ovulation has taken place, the ruptured follicle undergoes a transformation, taking the form of a solid, yellow mass of cells known as the *corpus luteum*, or "yellow body." If the ovum is not fertilized, the corpus luteum will grow for twelve to fourteen days and then degenerate. If conception does occur, the corpus luteum will continue to grow and secrete hormones for about twelve weeks, then the placental hormones take over the support of the pregnancy.

Uterine Changes: In its contracted state, the uterus, or womb, is about the size of a pear. Its walls, or *myometrium*, form one of the strongest muscles in the body enabling the uterus to expand dramatically during pregnancy to accommodate the growing baby.

The internal lining of the uterus, known as the *endometrium*, undergoes a series of changes during the menstrual cycle. While the follicle is maturing in the ovary, the cells of the endometrium multiply, causing it to grow much thicker. The mucus glands in the endometrium also grow and new blood vessels develop as the lining prepares itself to receive the fertilized ovum.

After ovulation, the lining of the uterus continues to thicken and the glands and blood vessels in it proliferate. The mucus glands also produce a thick secretion during what is know as the *secretory phase*. If fertilization has taken place, the endometrium will remain in this condition throughout pregnancy. If not, the upper layers deteriorate and are discharged through menstruation. Menstruation normally takes three to five days, depending upon the woman's condition and the foods that she is eating.

The uterine changes that occur during the menstrual cycle correlate with changes taking place in the ovaries and are influenced by hormones such as:

1) *Follicular, or estrogenic hormones:* Estrogens are more yin hormones produced by maturing follicles. Their influence is felt more during the first half of the menstrual cycle called the *follicular phase*, during which the uterus prepares itself to receive a fertilized ovum. The secretion of estrogens declines after ovulation.

2) *Corpus luteum hormone (progesterone):* Progesterone, a more yang hormone, is produced by the corpus luteum during the second half of the menstrual cycle, the secretory phase. It influences the changes in the uterine lining that follow ovulation. How the uterine lining changes depends upon whether or not an egg has been fertilized. If the ovum has not been fertilized, the corpus luteum regresses and is discharged together with the egg in the menstrual flow. If conception has occurred, the ovum will embed itself in the

The Menstrual Cycle

Period	Duration in Days	Day of Cycle	Changes in Uterine Mucosa	Changes in Ovaries
Menstruation	5	1st to 5th	Endometrial cells undergo necrosis; desquamation occurs; glands release secretions, blood vessels rupture, menstrual flow occurs	Corpus luteum continues to degenerate New follicle begins development
Repair and regeneration	2	5th to 7th	Uterine mucosa is restored	Follicle develops
Proliferative phase	8	7th to 15th	Endometrium grows, stroma becomes thicker, more vascular; glands become longer, but remain straight	Follicle matures and develops Estrogens are secreated Ovulation marks end of stage
Premenstrual, secretory, progestational or progravid phase	13	16th to 28th	Endometrium continues to grow; glands become longer, more tortuous and coiled. Cells enter secretory phase, secrete glycogen, mucoid material, and fat	Corpus luteum develops, matures, and begins to retrogress Secretes progesterone

(In long cycles of 30 to 35 days, a period of rest intervenes between the first and second stages shown in the table.)

Source: Anatomy and Physiology, Vol. 2 by Stern and montagu. Barnes and Noble, 1959.

uterine lining and continue to develop, while the corpus luteum develops as the corpus luteum of pregnancy. Throughout pregnancy, the corpus luteum secretes progesterone, which prevents ovulation and aids in the development of the placenta and embryonic membranes.

Diet, Environment, and the Menstrual Cycle

If a woman is healthy, her menstrual cycle will correspond to the monthly phases of the moon. The amount of time needed for each stage is strongly influenced by diet. Women who eat more extreme diets, for example those including eggs, meat, dairy products, and sugar, often need more time to discharge excess fat, protein, and water. Women who eat whole-grain and vegetable-based diets usually finish their menstrual period within three days, compared to the average of five days for women in the United States. Similarly, a woman who eats a balanced diet can accomplish the repair of her endometrium in only one day.

The menstrual cycle consists of two complementary phases, which correspond to the alternating atmospheric influence of heaven and earth's forces. During the more yang phase, which is governed by heaven's force, the lining of the womb repairs and regenerates itself, the follicle reaches maturity, and the ovum completes its formation. The body concentrates energy, blood, cells, and bodily fluids in toward the developing egg at this time. This more yang phase culminates in ovulation. It proceeds much more smoothly when atmospheric conditions become darker and heavier, as they do every month from the full to the new moon. During the more yin phase, the ovum is released and the lining of the uterus prepares to receive it. If fertilization does not occur, this process culminates in menstruation. The more yin part of the cycle progresses more smoothly when earth's force becomes stronger and the atmosphere becomes brighter and lighter, as it does from the new to the full moon.

Fig. 1 Correlation between the monthly lunar and menstrual cycles.

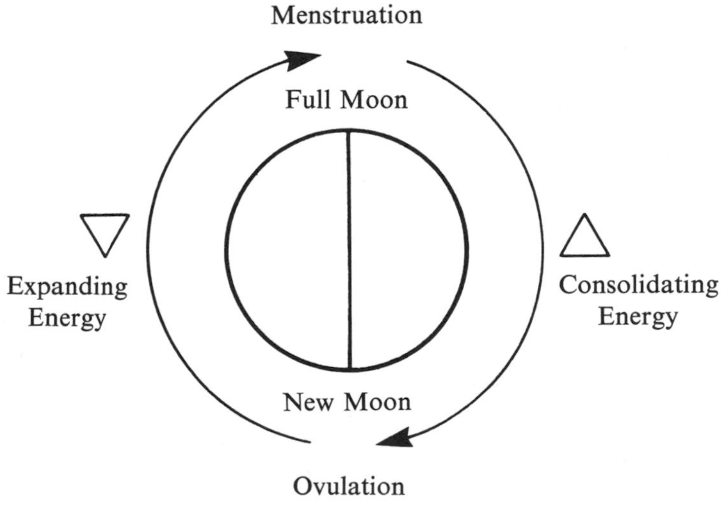

The intake of sugar, milk, ice cream, tropical fruits and other more yin foods can easily offset the more contracting tendency of the first half of the menstrual cycle. The result is often pain at the time of ovulation. Conversely, the excessive intake of salt, eggs, meat, poultry, and other animal foods often results in menstrual cramps, since these more yang foods frequently offset the more expansive changes which occur in a woman's body during the second half of the menstrual cycle. Both categories of problems can be remedied by avoiding extremes and by eating a more centrally balanced diet. (See Chapter 3 for more specific recommendations.) To recover a more natural balance, it is better for women who suffer from menstrual cramps to avoid animal products entirely, while women who experience pain during ovulation need to reduce or avoid foods which are extremely yin.

Yin and Yang in Daily Foods

Strong Yang Foods

Refined Salt	Poultry
Eggs	Fish
Meat	Seafood
Cheese	

Balanced Foods

Whole Cereal Grains	Root, Round, and Leafy
Seeds	Vegetables
Beans and Bean Products	Spring or Well Water
Nuts	Nonaromatic, Nonstimulant Teas
Sea Vegetables	Natural Sea Salt

Strong Yin Foods

Temperate Climate Fruit	Honey, Sugar, and Refined
White Rice, White Flour	Sweeteners
Tropical Fruits and Vegetables	Alcohol
Milk, Cream, Yogurt	Foods containing Chemicals,
Oils	Preservatives, Dyes,
Spices (pepper, curry, nutmeg, etc.)	Pesticides
	Drugs (marijuana, cocaine, etc.)
Aromatic and Stimulant Beverages (coffee, black tea, mint tea, etc.)	Medications (tranquilizers, antidepressants, etc.)

The Male Reproductive System

The male reproductive system and the characteristics associated with the male sex are created and energized by the downward flow of energy from heaven to earth. As a result, a man's primary reproductive organs are outside and below the body cavity.

The male reproductive organs include: 1) the testes; 2) the *scrotum*, the sac which contains the testes; 3) a system of tubes for transporting and ejecting sperm, including the *epididymis*, *seminal ducts* (also called the *vas deferens*), and the *urethra*; 4) glands, such as the *prostate*, which aid in the formation of the seminal fluid used to transport sperm; and 5) the penis.

The inner part of the testes is divided into many small chambers, or *lobules*. Each chamber contains from one to three tiny, tightly wound tubes known as *seminiferous tubules*. The cells which line the seminiferous tubules produce millions of sperm. Within each tubule, sperm cells can be found in various stages of development.

At maturity, sperm cells travel to the epididymis, where they are stored temporarily. During ejaculation, they pass through the vas deferens into the urethra and out via the penis. Sperm are carried in the seminal fluid, or *semen*, which is produced by the seminal vesicles and the prostate and *bulbourethral glands*. An average ejaculation contains as many as 200 to 400 million sperm and amounts to about two to three cubic centimeters of semen.

The testes also secrete hormones known as *androgens*, of which *testosterone* is the principal one. Testosterone is a more yang hormone which influences the secondary sex characteristics which develop at puberty, such as the growth of facial and pubic hair, enlargement of the vocal cords, the development of male stature and form, and the emergence of sexual libido.

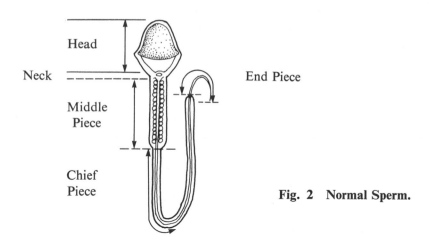

Fig. 2   Normal Sperm.

Sexual Health

Without sex, there would be no continuation of the human species. Good physical health is a primary condition for the maintenance of our reproductive ability. When the energies of heaven and earth stream freely throughout the body, their electromagnetic current charges the trillions of body cells, illuminating and irradiating them with energy. The active charge of heaven and earth's forces produces a vitality, a living energy that animates our entire life. Health, and therefore sexuality, is the overflow and reflection of this vitality.

To achieve sexual health, any blockages or toxic accumulations which impede the flow of this energy must be dissolved; to maintain sexual vitality the factors that produce these blockages should be eliminated. Today, most people suffer from various degrees of stagnation. This can be found in the intestinal region, the nasal cavity, within and around the reproductive organs and in many other locations throughout the body. Stagnation is caused primarily by a diet and way of life that produces mucus and fat deposits in the body. These accumulations interfere with and diminish the quality and intensity of our life charge. When this situation exists, sexual activity and desire are dulled.

Our daily diet is the single most important factor that influences our sexual happiness. A naturally balanced, well prepared diet will contribute toward the sound physical and mental condition that underlies a happy sexual life. A chaotic or unbalanced diet, on the other hand, contributes to a variety of problems that affect our health and therefore our sexuality.

For thousands of years, the majority of people achieved sexual satisfaction in a simple and natural fashion without any particular concern or effort. But today, many people cannot reach complete enjoyment since they are unable to generate a sufficient charge of life energy, especially along the primary channel. The lack of sexual fulfillment is one of the major reasons why so many couples separate or divorce. Although problems with the primary channel are the underlying cause, sexual problems can manifest in any of a number of ways. For example:

Frigidity: The term "frigidity" is used to describe the inability to experience pleasure from sexual activity and the absence of sexual feelings. A frigid person is icy cold, and no matter what is tried the body temperature will not rise and sufficient energy cannot be generated to make the spark of sex flow. But what makes people cold? The answer lies in what they are eating. If people are cold, then something they are eating is making them that way, especially foods such as ice cream, soft drinks, sugar, tropical fruits, fruit juices, too many salads and other more yin or expansive items.

Impotence: If a man eats too many extremely yin foods such as those mentioned above, his overall condition weakens and his sexual charge cannot be actively generated. This problem is commonly called impotence. *Erectile impotence* is the condition in which a man can't achieve an erection, while *ejaculatory impotence* describes the inability to achieve orgasm following erection.

Hardening of the Primary Channel: Besides the coldness that leads to impotence and frigidity, sexual problems also arise when heaven and earth's forces do not run smoothly through the body as a result of hardness along the primary channel. To check yourself for this condition, lie on your back with your knees bent and your feet on the floor, shoulder width apart, toward the buttocks. Place your hands above the abdominal region, and extend your fingers downward. As you exhale, push deeply but gently. Rigidity, hardness, or pain are signs that your primary channel has become hard because of the accumulation of fat and mucus. These deposits are caused by dairy foods such as cheese, butter and milk; animal fats from meat and eggs; sugar and soft drinks; overeating; and eating too many flour products, baked foods, or oily and greasy foods.

Looseness or Weakening of the Primary Channel: Another category of sexual problems results from weakness or looseness in the primary channel and *chakras*. Extremely yin foods, such as sugar, honey, and spices, and marijuana and other drugs and medications create a general weakening of the entire body.

Medical procedures also contribute to a diminishing of overall vitality. When a woman conceives, for example, there is a great concentration of energy in the depths of the womb in the region corresponding to the *hara chakra*, or abdominal energy center. If she then has an abortion, this energy suddenly disperses and the abdominal energy center becomes very weak and loose, affecting the entire primary channel. This also causes the legs to become weaker and can create an overall run-down condition.

But besides eating poorly or having an abortion, many people have their tonsils and adenoids removed under the guidance of their doctors. However, as we have seen, removal of these glands is not unlike having the ovaries or testes removed. The result is a loss of vitality, endurance, and patience, and a weakening of resistance to disease. People who have had such surgery also often experience a general reduction of sexual vitality. Perhaps as many as 80 percent of the American population have had either surgery to remove glands or organs, or have had at least one abortion. Although these people were born with perfect conditions, they now must live with bodies weakened by man-made procedures.

However, you need not worry if you have any of these disadvantages. By eating properly, you can compensate to the maximum degree. You may not be able to regain 100 percent ability, but you should be able to compensate by as much as 80 to 90 percent. Problems of sexual weakness can usually be easily solved with the standard macrobiotic diet, adjusted to fit the individual's needs. It may take months, or in some cases even a year, but definitely, in most cases, it can be done. For those who have damaged their energy centers with drugs and medications, recovery might take longer, perhaps up to three or four years, but eventually health and vitality will return.

How Sex is Determined

Our reproductive cells—the egg and sperm—are the highly compacted essence of a universal process of creation that includes the entire realm of biological life. Reproductive cells come from the blood, which in turn comes from the foods that are eaten. Food is produced by the transformation of inorganic factors—air, water, minerals, and sunlight, and various forms of radiation—into vegetable life. Inorganic elements and energy manifestations come from the world of vibrations and, ultimately, from the world of polarization, or yin and yang. Yin and yang originate within the oneness of the infinite universe. Everyone carries the memory of their infinite origin deep within their consciousness, together with the endless dream of returning to this universal source.

Each of the follicle cells in the ovary develops in a spiral pattern. As an egg cell matures, it gradually passes through these follicles, beginning at the peripheral regions and slowly moving toward the center. When a mature egg reaches the center, it bursts out of the follicle. The process of maturation is governed by the more yang, centripetal force.

Sperm mature through an opposite process. Growth occurs through the more yin process of differentiation, in which millions of sperm are formed at one time. The egg and sperm therefore carry complementary electromagnetic charges. The egg carries a more yang charge and sperm carry a more yin charge.

Fig. 3   The spiral formation of the egg and sperm.

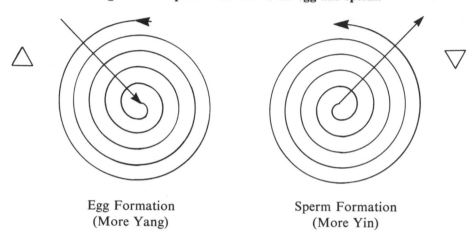

Egg Formation
(More Yang)

Sperm Formation
(More Yin)

Reproductive cells combine through the universal process that causes positively and negatively charged particles or objects to meet. Because of its nature, the egg cell moves more easily in a downward direction, while sperm move upward more easily. The more yang egg also becomes the focus around which sperm are attracted, similar to the way that a nucleus acts as the central focus for orbiting electrons of an atom.

The complementary charged egg and sperm never neutralize each other. A fertilized ovum will either have a slightly more yin charge, as a result of the predominating influence of the father's sperm, or a slightly more yang charge, due to the predominance of the mother's egg. The charge of the ovum influences the quality of nourishment that it takes in during the nine months of pregnancy.

All of the nutrients absorbed by the embryo—the amino acids, lipids, carbohydrates, and minerals—can be divided into yin and yang. Even if all fertilized eggs were nourished from an identical bloodstream, no two cells would attract and absorb an identical proportion of nutrients.

If the ovum's yang charge is stronger than the sperm's yin charge, the fertilized ovum will be more yangly charged and will attract an opposite, or more yin quality nourishment from the mother's blood. During pregnancy, the cell, originally more yang, then becomes more yin. As a result, the reproductive organs develop externally, expanding outward from the body, and creating a boy.

In the opposite case, the ovum has a more yin charge as a result of the predominance of the sperm at the time of conception. A more yin ovum attracts a more yang quality of nourishment during pregnancy, which in turn creates a more compacted physical structure in which the sexual organs are held inside the body. These developments indicate that the baby is a girl.

Even though the sexual organs do not actually develop until later in pregnancy, the baby's sex is determined by the quality of the egg and sperm which unite at conception. If, at the time of conception, a woman generally is stronger, healthier, and more active than her partner, the fertilized ovum will develop into a boy. If the man is generally healthier and more active, a girl will be born.

According to Oriental and macrobiotic understanding, if there are more boys than girls in a particular family, then the mother is thought to be the stronger of the parents. More girls customarily indicate that the father is stronger. During periods when the father is stronger, girls are produced, while boys are born when the mother is stronger. The birth of children thus helps create balance in a family. Also it is said that more richly prepared food tends to create females and simpler food tends to produce males.

Animal foods conduct more of heaven's force than vegetables do. They strengthen a man's conductivity of heaven's force and weaken a woman's natural conductivity of earth's force. A diet rich in animal proteins can easily make a man's sperm more active and highly charged while at the same time weakening the quality and charge of the egg.

However, keep in mind that the quality of our blood and of our reproductive cells changes moment by moment as a result of what we eat. Even one piece of pie or a glass of beer changes the quality of our blood and in turn influences these cells. When our eating becomes chaotic, as it is in most societies today, it is difficult to predict accurately what the sex of a child will be. As people begin to eat according to macrobiotic principles, however, the birth of children occurs more in accord with the natural order.

Infertility

The problem of infertility is becoming increasingly common today. According to some estimates, as many as 3.5 million American couples, or one couple out of every six, are unable to have children. When taken together with related trends, it appears that modern people are losing the ability to reproduce themselves. Consider, for example:

1) Approximately 800,000 women in the United States have their ovaries and uterus removed every year. Fifty percent of all American women have had a *hysterectomy* (the surgical removal of the uterus) by the age of sixty-five.
2) A recent study found that average sperm counts were almost 40 percent lower than they were in 1920.
3) In one survey of college students, 23 percent were found to be functionally sterile.
4) The current increase in the number of births in the United States is due to more women entering childbearing age and not to an increase in the actual

birth rate. Birth expectations among married women in the prime of their childbearing years are at an all-time low.

Modern medicine deals with the problem of infertility on a symptomatic level which ignores the underlying cause. An array of drugs, surgical techniques, and sensational new approaches are being tried, including *in vitro* fertilization, or IVF (commonly known as the "test tube" baby), artificial insemination, and "surrogate mothers," in which a woman is hired to become pregnant using sperm from the husband of an infertile wife.

Couples are considered infertile if they try to conceive for one year without success. In many infertile couples, possibly as many as 20 percent, no apparent medical cause is found. In another 30 percent to 40 percent, the problem is the result of abnormalities in the production or transport of the husband's sperm. In the remaining cases, infertility usually results from a failure to ovulate, problems with the transport of released eggs, or problems with the quality of mucus in the cervix.

Let us consider each factor in more detail.

Male Factors

1) *Faulty semen:* Normally, men produce 75 to 125 million sperm in each cubic centimeter of semen, and discharge two to three cubic centimeters of semen with each ejaculation. If the number of sperm goes below 50 million per cubic centimeter, fertilization becomes difficult. Counts of 25 million usually mean infertility and if the number drops as low as 5 to 10 million, conception is highly unlikely. Infertility can also arise when not enough healthy sperm are produced; the sperm are either too weak to propel themselves through the female reproductive tract or are not fully developed. A man is considered fertile if at least 60 percent of his sperm cells have mature, oval heads and the ability to move actively.

Fig. 4 Abnormal sperm.

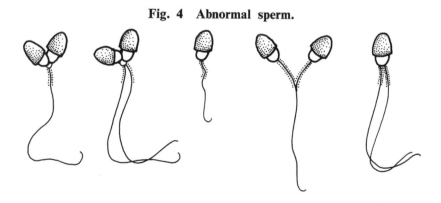

The inability to produce enough high quality sperm can result from injury or from inflammation, such as that associated with severe cases of mumps. However, in the majority of cases, there is no apparent reason for the inability to produce an adequate number and quality of sperm. Like the sexual disorders discussed earlier, problems related to the production of sperm have an underlying dietary cause, specifically the overconsumption of extremely yin items, including chemicals, drugs, medications, coffee, soft drinks, sugar, fruit and fruit juice, chocolate, carob, spices, alcohol, and various aromatic or stimulant foods and beverages. Recently, chemical toxins, including those in the environment, are also being implicated.

2) *Varicocele:* Poor sperm production can also be traced to varicoceles, or varicose veins in the scrotum. About half of the men with this condition have diminished sperm counts, weak sperm motility, or problems with their semen. The enlargement of the veins of the spermatic cord, which may develop with this condition, can cause blood from the abdomen to collect in the scrotum. An increase in the temperature in the scrotum often destroys sperm. Varicoceles result from a diet rich in extremes of both yin and yang, including items such as protein and saturated fat, especially that found in the more heavy dairy foods such as cheese, sugar and other sweets, drugs, soft drinks, coffee and other stimulant beverages, and fruit and fruit juice, especially those of tropical origin.

3) *Duct blockage:* A less common problem occurs when the production of sperm is normal but their movement through the tubes which convey them from the testes to the penis is blocked. Duct blockage can result from a previous vasectomy or gonorrheal infection or from the accumulation of protein and fat in the vas deferens. Foods such as dairy products, fatty, oily, and greasy foods, animal fats and proteins, and sugar and sugared products contribute to the formation of these blockages in the male genital ducts.

Female Factors

1) *Failure to ovulate:* About 20 percent of female infertility comes from the inability of the ovaries to produce a normal egg cell each month. *Anovulation,* or the inability to produce an egg cell, is frequently accompanied by hormonal imbalance. Underlying this problem is a diet based on extremes of both yin and yang, especially the overconsumption of fruits, fruit juices, sugar and other sweets, and chemicals and drugs, in combination with an excessive intake of fatty animal foods such as eggs, cheese, and meat. Greasy, high- fat items especially aggravate this condition, while the predominant cause is the excessive intake of extreme yin items.

In some instances, these extremes cause the ovaries to wither and age prematurely, and no eggs remain to mature, while in others, the surface of the ovary thickens and ovulation occurs infrequently. Other factors which have some influence on ovulation are extremes in body fat—either too much or too little—and severe physical or psychological stress.

2) *Endometriosis:* When a woman develops endometriosis, portions of the endometrium, or lining of the womb, break away from the uterus and start to grow in other parts of the pelvis, for example, in the Fallopian tubes,

ovaries, or on the surface of the bladder or rectum. These tissues frequently block the reproductive tract and can cause sterility. Even in mild cases this condition may contribute to infertility by affecting hormonal balance. Endometriosis may or may not produce discomfort in the pelvic region. The most common symptom is pain which begins several days before the start of a menstrual period, most probably caused when the endometrial tissue in various other locations undergoes changes similar to those occurring in the uterine lining.

Endometriosis, which appears to be increasing in incidence, is caused by an excessive diet, especially the repeated overconsumption of animal products—including fatty, oily and greasy foods such as pizza, hamburger, bacon, fried chicken, and others—plus the overintake of sugar and sweets, fruits, flour products, stimulants, aromatic foods and beverages, alcohol, and drugs and chemicals.

3) *Fallopian tube blockage:*   Blockage of the Fallopian tubes is a common problem in female infertility. It may result from endometriosis or from pelvic inflammations such as those which occur in severe cases of gonorrhea or with the use of an IUD. However, many of these blockages have no apparent cause.

An improper diet underlies the majority of Fallopian tube blockages, even those which develop following severe pelvic inflammation. With gonorrhea, for example, the types of foods that a woman is eating largely determines whether or not exposure to the bacteria will produce an infection that is severe enough to cause sterility. Even congenital abnormalities in the Fallopian tubes can be traced to foods eaten by the mother during pregnancy. (See the discussion of uterine anomalies in Chapter 4.)

In most cases, blockages of the Fallopian tubes develop through a mechanism that is similar to that presented in Chapter 4 in our discussion of *fibroids*. The overconsumption of foods rich in protein, fat, and salts—such as meat and cheese, plus other fatty, oily, and greasy foods—along with foods such as sugar, sweets, soft drinks, chemicals, and flour products, combine to create deposits of fat and mucus throughout the body. When these deposits interfere with the passage of eggs through the Fallopian tubes, infertility is the result.

In some cases, an improper diet, especially the overconsumption of greasy or oily foods, including animal fats and dairy, causes toxic factors to accumulate in the cervical mucus. If the cervical mucus becomes toxic enough, it can actually kill any sperm cells that come in contact with it. This condition is known as *hostile cervical mucus* and is the cause of about 10 percent of the cases of infertility in women.

The use of intrauterine contraceptive devices (IUDs) and previous abortions can also diminish fertility. Many women with IUDs develop chronic low grade infections while some develop acute infections or pelvic abscesses. Pelvic infections sometimes develop following abortion, while pelvic adhesions, which can also block the passage of the egg, may occur following the removal of fibroids, ovarian cysts, tubal pregnancies, or after pelvic surgery.

Fibroids which distort the shape of the uterus also cause infertility, as do congenital anomalies such as those found in the daughters of women who took the drug *diethylstilbesterol* (DES) during pregnancy.

The macrobiotic approach to infertility: It is based on correcting the underlying dietary cause of the problem. A large number of infertile couples could recover their ability to have children by eating according to the standard macrobiotic diet, with specific modifications for each circumstance. If the problem results from a low sperm count, for example, slightly stronger cooking methods can be emphasized, and dishes which are a little more strongly seasoned with sea salt, *miso*, or *tamari* soy sauce can be served more often. More yin items such as salad, fruit, fruit juice, or nuts may need to be minimized or avoided for several months.

Varicoceles and blockages of the sperm ducts can also be remedied with the standard macrobiotic diet while minimizing or avoiding the intake of foods that lead to the development of mucus and fat, including animal foods, flour products, oil, nuts and their products, and fruits and fruit juices. The moderate use of macrobiotic seasonings would be more appropriate, while beans and bean products, which contain protein and fats, are best eaten in moderate amounts only. A variety of special dishes—such as cooked *daikon*, *daikon* greens, and *kombu* or shredded *daikon* cooked with *kombu* and *tamari*—are helpful in discharging fat and mucus from the body and can be eaten regularly by persons with these conditions.

The standard macrobiotic approach is also recommended for women who cannot ovulate. The drugs used to induce ovulation frequently overstimulate the ovaries and cause them to release more than one egg at a time, resulting in multiple births. In most cases, the dietary recommendations presented in Chapter 4 for fibroids and vaginal discharges may be observed. The special treatments presented for those conditions may also be used.

In a large number of cases, blockages of the Fallopian tubes can also be corrected with the standard macrobiotic diet. The specific recommendations presented in the discussion of fibroids, including the external treatments, can be applied.

Birth Control

The various methods of birth control can create their own set of problems, affecting not only the reproductive system, but the overall physical and mental condition as well. Let us review the more commonly used methods of birth control.

Oral Contraceptives (OC's) or the Birth Control Pill: Despite repeated warnings of serious side effects, the birth control pill, first made available in 1959, is still the most widely used form of contraception in the United States. There are a variety of OC's on the market. These differ in the type and dosage of hormone used. However, the most commonly used types can be divided into two major categories; the combination pill that contains both a synthetic estrogen and a synthetic progestogen and the synthetic progestogen only pill.

Excessive doses of estrogen, a more yin female hormone, hinder the formation of eggs, which are made by the more yang, inward motion of follicles in the ovaries. Also a variety of more yin effects can be produced in the body when repeated doses, beyond the amount usually produced by the ovaries, are taken. This happens because estrogen is carried throughout the body by the circulation of the blood and body fluids. These effects include headaches due to expansion of the brain cells; loss of mental clarity, caused by gradual expansion of the inner midbrain region; irregular heart palpitation, caused by a gradual expansion of the heart and blood vessels; gradual weakening of the functions of more contracted organs such as the liver, kidneys, and spleen; gradual irritation of the parasympathetic nerve function; and other similar effects. These more yin conditions may manifest differently and to varying degrees from person to person, because of differences in constitution, dietary practice, and living conditions.

When the more yang progestogen based pill is used, a woman's condition may become progressively more constricted or tight, and various more yang symptoms may develop. However, even if no symptoms appear, the use of oral contraceptives can have a gradually accumulating negative affect on the individual's overall condition. For this reason, we recommend that women avoid all forms of oral contraceptives as a method of birth control.

A variety of recent studies have confirmed that users of the pill have an increased risk of degenerative disorders. Most experts agree that users of the pill have a higher than average risk of strokes due to the development of blood clots, while some studies have suggested that women over forty who use the pill have a higher risk of heart attack. Other research has shown that certain female hormones may cause changes in the tissues of the uterus and breast. Estrogen dependent breast tumors also occur, while a number of studies have correlated the long term use of oral contraceptives with tumors of the liver. These tumors, known as *adenomas*, have a tendency to bleed into the abdominal cavity and can be fatal.

Intra-Uterine Device (IUD):   IUDs are plastic or metal objects of various shapes and sizes which are inserted through the cervix into the uterus. Within the uterus, a constant flow of electromagnetic energy is generated around the abdominal energy center, located in women in the inner depths of the uterus. This energy flow charges the fertilized egg and keeps the embryo alive and growing. An IUD disturbs the normal pattern of this electromagnetic flow and as a result, interferes with implantation and embryonic growth. Moreover, IUDs also disturb the electromagnetic current flowing through the entire body, including the movement of energy along the meridians. The functions of the various organs, which are governed by electromagnetic energy, are also directly and indirectly disturbed. When the flow of electromagnetic energy is disrupted general fatigue and emotional irritability are often the result. Also, the natural mechanical response of the body is to try to eliminate unnatural obstacles from the uterus. This impulse causes physical and emotional tension and disharmony, as long as the IUD remains in place. To maintain a peaceful and harmonious physical and emotional balance, we recommend that you avoid using an IUD.

IUDs were first popularized in the 1960s and are now used by an estimated 15 to 20-million women throughout the world. It is estimated that more than 2 million women in the United States use them. However, a growing number of people now realize that IUDs are often neither safe nor effective. About 3 percent of women with IUDs become pregnant, and there is a higher incidence of tubal pregnancy in this case than in the overall population. Some of the other recognized dangers of IUD use include:

1) *Bleeding and cramping in the uterus:* At least 20 percent of IUD users report bleeding and cramping following insertion of the device. A similar percentage of users have their IUDs removed within the first year because of these complications.

2) *Pelvic infections:* A recent article in the *Journal of the American Medical Association* stated that the risk of pelvic inflammatory disease is nine times greater among IUD users than among women who use other forms of contraception. Pelvic disease is a common cause of infertility among women and, in rare cases, can cause death. This was especially so with the Dalkon Shield IUD that was removed from the market in 1975. Doctors have reported a sharp increase in infertility during the years of IUD use.

Diaphragm with Spermicidal Agent: The use of a diaphragm is much safer than the above two methods of birth control. A diaphragm is used in combination with a sperm killing agent such as a jelly or cream which is applied to both sides of the device. However, the use of chemically synthesized jellies or creams causes undesirable effects. These extremely yin substances are absorbed through the wall of the vagina and uterus and into the body fluid and bloodstream. Although such effects are minor, frequent use could create an allergic reaction and eventually nervousness and fatigue. It is advisable to douche with warm salt water after using a diaphragm with a spermicidal agent. A number of women experience irritation in the vagina and surrounding tissues as a result of using these agents.

Condom: Condoms are used primarily to prevent ejaculated sperm from entering the vagina. They are the most commonly used method of birth control throughout the world and, healthwise, are much safer than the previously discussed methods, especially for women. However, the drawback of this method is that it is distracting and interferes with both partners' complete physical and emotional satisfaction during intercourse. Condoms prevent the man's ejaculated stream of sperm and sexual fluids from stimulating the sensitive inner walls of the vagina and uterus. They also limit the flow of energy between the couple.

Natural Birth Control: Based on the natural cycle of ovulation, natural birth control is by far the safest method in terms of mental and physical health. In this method, a few days before and after ovulation, intercourse is avoided since the fertilizing ability of the sperm is generally two days, although they may survive in the womb for as long as 14 days. In order to practice this method, however, a couple must know the exact time of ovulation. Through the macrobiotic diet and way of life, a woman can establish a regular menstrual cycle that is in exact accordance with the 28-day cycle of the moon. Therefore, it is easier to practice natural birth control within a macrobiotic way of life.

Other Artificial Birth Control Methods: Because of the harmful side effects produced by birth control pills, IUDs, and other methods, researchers are constantly searching for safer alternatives. However, any artificial method other than natural birth control will produce some degree of side effects, either short or long term. Immunization, tubal interruption, vasectomy, the once-a-month or "morning after" pill, or periodic hormone injections—all of these methods, as well as any that may be developed in the future—will have side effects, simply because they are unnatural and foreign to the human metabolism.

Abortion

It is estimated that 1.5 million induced abortions are performed every year in the United States. Contrary to popular belief, the majority of American women seeking abortions are not unwed mothers. As many as four out of five are married and have children. Induced abortion is used widely throughout the world as a means of birth control.

Many of the physical effects of abortion are not yet fully recognized by the medical profession. If the procedure is performed without injury, if bleeding and infection are kept to a minimun, and if the uterus heals within a given period of time, the abortion is considered a success. Of course, the emotional impact is also taken into consideration, but the effects of an abortion—physical, mental and spiritual—are far greater than most people realize.

To better understand the effects an abortion has on a woman we can use the analogy of a plant. The flower of the plant produces fruit which contains seeds, which are the offspring of the plant. Abortion is similar to cutting the flower from the plant. A long recovery time must pass although it seems little physical damage has been done.

After fertilization, a woman's body begins concentrating blood and energy toward the depths of the womb. The embryo begins to develop as a result of the intense generation of heaven and earth's force in the area corresponding to the *hara chakra*, or abdominal energy center. If the embryo is artificially removed, these inward gathering energies are dispersed throughout the body, substantially weakening the charge of life force in the abdominal energy center and along the entire primary channel. All of the body's organs, glands, tissues, and cells are dependent on the primary channel for a continual supply of life energy, and their functioning is thus also weakened by this procedure. The organs in the lower abdomen, which receive their supply of life energy directly from the abdominal energy center, are especially affected. Abortion weakens the vitality and functioning of the small and large intestines, the kidneys, adrenal glands, bladder, and ovaries and uterus. At the same time, the charge of life energy that is distributed from this center downward to the legs is diminished, causing a weakening of the leg muscles. In a related way, induced abortion can increase the likelihood of such disorders as chronic indigestion, constipation, poor absorption of nutrients, anemia, fatigue, poor circulation, urinary infection, kidney stones, menstrual irregularity, vaginal discharge, fibroid tumors, increased susceptibility to infection, ovarian cysts, and a variety of others. When combined with a chronically poor diet, abortion can also contribute to the development of serious degenerative conditions, including multiple sclerosis and cancer.

Because abortion is so drastic, it may require up to three years for a woman to overcome its adverse physical effects. The speed of recovery depends on the overall state of a woman's health and the quality of her diet. If she eats a well balanced diet and maintains the appropriate activity, she will be able to recover to the maximum degree, although some weakness may remain throughout life. The dietary recommendations presented in Chapter 4 for miscarriage can be applied immediately following an abortion in order to aid the process of recovery. The way of life recommendations presented in Chapter 3 are also important in the recovery process. It is especially recommended that women recovering from abortion avoid taking long hot baths or showers, avoid wearing synthetic clothing, and refrain from using blankets, pillowcases, and other sleeping materials made of synthetic fabrics. The practice of scrubbing the entire body daily with a hot moist towel is especially recommended as a means of activating circulation and restoring vitality.

The psychological effects of abortion are also considerable. Many women experience a sense of sorrow and loss following their decision to terminate the life of their unborn child. As time passes and a woman gains a deeper understanding of life, the psychological impact of abortion often grows in importance, frequently in the form of sadness and regret over what cannot be undone.

The process through which children are born on this earth occurs according to the order of the universe or natural law. Induced abortion represents an artificial attempt to block or interfere with the natural process in which all beings and phenomena come into existence. Abortion for the sake of the future parents is therefore more egocentric compared to the acceptance of the natural order and appreciation for life. Since nature and the universe are infinitely more powerful than the immediate concerns of individuals or society, such artificial procedures can easily increase our separation from natural happiness.

As in any attempt to bend the laws of nature to our own purpose, unforeseen problems of many kinds may arise following an abortion. Therefore, if such a drastic step is being considered, deep self reflection is recommended as a means to gain an appreciation for the meaning and the purpose of life.

2|From Conception to Birth

Conception, or the fusion of egg and sperm, marks the completion of a universal process of creation and the beginning of new life. In this chapter we will trace the progression of human life from the moment of conception until the time of birth.

For seven days following conception, the various yin and yang factors within the fertilized ovum begin to differentiate through a process known as system formation. The major bodily systems begin as two spirallic energy matrixes—one, a more yin spiral, expands outward from the center to the periphery; the other, a more yang spiral, coils inward from the periphery to the center. The more yin spiral develops toward the front of the ovum and eventually becomes the digestive and respiratory systems. The more yang spiral develops toward the back and later becomes the nervous system. A third spiral, at the center of which the heart will eventually develop, also materializes and becomes the circulatory and excretory systems.

It takes the fertilized egg about seven days to travel the length of the Fallopian tube and implant itself in the lining of the uterus. During this time the two primary spiral formations give rise to the primary germ layers from which the embryo develops.

Fig. 5   Spiral development in the human embryo (schematic).

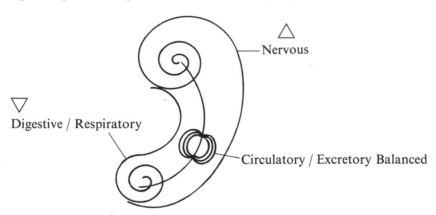

The more yang spiral begins to develop as a peripheral layer of cells known as the *ectoderm*, while the more yin spiral begins to materialize as an inner layer known as the *endoderm*. Following development of these two primary layers, the third, or middle spiral materializes as another germ layer, the *mesoderm*, which occupies the space between the two primary layers.

The ectoderm eventually develops into the nervous system, including the brain, spinal cord, nerves, and nerve endings, while the endoderm eventually becomes the digestive system, including the organs of the alimentary canal and glands such as the liver, gallbladder, and pancreas. The respiratory system also arises from this inner layer of cells. The third, or middle layer, gives rise to the circulatory system, together with the excretory and reproductive systems.

The human body is created from the initial polarization of the fertilized ovum into yin and yang, and the subsequent development of spirallic systems, organs, tissues and cells. A figure showing the primary derivatives of each of the three spirallic germ layers is presented below.

Fig. 6 Germ layer derivatives.

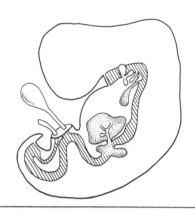 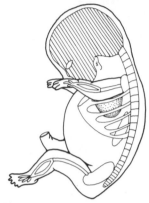 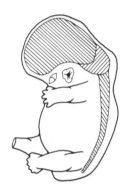

ENDODERM	MESODERM	ECTODERM
General Derivatives:	*General Derivatives:*	*General Derivatives:*
Digestive and respiratory systems, certain excretory and reproductive ducts	Muscular, skeletal, circulatory, excretory, and reproductive systems	Nervous system, sense organs, mouth cavity, skin
Specific Derivatives:	*Specific Derivatives:*	*Specific Derivatives:*
Lining of alimentary canal (except terminal portions), including pharynx and derivatives (auditory tubes, tympanic cavity, thyroid, parathyroids)	All muscle tissues (smooth, striated, cardiac)	Epidermis of skin and its derivatives (hair, nails, and sebaceous, sweat, and mammary glands)
Epithelium of digestive glands and their ducts (liver, pancreas, gallbladder, bile duct)	All connective tissues (bone, cartilage, ligaments, tendons)	Brain, spinal cord, ganglia, nerves
Lining of respiratory organs (except nasal cavity), including larynx, trachea, bronchial tree, lungs	All circulatory organs (heart, blood and lymph vessels, lymphatic organs, blood and blood-forming organs)	Lens, conjunctiva, retina, external and internal ear
Bladder (except trigone)	Excretory organs (kidney, ureter, trigone of bladder)	Lining of buccal and nasal cavities and parts of the pharynx and the paranasal sinuses
Female urethra and vestibular glands	Reproductive organs (testes, ductus deferens, seminal vesicles, ovaries, uterine tubes, vagina)	Epithelium of the salivary glands and enamel of the teeth
Male urethra (proximal portion), prostate, and bulbo-urethral glands	Serous membranes (pleurae, pericardium, peritoneum)	Hypophysis cerebri
	Pulp, dentine, and cementum of teeth	Anus and distal portion of male urethra
	Cortex of the adrenal gland	Medulla of adrenal gland

The developments that follow conception reflect the spiral pattern in which the universe itself is created. The genesis of the universe was described more than 2,500 years ago by the Chinese philosopher, Lao Tzu, when he wrote, "One gave birth to two; two gave birth to three; and three gave birth to all the myriad things." In this passage he describes the polarization of one infinity into two, yin and yang, and, through the spirallic interaction of the two basic forces, the never-ending creation of countless individual beings.

A similar pattern also governs the formation and development of each human being. The single ovum differentiates into two cells, then into two primary spirallic layers, then into three layers, and finally into the organs, tissues, glands, and trillions of cells that comprise the human body.

The differentiation of the layers into primitive organs occurs during the next period of pregnancy which lasts approximately 21 days. The excretory and respiratory systems also differentiate during this period. More minute structures such as the endocrine glands and sexual organs develop during the following period, which lasts for about 63 days. The organs and systems which appear during the first two periods also continue to grow and mature during this stage.

The first three periods of pregnancy (7 days, 21 days, 63 days) total approximately 91 days, or about three months. Therefore, the first trimester of pregnancy is the time during which the foundation of our physical structure is created. During the second trimester, the physical constitution with basic organs is strengthened and more peripheral structures develop. Coordination among the various systems, organs, and glands is established during the final trimester, as the fetus prepares itself for independent life.

Conception

Mature sperm are the smallest cells in the human body. However, because they are so highly charged with electromagnetic energy, they are also the most motile of the body's cells. Sperm consist of an oval shaped head, which carries the male chromosomes, and a long slender tail, which vibrates back and forth to produce movement. They are able to travel about one inch in 20 minutes.

Before leaving the penis, sperm travel more than 20 feet through the coiled sex ducts of the male. Being more yin, they move more easily in an upward direction. After being deposited in the vagina, sperm are aided in their upward motion by the rhythmic contractions of the female sex ducts and by the invisible, upward current of electromagnetic energy, or earth's force, which continuously enters the female body through the sexual organs. During their journey, sperm travel upward through the vagina, the uterus and into the Fallopian tubes. If a mature egg has been discharged by the ovary, fertilization may occur in the upper end of the tube.

Actually, only a small number of the millions of sperm contained in an average ejaculation travel the entire length of the Fallopian tubes. It is not known exactly how long sperm live in the female sex ducts but studies suggest that they may survive for up to 14 days, although three days is about the average. The quality of the cervical mucus and the vitality of sperm determine how long the sperm survive once they enter the vagina.

After being released from the ovary, the mature egg passes through the Fallopian tube en route to the uterus. If, during its passage through the tube, it is met and entered by a sperm, this newly fertilized ovum begins to undergo rapid change.

The fertilized ovum is a replica of the earth. Like the earth, it rotates and produces electromagnetic belts which radiate from its central core. The egg also undergoes a repeated shifting of its vertical axis—something the earth has also done many times in the past.

The dual forces of heaven and earth that pass through the mother's body nourish the egg with a constant stream of electromagnetic energy. Heaven and earth's forces meet in the uterus, specifically in the region of the abdominal energy center called the *hara* which is located deep within the womb. The life energy which streams along the mother's primary channel generates rapid growth and cell division in the newly fertilized ovum (see Chapter 1).

The fertilized ovum carries within it an unlimited potential for future development. The egg and sperm both contain a complete record of the evolution of life, together with a vision of, and aspiration toward, an unending future. At the moment of conception, a new human being is created that embodies both of these aspects.

Fig. 7   Fertilization.

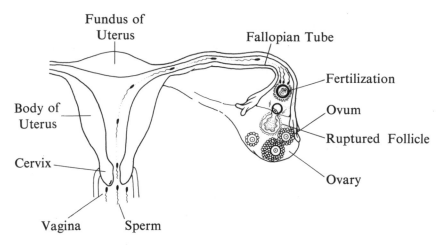

Of the several hundred million sperm deposited in the vagina during intercourse, only three to five hundred reach the egg at the far end of the Fallopian tube. Only one will fertilize the egg.

The First Month

The fertilized human ovum is about 1/200th of an inch across and barely visible to the naked eye. By the end of the first month, it has already developed into a young human embryo which is about 1/4th of an inch long.

During the first 30 days, the tiny, round egg cell develops toward a more human form with a head and body and the beginnings of eyes and ears, arms and legs, brain and stomach. The heart also forms during this period, as does blood which begins to circulate. Almost all of the major organs begin their development during this stage.

Implantation: After being fertilized, the egg travels through the Fallopian tube to the uterus. During this journey it rapidly divides into 2 cells, then into 4, 8, 16, 32, 64, and so on, until it takes the form of a small ball of about one hundred cells. It is this tiny mass of cells, known as the *morula*, which slowly travels through the uterine tube and into the uterus.

When fertilization occurs, the ovum begins to shake as in an earthquake, as its charge of life energy intensifies. It is then attracted to the stream of electromagnetic energy which charges the mother's primary channel, in order to provide itself with the energy necessary to continue its rapid growth and cell division.

Fig. 8   The first seven days of development

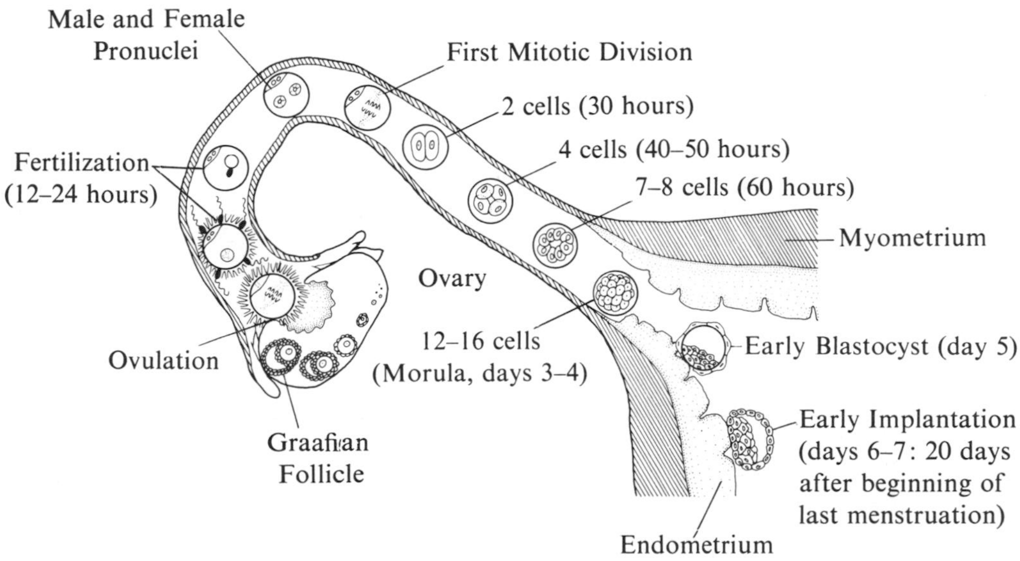

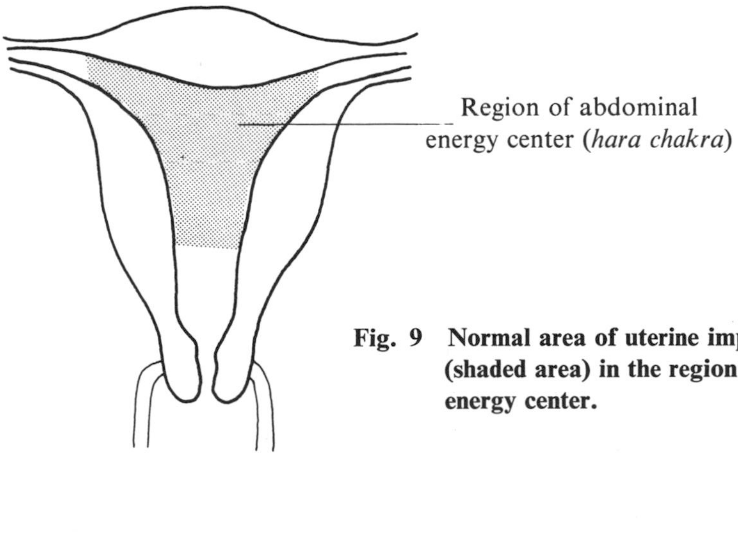

Fig. 9   Normal area of uterine implantation (shaded area) in the region of the abdominal energy center.

Following the development of the morula, a small cavity begins to form in the center of this mass of cells. The morula then develops into a hollow ball of cells known as the *blastocyst*. Around the seventh day after conception the ovum enters the uterine cavity and begins to attach itself to the lining of the uterus. The developing egg is usually completely embedded within these tissues by the end of the second week. Implantation normally occurs in the upper part of the womb in the area around the highly charged abdominal energy center.

Around the sixth day after conception, a thin layer of surface cells separates from the inner mass of the blastocyst. They are called *extra-embryonic trophoblast cells* and they grow very quickly during the second week until they form a velvety covering of treelike, branching tissues which cover the surface of the blastocyst. The trophoblast cells that later will form part of the placenta send out fingerlike projections, or villi, which burrow into the uterine tissues in order to obtain nutrients.

The tissues of the uterine lining are prepared for the arrival of the ovum by hormones secreted by the ovaries in coordination with the function of the pituitary gland. The uterine lining, now known as the *decidua*, is in a very active state—rich in blood with glands ready for secretion. Implantation takes place through a process in which the trophoblast cells take root in, engulf, and eventually dissolve the cells of the endometrium. As this happens, the blood vessels of the uterine lining rupture, causing a pool of blood to form around the ovum. It is from this blood that the trophoblast cells begin to absorb the oxygen, water, and nutrients necessary for the growth of the embryo. A protective wall of tissue gradually develops around the area of implantation, and it is here that the maternal and trophoblast cells cooperate in forming the placenta.

As they continue to grow, the trophoblast cells secrete *chorionic gonadotropic hormone*, also known as *placental hormone*, into the mother's bloodstream. The placental hormone prevents further menstruation and promotes adjustment of the mother's body to pregnancy. It is the presence of this hormone in the mother's blood or urine which makes it possible to confirm whether a woman is pregnant within three to four weeks after fertilization. Newer serum pregnancy tests make it possible to tell within five to six days after conception.

Other Developments: Following development of the three spirallic germ layers, organs such as the brain and heart begin to form. The ovum also changes from a hollow ball of cells into a flat, double-layered disc, and then into a definitely structured form with a clear distinction between the head and tail and left and right sides.

The *neural plate*, which is an early form of the nervous system, also develops within the outermost layer of cells. The periphery of the embryo eventually becomes the back of the body, leading to a further differentiation into yin and yang with the formation of parallel ridges on the left and right sides. These ridges bend toward each other and then fuse, changing the flat embryonic disc into a closed tube. The front portion then thickens and expands into the brain and the rear portion develops as the compact spinal cord.

The heart and blood vessels also develop during this period. Around the sixteenth day, groups of cells appear in the tissue that lies between the three germinal layers. These cells grow and develop into the first blood cells and vessels. As more of these cells form, those in the upper region grow into two tubes, one conducting heaven's force and the other earth's force. By the twenty-second day, heaven and earth's forces merge along the baby's primary channel, causing the tubes to fuse into a single heart tube.

The primitive heart then begins to beat in response to the rhythmic pulsation of heaven and earth's forces. The heartbeat commences on about the twenty-fourth day, causing blood to circulate throughout the embryonic disc and primitive placenta.

From the twentieth to the thirtieth day, tiny paired blocks of tissue, known as *somites*, arise along the back, molding the skin on either side of the future spinal cord into parallel rows of small bumps. The somites eventually develop into all of the body's muscles and bones.

During the third and fourth weeks, the embryo changes more rapidly than at any other period of life. The digestive system begins to form at this time, as the innermost germinal layer differentiates into two regions, the *foregut*, which lies more toward the front of the body, and the *hindgut*, which develops more toward the rear of the body.

During the fourth week, the embryo triples its size in seven days and changes from a straight tube to a curved spiral form with a head and tail portion. The formation of the brain and heart progresses rapidly and both organs create bulges in the front of the body. The eyes and ears also begin to develop.

Life in the womb is a repetition of evolutionary developments on earth, from the first appearance of single-celled organisms through the development of fish and other forms of marine life. Birth corresponds to the transition from water to land life which occurred hundreds of millions of years ago. An example of this evolutionary repetition occurs during the fourth week of pregnancy when a series of three grooves and ridges appear below the head on either side of the future neck. The grooves are similar to the gill slits in fish, while the ridges are like the gill bars in the neck of the fish. The ridges later develop into the baby's face and neck.

The kidneys present another example of the recapitulation of evolutionary history. The kidneys develop in stages; the first to develop is a type of kidney similar to that found in primitive fish and eels. The first kidney degenerates soon after being formed. By the end of the fourth week, it is replaced by the middle kidney, or *mesonephros*, a long, slender organ with many coiled tubules, which lies between the spinal cord and intestine. During the second month, the tubules develop into the ducts of the male reproductive system. In the meantime, at the end of the first month, the third and final form of the kidney begins to develop near the tail end of the body.

By the end of the first month, the embryo has increased about eight thousand times in weight. Although only about a quarter of an inch long, the embryo has now passed through the equivalent of hundreds of millions of years of evolutionary history and has completed the foundation for life toward a human being.

Fig. 10 Development of the internal organs during the fourth week.

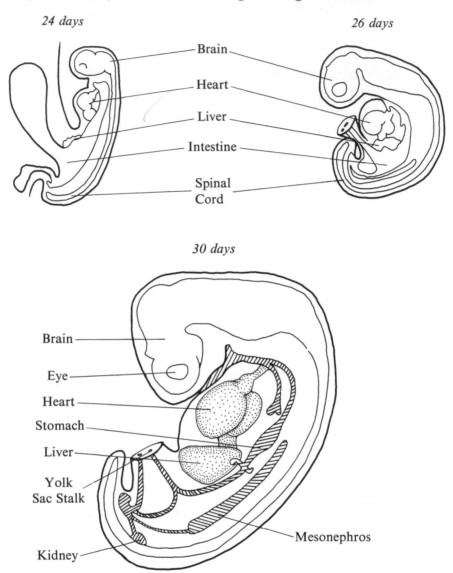

The three embryos are drawn to the same scale and show the rapid growth that occurs in the brain, heart, liver, and other organs.

The Extra-Embryonic Membranes: Soon after fertilization, the cells within the blastocyst divide into two complementary groups: those which develop as part of the human body and those which produce the various structures which protect, nourish, and sustain the developing baby. Structures which are located outside the body and discarded at birth include: 1) the placenta, 2) the amniotic sac, 3) the yolk sac, 4) the allantois, 5) the chorion and 6) the umbilical cord.

Fig. 11 Uterine / fetal relationships.

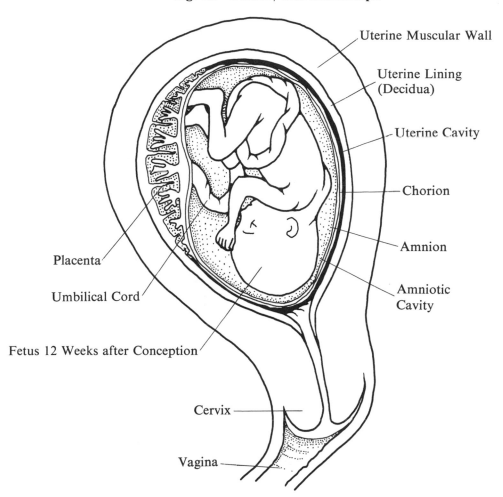

Uterine Muscular Wall

Uterine Lining (Decidua)

Uterine Cavity

Chorion

Amnion

Amniotic Cavity

Placenta

Umbilical Cord

Fetus 12 Weeks after Conception

Cervix

Vagina

1) *The placenta:* The placenta, or afterbirth, contains both maternal and embryonic portions. At birth, it is a flat, disc-shaped structure about seven or eight inches in diameter and about an inch thick. It usually weighs about one pound and is composed of millions of tiny projections known as *chorionic villi.*

The placental villi are part of the embryonic circulatory system. All of the minerals, proteins, carbohydrates, fats, and other substances which the baby needs are carried to the placenta by the blood and tissues of the mother. Nutrients are absorbed by the villi, resynthesized according to the baby's needs, and passed into the baby's circulatory system through the umbilical cord.

The placenta acts as a filter. Only certain particles pass from mother to baby through the membranes of the villi. The substances that pass through are attracted to certain regions of the developing embryonic body according

Fig. 12   The placenta.

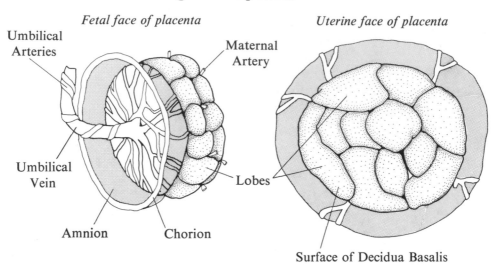

Fetal face of placenta

Uterine face of placenta

Umbilical
Arteries

Maternal
Artery

Umbilical
Vein

Lobes

Amnion

Chorion

Surface of Decidua Basalis

to their yin and yang qualities. Calcium, minerals, and other more yang nutrients are attracted more toward the back of the body. Here, more dense masses of tissue form, for example, the brain, spinal cord, and somites, from which the spine and skeleton eventually develop. The contracting and expanding influences provided by minerals and other nutrients, together with polarized electromagnetic charges, also cause the embryo to change shape. Initially, the embryo assumes the form of a more or less straight tube which reflects the vertical charge of heaven and earth's forces. By the fourth week, these combined influences cause the embryo to curve inward, with the tail nearly touching the head.

The more yin nutrients absorbed by the embryo—especially proteins and fats—gather more toward the inner or frontal regions of the body, causing the softer tissues of the major organs to develop and expand. The more yin effect of these nutrients becomes apparent during the first month when a bulge develops in the area of the heart. Through the remainder of pregnancy, the softer, more expanded structures that develop in the front of the body contrast markedly with the tighter and more compact structures that develop along the back of the body.

Once the heart and blood vessels begin to function, blood circulates through the embryonic body and out through the umbilical cord to the placenta. The nutrients, oxygen, hormones, and antibodies that have been absorbed by the villi are carried back to the baby with the returning blood. Conversely, waste products from the baby's metabolism, including *urea*, the waste product of protein metabolism, carbon dioxide, and water, are carried out to the placenta. Waste products diffuse into the mother's blood and are eventually discharged from her body. The blood of the mother and that of the baby flow past each other in separate channels and are separated by a thin layer of cells that cover the villi. There is no intermingling of the two bloodstreams during pregnancy.

Fig. 13   Exchange between the placental villi and lining of the uterus.

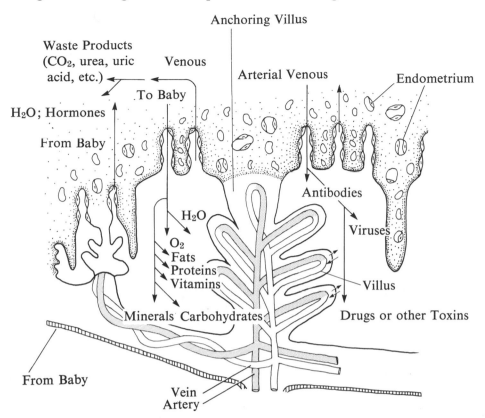

The placenta is structurally similar to the liver. Both organs contain many branched and highly differentiated blood vessels and ducts. The mammary glands also have a similar structure. During pregnancy, the mother's breasts start to grow and the tips become very sensitive and, in some cases, painful. The nipples also change from their normally more yang, pinkish red color, to a dark brown color which is more yin. During pregnancy, the upper regions of a woman's body become more yin or expanded, while energy, blood, and nutrients gather toward the depths of the womb, making the lower part of her body more yang.

The breasts and the placenta provide complementary forms of nourishment for the baby. The placenta filters blood to produce a highly concentrated, more yang form of nourishment. After birth, the mammary glands filter blood in order to create a form of nourishment that is sweeter and more yin than that provided by the placenta.

Both placenta and embryo develop in a manner which is similar to the structure of a tree. The trunk of the placental tree is the umbilical cord in which several large umbilical blood vessels develop. The blood vessels split into smaller and smaller branches, similar to the way that the trunk of a tree gives rise to branches. The leaves of the tree are the numerous chorionic villi which implant themselves in the lining of the uterus. By the time they reach the villi, vessels differentiate into millions of tiny capillaries through which oxygen and nutrients are absorbed.

The embryonic tree has a complementary structure. In this case, the millions of chorionic villi serve as the roots of the tree. Blood bathes the villi similar to the way that the roots of a tree are bathed by water in the soil. Like the roots of a tree, the villi absorb nutrients through their cellular membranes. The umbilical cord, through which these nutrients pass, comprises the trunk of the embryonic tree. The branches are made up by the blood vessels which branch from the umbilical cord throughout the baby's entire body. The leaves of this tree are the body cells themselves. After birth, the internal organs assume the various functions of the placental villi; the intestinal villi begin to absorb nutrients, the lungs absorb oxygen, and the respiratory and excretory organs discharge waste products.

As the baby grows, so does the placenta; it eventually covers about one-third of the inner surface of the uterus. During the first four months, the placenta is larger and heavier than the baby, while the baby grows more actively than the placenta during the remainder of pregnancy. The placenta also produces hormones that act on the womb, breasts, and blood to produce many of the physical and emotional changes which occur during pregnancy—changes which involve practically every organ and system in the mother's body.

2) *The amniotic sac:*   The amniotic sac, or *amnion*, surrounds the baby and contains the fluid in which the baby floats. The amniotic fluid provides a watery environment replicating the ancient ocean in which life evolved for billions of years. It also provides a protective envelope that surrounds the baby, cushioning any shocks or sudden movements that the mother may experience. The amniotic fluid also permits the baby to move about with relative freedom.

At birth, uterine contractions push the amniotic sac into the cervical canal, aiding the dilation of the cervix. The amnion normally ruptures just before birth, and this "flow of waters" passes through the vagina ahead of the infant, lubricating and disinfecting the birth canal.

3) *The yolk sac:*   The yolk sac develops shortly after conception and hangs from the belly of the embryo. It does not contain any yolk and is another example of the recapitulation of earlier stages of evolution during pregnancy. In other species, the yolk sac provides nourishment for the embryo, while in humans it is incorporated into the umbilical cord and the digestive tract.

4) *The allantois:*   The allantois is a small growth which appears at the tail end of the embryo. After about the fourth week, it becomes a part of the umbilical cord. Like the yolk sac, the allantois is a vestige of an earlier stage of biological evolution. The allantois plays a much more important role in the embryonic development of other species, where it serves both as a respiratory and nutritive organ.

5) *The chorion:* The chorion is an important embryonic membrane that develops from the outer layer of the trophoblast. It forms the outer wall of the blastocyst from which the placental villi develop. Together with the placenta, the chorion functions primarily in providing nutrients for the baby.

6) *The umbilical cord:* As the more yin digestive system spiral begins to develop, it causes a portion of the body wall to project outward, eventually developing into the spirally coiled tube known as the umbilical cord. The cord contains two umbilical arteries which carry nutrient rich blood to the baby and one vein which carries the waste products of fetal metabolism out to the placenta. The expanding force generated by the developing spiral of the digestive tract pushes part of the long, coiled intestine out into the opening where the umbilical cord attaches to the body wall. These tissues comprise what is known as an *umbilical hernia.* By the fourth month, the intestines are withdrawn back into the abdomen. At birth, the umbilical cord is spirally twisted and extends about two feet. Longer cords are generally the result of an overconsumption of more yin foods by the mother, while shorter cords result when the mother's diet is generally more yang.

The Second Month

During the second month of life, the embryo continues to grow rapidly, passing through the equivalent of hundreds of millions of years of biological evolution. By the end of the second month, the embryo weighs about one gram and is about one inch in length. At the beginning of the second month, the head comprises about one third of the body. In the weeks that follow, the face, which initially resembles that of a fish or tadpole, becomes more distinctly human.

Fig. 14 Development of the embryo during the second month of life.

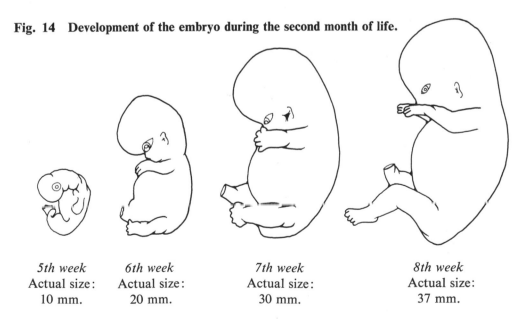

5th week	*6th week*	*7th week*	*8th week*
Actual size:	Actual size:	Actual size:	Actual size:
10 mm.	20 mm.	30 mm.	37 mm.

The Face and Internal Organs: The development of the face reflects the recapitulation of biological evolution and also corresponds to the development of the internal organs. Therefore, each of the facial features develop together with one or several of the internal organs. Several of these correspondences are presented below.*

1)   *The heart/nose and face as a whole:*   At the beginning of the second month, the nose consists of two shallow pits of specialized skin which overlie the front end of the brain. The nasal pits deepen during the second month to form the nasal cavities. They are originally located far out on either side of the face but through a gradual process of contraction grow closer together until they are enclosed in the ridge of tissue that becomes the nose.
A similar contracting process takes place in the heart, which begins as two separate tubes which fuse into a single organ. By the end of the second month, the nose has a broad, flat shape with the nostrils pointing forward. The heart also changes from a simple bent tube to the normal adult form with four internal sections—two atria and two ventricles—separated by partitions known as septa.

The sixth and seventh weeks are especially important for the developing heart. It is then that the septum which divides the ventricles grows rapidly and closes off the opening between these two chambers. If the mother's diet is deficient in minerals or complex carbohydrates in early pregnancy, or if she consumes too much simple sugar, fruit, fruit juice, soft drinks, or other items that deprive the body of minerals and complex sugars, the closure can be delayed or prevented from occurring. The result is often the persistence of an opening through which blood leaks from the right to the left ventricle when the heart contracts. A hole in the septum can cause serious problems for the infant after birth.

If the maternal diet is less extreme than mentioned above but still lacking in sufficient minerals and other more yang nutrients, the right and left chambers of the heart may not fuse properly, resulting in a lack of coordination in the heartbeat which manifests as a heart murmur. Heart murmurs are often accompanied by a cleft in the tip of the nose, also a sign that the maternal diet was lacking in minerals and other more contractive foods.

The septum that separates the left and right atria also has an opening in it, but this is normal in the fetus as it allows some of the blood pumped by the heart to bypass the lungs which do not function in the womb. In most cases, the opening closes soon after birth. However, if the mother has consumed an excessive quantity of more yin foods during her pregnancy and has not eaten an adequate balance of minerals and complex sugars, it may not close properly. (Please see Chapter 7 for further discussion of congenital heart defects.)

---

* A more complete explanation of the relationship between the internal organs and the facial features is presented in *How to See Your Health: the Book of Oriental Diagnosis* (Japan Publications, Inc.) and in *Your Face Never Lies* (Avery Publishing Group), by Michio Kushi.

2) *The digestive tract/mouth:* At the beginning of the second month, the mouth resembles a wide gaping hole. During the second month, the lower and upper jaws differentiate and develop, and the mouth becomes progressively more yang or contracted, although it is still much wider than at birth. After the second month of pregnancy, the jaws fuse at the proper place, the cheeks and lips begin to develop more clearly, and the mouth narrows to a more normal width.

Rapid developments occur in the digestive tract, as the tongue, taste buds, lips, and precursers of teeth begin to form, together with the esophagus, stomach, small and large intestines, and rectum. The inner lining of the intestines, where the intestinal villi develop, also forms during this period.

If during pregnancy the mother consumes a large volume of tropical fruits, fruit juice, sugar, soft drinks, more acidic vegetables such as tomatoes, eggplant, and potatoes, oil and fat, and coffee and other stimulants, the embryo will lack the contracting power necessary to cause the mouth to tighten and narrow sufficiently. A wide mouth is an indication that on the whole, the digestive system is natively weaker in its function. An ideal mouth, which indicates a strong and vital digestive system, is one that has the same or a narrower width than the nostrils. Narrower mouths were prevalent in the past when people ate traditionally based diets, prior to the widespread use of industrialized and processed foods.

Fig. 15 Development of the face during the second month.

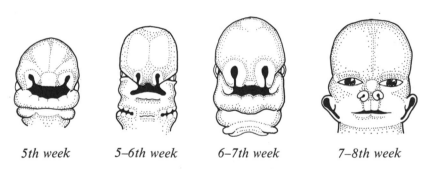

5th week	*5–6th week*	*6–7th week*	*7–8th week*

3) *The kidneys/ears:* The ears develop from the fusion of the nodules that appear around the largest of the primitive gill-like grooves in the neck region. The nodules develop into the external ear, while the groove itself develops into the ear cavity and canal.

During the second month, the ears migrate from a lower position, almost in the neck region, to a higher position on the sides of the head. The position and shape of the ears reflect the baby's whole physical and mental constitution, in addition to reflecting the development and condition of the kidneys. In general, a normal, healthy constitution, including strong kidneys, is reflected in large, well developed ears that begin at eye-level and extend down to the mouth. Large, well developed ears result from a maternal diet which contains the proper balance of minerals, proteins, and complex carbohydrates. Small ears, ears that develop high up on the head, or ears that possess little or no lobe show that a baby's overall constitution is weaker. A weaker constitution results from an unbalanced diet during pregnancy, especially a diet lacking in sufficient minerals or one that is too high in protein, especially animal protein such as meat, eggs, poultry, and fish. The left ear reflects the development of the left kidney, while the right ear reflects the right kidney.

4) *The centrally located organs/eyes:* The left eye reflects the development and condition of the spleen and pancreas, while the right eye corresponds to the liver and gallbladder.

At the beginning of the second month, the eyes lie far apart on the opposite sides of the head. During the weeks that follow, the contracting force that molds the face causes the eyes to migrate from the sides toward the center and front of the face. By the end of the second month, the eyes are much closer together, although they are still farther apart than they will be at birth. During the seventh week of life, folds of skin develop above the eyes and become the eyelids. They close soon afterward and remain closed for the next three months.

The distance between the eyes is determined by the type of food eaten by the mother during pregnancy. Eyes that are very close together show that the mother ate strong yang foods, especially animal products, and indicate that the baby has a tendency to develop a more aggressive, and perhaps stubborn, personality. Eyes that are far apart result from a more yin diet, with a larger consumption of foods such as sugar, fruit, fruit juice, salad, and more watery foods. A baby born with more widely set eyes has a tendency to develop a more gentle, and perhaps timid, or indecisive character.

Additional correlations between the organs and facial features are as follows:

1. The lungs—cheeks.
2. The bronchi—nostrils.
3. The stomach—the middle part of the nose.
4. The pancreas—upper middle part of the nose.
5. The kidneys and sexual organs—eyes. In girls the eyes reflect the ovaries and in boys, the testes.
6. The liver—the region of the face between the eyebrows.
7. The spleen—the temples on both sides of the face, as well as the whole part of the nose pillar.
8. The intestines—the forehead as well as the mouth.
9. The bladder—the uppermost region of the forehead around the hairline.
10. The sexual organs—the area around the mouth.

The forces generated by the growth of the body's three major spirallic systems converge in the face and exert a contracting influence. The force generated by the development of the digestive system begins at the central region of the small intestine, in the abdominal energy center (*hara chakra*), and expands outward and upward, differentiating into the respiratory organs. It continues upward and influences the formation of the lower part of the face around the mouth. The influence of the digestive system extends upward to the lines which in adults flow down from the sides of the nose (see Fig. 16). The lips, tongue, and mouth cavity are included in this area.

Fig. 16   Face and major system correlations.

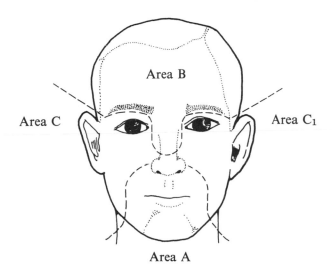

Area B

Area C

Area C₁

Area A

Area A: The condition of the mouth, lips, tongue, mouth cavity, and area around the mouth, show the digestive functions as a whole. This area also relates partially to the respiratory function, especially at its peripheral area.

Area B: The condition of the forehead and its periphery, including the temples and eyebrows, represent the condition of the nervous system as a whole.

Areas C and C₁: The side facial areas, including both eyes, cheeks and ears, represent the condition and function of the circulatory and excretory systems as a whole.

The upper part of the face is influenced primarily by the nervous system and brain. The area influenced by the nervous system extends down the front of the face and includes the forehead, temples, eyebrows, and nose. The spiral of the circulatory and excretory systems influences the formation of the side areas of the face, including both cheeks, eyes, and ears.

The Arms and Legs: The arms and legs develop from small buds that project from the sides of the body. During the fifth week, the limb buds flatten into paddle-like ridges, in which four parallel grooves appear, marking off five digits. As the grooves deepen, the fingers and toes begin to take form. Nail beds appear several weeks later, leading to the development of nails during the fifth month.

Fig. 17   Development of the hands and feet, fingers and toes during the second and third months.

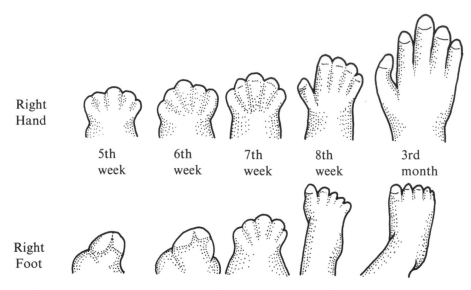

The fingers and toes develop together with the internal organs and bodily functions. The fingers and fingernails correspond to the internal organs and bodily functions in the following manner:

1)   Thumb—lungs and respiratory organs.
2)   Index finger—large intestine.
3)   Middle finger—the function of blood and energy circulation which is centered mostly around the heart and the reproductive organs.
4)   Ring finger—the function of eliminating excessive energy from the heart, stomach, and intestinal region and the regulation of the body's metabolism.
5)   Little finger—the heart and small intestine.

The toes and toenails correspond to the internal organs and their respective functions as follows:

1)   First toe (outer region in the same direction as the arch of the foot)—spleen.
2)   First toe (inner region toward the second toe)—liver.
3)   Second and third toes—stomach. (The second toe corresponds more to the body of the stomach and the third toe to the sphincter and duodenum.)
4)   Fourth toe—gallbladder.
5)   Fifth toe—bladder.

To understand how these developments are connected, we need to understand the way in which the energy of heaven and earth influences the embryo and its environment.

The uterus contains a series of invisible energy ridges that resemble the vertical ridges of a pumpkin. The uterine ridges, or meridians, carry a strong electromagnetic charge and provide the developing embryo with a continual supply of energy. There are twelve meridians running along the surface of the inner wall of the uterus.

Since the fertilized ovum continually rotates, energy from the uterine meridians assumes a curved, or spiral path as it channels in toward the central regions of the ovum. The twelve major channels of energy collect in the form of densely compacted spirals deep within the ovum. When similar energy spirals are created in fruits and vegetables, they develop into seeds. When they are created in the human body, they become the internal organs. Energy is then discharged through two pairs of streams, one pair spiralling upward and the other downward.

The upward spirals give rise to the arms, hands, and fingers. The lower spirals produce the legs, feet, and toes. The internal organs are not separate from these spiral streams; both are aspects of the same energy continuum. It is for this reason that developments in the internal organs parallel developments in the fingers and toes.

Fig. 18 Schematic energy flow within the embryo connecting the internal organs with the arms and legs, fingers and toes.

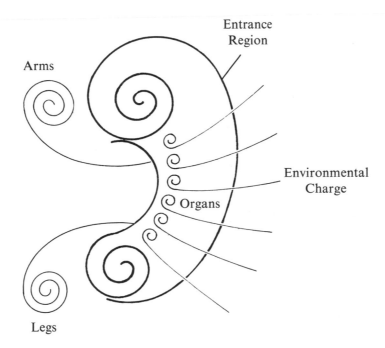

Energy from the environment enters the developing embryo through the back, creates the internal organs, and exits through the front of the body along the arms and legs.

The energy that creates the internal organs originates with the twelve meridians of the mother's uterus, which in turn are nourished by the twelve meridians running along the surface of her body. The mother's surface meridians receive a constant supply of energy from the environment and ultimately from the twelve constellations which circle the earth in far distant space. Throughout life, the meridians and organs are constantly influenced by the activity of these twelve constellations.

During the second month, the arms and legs elongate and are subdivided by joints in the elbows, wrists, knees, and ankles. Joints mark the orbits of the arm and leg spirals, both of which eventually form seven complete orbits. Bones and muscles begin to form within the arms and legs during the latter part of the second month, guided by the invisible energy blueprint laid out by the limb spirals.

The formation of the arms and legs depends on the quality of nourishment provided by the mother's bloodstream. The quality of the mother's blood is determined by what she consumes daily. The thalidomide tragedies that occurred about twenty years ago illustrate the influence that the products a pregnant woman consumes has on her rapidly growing baby. Thalidomide, an extremely yin drug, arrested the development of the limb buds. If taken by the mother at the time when the limb buds were developing, growth stopped at the limb bud stage and the baby was born with rudimentary arms and legs. The drug prevented the full seven orbits of spirallic development from occurring.

The Muscles and Bones: By the end of the second month, all of the large muscles of the body have formed, including those of the arms and legs. The bones also begin to develop at this time. The bones of the head develop in a manner that is complementary to the formation of bones in the rest of the body. The bones in the head develop directly as hard bone, while those in the body develop through a process in which primary models, or *templates*, are initially set in softer cartilage and then are gradually replaced by more rigid, bony tissue. During the second month, the cartilage model of the entire skeleton develops. The growth of cartilage and its transformation into bone begins during the second month and continues after birth until full physical maturity is accomplished.

The transformation of cartilage into bone is known as *ossification*. A thin sheet of bone develops like a collar around the middle of each cartilage template. Bony covering then spreads over the surface of the model and also penetrates the underlying layers, while the original cartilage stops growing and eventually disappears.

The embryonic stage draws to a close at the end of the second month, as the face and organs, arms and legs, hands and feet, and muscles and bones develop. Through the remainder of pregnancy, the developing baby is referred to as a fetus.

The Third Month

During the third month, many of the organs begin to function and more highly specialized structures begin to form. The fetus grows to about three inches in length and about fourteen grams in weight. The sex of the baby becomes distinguishable, and the fetus begins preparing itself for life outside the womb.

The Development of Sex: The sexual organs begin to develop during the sixth week when a primitive gonad appears within the mesonephros, or middle kidney. The gonad has the capacity to differentiate into either the testes or ovaries. By the end of the third month, the surface of the gonad differentiates into cords of cells that are the forerunners of the sperm-producing tubules of the testes. In girls, the cords are abandoned during the third month and a second set of sexual cells develop, which eventually become the sex cells of the ovary.

The genital ducts also develop from common predecessors. At two months, males and females both possess two complete sets of ducts which develop near the gonads. These are known as the *Wolffian ducts*, which are part of the mesonephros, and the *Mullerian ducts*, which develop alongside the first set of ducts and grow downward toward the bladder. The right and left Mullerian ducts fuse in the lower ... t.

... ex ducts of the indifferent period into

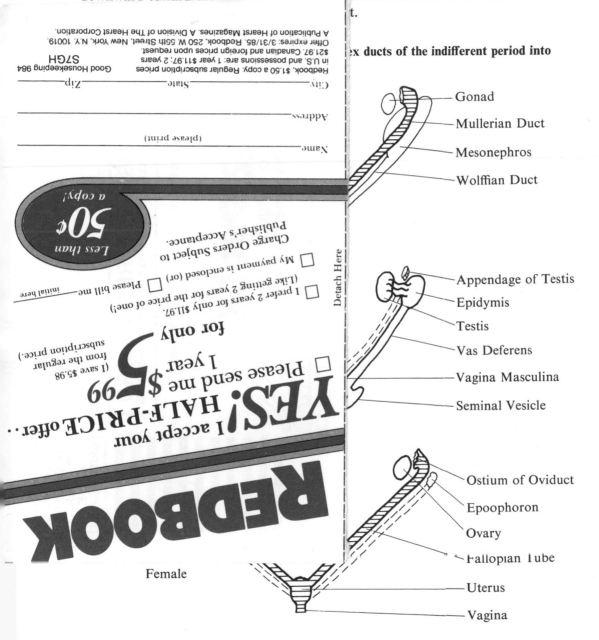

Gonad
Mullerian Duct
Mesonephros
Wolffian Duct

Appendage of Testis
Epidymis
Testis
Vas Deferens
Vagina Masculina
Seminal Vesicle

Female

Ostium of Oviduct
Epoophoron
Ovary
Fallopian Tube
Uterus
Vagina

If the indifferent gonads develop into testes, the Mullerian ducts begin to degenerate. The Wolffian ducts enlarge and become the vas deferens, which extend from the testes down toward the bladder, emptying into a little mound known as the *genital tubercle.*

The genital tubercle is located on the belly wall between the umbilical cord and legs. All fetuses develop this feature. On the underside of the tubercle lies an opening into which the urinary ducts from the bladder empty, together with the Wolffian and Mullerian ducts. The opening appears as a long groove and is known as the *urogenital sinus.* As the testes begin to develop, the genital tubercle grows and becomes the penis.

The opening is surrounded by two parallel folds of skin, which eventually fuse, leaving only a small opening at the tip of the penis. Surrounding the genital folds are additional mounds of skin known as the *genital swellings.* The swellings continue to expand until they form two pouches that fuse and develop into the scrotum. The testes enter the scrotum near the end of pregnancy after migrating from their original position near the kidneys.

In girls, the Mullerian duct develops into the Fallopian tubes, uterus, and most of the vagina, while the Wolffian duct degenerates. The upper section of the Mullerian duct develops into the Fallopian tubes, while the lower section fuses and develops a thick muscular wall which becomes the uterus and most of the vagina.

The development of the sexual organs is guided by the forces of centripetality and centrifugality, or yang and yin. In boys, a more yin, or centrifugal force causes the genital tubercle to enlarge and develop into the penis. It also causes the testes to migrate from the body cavity into the scrotum.

In girls, a more centripetal, or contracting force limits the growth of the genital tubercle; rather than enlarging, it remains small and develops as the clitoris. At the same time, the urogenital sinus remains open, forming the vestibule into which the vagina and urethra open. The genitals remain separate and form a pair of lips which surround the open sinus. The genital swellings do not expand as they do in boys. They remain small and develop into a second pair of lips, the labia majora, which surround the inner pair.

Other Developments: In the mouth, a series of tooth buds that secrete enamel and dentine develop into the upper and lower jaws. The tooth buds gradually develop into the twenty baby teeth that will break through the child's gums during the first three years of life.

The palate also develops during the second month. The palate is initially separated into halves which fuse and create a horizontal bridge separating the mouth and nasal cavity. Fusion of the palate is dependent on the quality of nutrients supplied by the mother, especially the proper quality and amount of minerals and vitamins. Foods such as refined sugar, soft drinks, tropical fruits and juices, spices, coffee, highly acidic vegetables such as tomatoes, potatoes, and eggplant, and drugs and medications often interfere with complete fusion of the palate. Extremely yin foods deplete minerals; if the lack of minerals becomes severe enough, the palate may not fuse completely, resulting in the more yin condition known as *cleft palate* (See Chapter 7).

If plenty of more yin foods are consumed when the bones and teeth are forming, the baby is often born with a weaker and more frail constitution, since the development of these structures depends largely on the supply of minerals. Foods such as whole grains, vegetables, and sea vegetables, which contain a proper balance of vitamins and minerals, are especially important in the formation of the bones and teeth and in the proper development of the palate. Sea vegetables such as *hijiki*, *arame*, *kombu*, and *wakame* and green leafy vegetables including *daikon* and turnip greens, kale, and watercress contain plenty of calcium and other minerals and are especially recommended during pregnancy.

The region around the mouth and the throat *chakra* or energy center, becomes active during the third month as the larynx, or voice box, begins to develop. The salivary glands begin to secrete a highly charged digestive liquid, saliva, and the gastric glands in the stomach begin to secrete mucus. During the following month, the salivary glands being secreting *pytalin*, an enzyme that is especially important in the breakdown of cereal grains, and the gastric glands begin to secrete *pepsin*.

The liver begins to assume some of the functions of the placenta, including the synthesis of certain chemicals needed for fetal growth. The liver also assumes a temporary role in the formation of red blood cells. During the following month, this function is shared by the spleen.

In the pancreas, two types of specialized cells differentiate and form clusters known as the *Islands of Langerhans*. The more yang type of cells within these clusters are known as *beta* cells, and they secrete *insulin*, a more yang hormone that controls the metabolism of sugar in the body. The more yin type of cells, known as *alpha* cells, secrete a hormone known as *glucagon*, or anti-insulin. These complementary hormones work throughout life to maintain the proper balance of sugar in the blood.

The final model of the kidney begins to function during the third month. (However, the kidneys do not complete their full development until about a month after birth.) The kidneys begin producing *amniotic fluid* at this stage, causing it to increase in volume. Amniotic fluid originates with the liquid taken in by the mother, which is passed through the placenta and into the baby's bloodstream. The circulation of amniotic fluid is established at this time, with old fluid being continually removed and new fluid added. As the baby's digestive organs begin to function, amniotic fluid is frequently swallowed and absorbed into the bloodstream through the digestive tract. Some of this swallowed liquid is passed back into the surrounding fluid by the baby's kidneys. At full term, a baby is surrounded by about one quart of amniotic fluid.

Much before the end of the third month, the baby begins to move, although it is rarely noticed by the mother because of the cushion provided by the amniotic fluid. A baby's basic constitution has been largely completed after the first three months of pregnancy. At that time, the mother often loses body weight. During the remainder of the pregnancy, the fundamental quality is strengthened in preparation for the life outside the womb.

The Fourth Month

The developments that occur at this stage are more subtle than those of the first three months of pregnancy. The rate of growth slows down; the baby triples in size during the third month but only doubles during the fourth. From the sixth to ninth months, the baby grows about an inch every ten days.

Clear patterns of movement and rest are established at this time, as the baby begins to stir, stretch, and thrust his or her arms and legs outward. These movements alternate with periods of quiet, motionless sleep and are initially felt by the mother as vague sensations which are like the fluttering of wings. However, the baby's movements soon become more forceful. These first movements have been traditionally referred to as the "quickening of life" in the womb.

The Fifth Month

During the fifth month, the skin becomes thicker, and flat, cornified cells develop in the peripheral layers. Dead skin cells are continually sloughed off and combine with oil from the skin glands to form the *vernix caseosa*, an oily substance that coats the baby's skin. Oil is a more yin substance, and serves to repel water, which is also yin. Therefore the vernix caseosa helps prevent the baby's skin from becoming waterlogged or overly soft or loose during the remaining time spent in the watery environment of the womb.

The Lines of the Palm: The skin on the palm and soles of the feet becomes thicker, and spirallic whorls and lines appear on the tips of the fingers and toes. The lines of the palm also form during this period. The palm lines correspond to the three primary germ layers from which the major bodily systems develop.

Fig. 20 Correlation between the lines of the palm and the major organ systems.

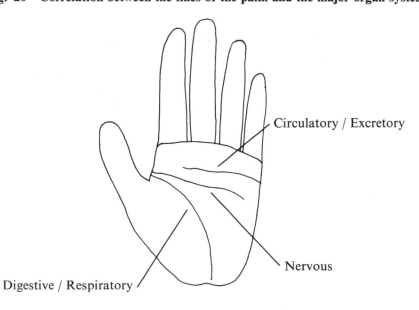

Circulatory / Excretory

Nervous

Digestive / Respiratory

The innermost line, often referred to as the "life line," reflects the development and formation of the digestive and respiratory systems. The middle line reflects the development of the nervous system, while the uppermost line reflects the development of the circulatory and excretory systems.

The three major lines also reflect the influence received from the parents. If they are deep and clear and the digestive/respiratory line is long and unbroken, the baby has a strong and balanced constitution, with all of the major systems coordinating smoothly with each other. If the lines on the baby's right palm are deeper and clearer than those on the left, the mother is the more healthy and active parent. If those on the left are more distinct, then the father is stronger.

The influence of the grandparents also leaves an imprint on the lines of the palm. When the major systems and organs first begin to develop, the embryo forms an almost closed circle with the tail nearly touching the head.* At two months, the back is about twice as long as the front. The back, which is in a more peripheral, yin location, is influenced more by the father's sperm, while the more yang, centrally located front, is influenced more by the mother's egg.

The brain and nervous system, which develop along the back, are therefore influenced primarily by the quality of the father's sperm cell, while the digestive and respiratory systems, which develop more toward the front, are influenced more by the quality of the mother's egg. The circulatory and excretory systems contain a more combined balance of both parents' influences.

Taken as a whole, the lines of the right palm reflect the mother's heritage. Within this overall correspondence, the digestive/respiratory line on the right hand reflects the influence received by the maternal grandmother. The nervous system line reflects the influence of the maternal grandfather. The circulatory/excretory line shows the combined influence of both maternal grandparents.

The left palm reflects the father's heritage. The digestive/respiratory line on the left hand reflects the influence of the father's mother; the nervous system line, that of the father's father; and the circulatory/excretory line, the combined influence of both the father's parents.

If a particular line is deep and clear, it means that the corresponding system is natively strong and well developed. If a line is less deep and clear, or if the digestive/respiratory line is short, the corresponding system is constitutionally weaker.

Head and Body Hair: By the end of the fifth month, some of the proteins, minerals, and fats that the baby takes in are discharged in the form of fine hair which covers the head, back, shoulders, and other parts of the body. As head hair develops, the hair spiral becomes visible, reflecting the spirallic development of the human body. The hair spiral traces the spiral path left by heaven's force as it enters the body at the top of the head. By the end of the fifth month, soft, fine hair, known as *lanugo*, appears on the back, arms, and legs. The lanugo hair creates a soft covering over the entire body. Most of it disappears before birth and is replaced by the sparser but heavier body hair of the infant.

---

* The tail grows rapidly until the second month, after which it regresses and is hidden by the growing buttocks. It is a remnant of an earlier stage of biological evolution.

The five-month-old fetus frequently swallows amniotic fluid which contains fatty vernix caseosa, dead skin cells, and lanugo hairs. Some of these materials are absorbed through the digestive tract and into the bloodstream. Undigestible portions accumulate in the large intestine in the form of a watery feces known as *meconium*. The secretion of bile into the intestinal tract causes the meconium to take on a dark green color. The meconium is usually held in the intestines throughout pregnancy and discharged shortly after birth.

The Sixth Month to Birth

During the sixth month, the baby reaches an average length of thirteen inches and an average weight of between one-and-one-half to two pounds. If born at this stage, most babies live for several hours but rarely survive. As the weeks go by, however, the baby's chances of surviving premature birth improve rapidly.

The eyelids open during the sixth month. Eyelashes and eyebrows appear and the lips become distinct. The body becomes better proportioned, and the fetus begins to resemble a human infant. Because the iris lacks pigment, all babies normally have dark, bluish grey eyes when born. It is not until after birth that pigment develops in the iris, giving the baby his or her characteristic eye color. During the seventh month, development has reached the point where most babies are able to live outside the womb. With favorable birth conditions, seven-month-old babies often survive premature birth.

The Brain and Nervous System: With the exception of the reproductive system, the brain and nervous system is the last system to achieve maturity. The brain develops in the form of a spiral which, once completed, contains seven full orbits. The *cerebral cortex*, which is the last part of the brain to develop, comprises the most peripheral part of the spiral and is a recent product of evolution. The inner parts of the brain, which deal more with the body's autonomic functions, are the first to develop and correspond to an earlier stage in the evolution of the nervous system. Through the process of evolution, which is repeated in the womb, the brain and nervous system have become increasingly complex, culminating in the development of the cerebral cortex. The increasing complexity of the brain and nervous system sets the stage for the evolution of consciousness from the most basic level of 1) mechanical response to the environment at birth, through 2) sensorial awareness, 3) emotional response, 4) analytical or rational thinking, 5) social awareness, 6) philosophical or ideological consciousness, and ultimately toward 7) universal, cosmic consciousness, as human life continues.

During the second and third months of embryonic life, long bundles of nerve fibers develop within the brain and spinal cord. These fibers connect all parts of the brain and spinal cord with each other. Gradually, the internal nerve fibers and external nerve branches begin to function, starting with those which have formed first.

At the beginning of the second month, the cerebral hemispheres take the form of two thin-walled sacs which develop outward from the front of the brain. During the remainder of pregnancy, and following birth, the cerebral hemispheres grow more rapidly than other parts of the brain, adding additional layers on top of the older and more primitive layers. Highly specialized nerve cells migrate to the periphery of the hemispheres, forming the tissue of the cerebral cortex. From the sixth month onward, the amount of cortex increases continuously as the many grooves and ridges of the brain develop.

During embryonic life, the nervous system functions automatically, in a manner similar to that of more primitive species. As more nerves and nerve tracts within the brain and spinal cord begin to function, a wider area of the body becomes sensitive and the brain gradually begins to regulate the autonomic functioning of the organs. The nervous system continues to mature after birth and throughout life as the sensory organs begin to function and as our level of consciousness develops and matures through the various levels.

The mother's diet during pregnancy and after birth when she is nursing plays a crucial role in the proper maturation of the nervous system. A proper diet provides the optimum foundation for the development of the nervous system and the growth of consciousness in its fullest dimensions.

Prematurity: Premature infants face a number of difficulties. The lungs, which are useful only in the ocean of air outside the womb, are poorly developed before the seventh month of life. Late in the first month, two lung buds appear and differentiate into the many bronchial tubes that carry air to the *alveoli*, or air sacs. By the end of the seventh month, only about two-thirds of the bronchial tubes and air sacs have formed. At birth, only about three-fourths have developed, and the lungs do not complete their development until the middle of childhood. By the seventh month, however, enough of the alveoli have formed to provide the baby with the oxygen needed for life. The muscles of the chest wall and diaphragm which cause the lungs to expand and contract during breathing also become functional at this time. However, in order for regular breathing to begin, the reflex centers of the brain which control these muscles must be sufficiently developed. Other problems faced by premature infants include maintaining proper body temperature and coordinating the muscles involved in swallowing.

Some infants are able to live after spending only two-thirds of the normal length of pregnancy in the womb. Each additional day or week in the womb beyond this time increases the probability of survival. Therefore, a mother must be very careful about her diet and activity during this time so as to minimize the possibility of premature delivery. After spending thirty weeks in the uterus, most babies weigh about three pounds, and their chance of surviving premature birth increases rapidly from this point on. If a baby remains in the womb for at least thirty-six weeks and reaches a weight of over five pounds, he or she has about the same chance of surviving as does the full term infant which averages between six and seven pounds at birth.

The Reproductive Organs: The reproductive organs develop rapidly during the final trimester of pregnancy. The testes migrate from their original position in the abdomen to the floor of the pelvic cavity and into the scrotum. The ovaries also migrate but are held inside the body and move outward only as far as the back wall of the pelvic cavity.

The intersection of heaven and earth's forces in the region of the heart energy center or *chakra* creates a pair of spirals which develop as the mammary glands. Mammary glands arise in both sexes during the second month and develop rapidly toward the end of pregnancy. At birth, the mammary glands and nipples are the same in both sexes. The glands become dormant until the female breasts begin to enlarge and develop at puberty.

Aging of the Placenta: During the final month of uterine life, the placenta begins to age, and its efficiency in providing food for the baby decreases. The placenta reaches peak activity at about thirty-four to thirty-five weeks of pregnancy, after which its activity begins to decline. As the placental barrier deteriorates, substances that previously did not pass through the placenta now pass back and forth between mother and baby. The mother and baby may begin to exchange blood cells. If the blood of the mother is incompatible with that of the fetus, the presence of fetal blood cells in the mother's bloodstream may cause antibodies to develop. If these antibodies pass through the placenta and into the baby's bloodstream, they begin to attack and destroy the baby's blood cells. However, this is rare; most fetal-maternal bleeding or blood exchange takes place at delivery if at all. (See the discussion of the Rh problem in Chapter 4.)

In most cases, it is to the baby's advantage to receive maternal antibodies, as they provide the newborn with natural immunity against a variety of diseases. Maternal antibodies are especially needed during the first several months after birth when the baby's natural resistance is only beginning to develop.

The aging of the placenta signals the approaching end of the baby's existence in the dark, watery environment of the womb. The new human being is now ready to be born into a much wider and brighter world.

3 | A Healthy Pregnancy

There is no mystery about the factors that contribute to a comfortable pregnancy, a safe and trouble free labor and the birth of a healthy child. Just as conception results from the natural attraction between a couple, pregnancy and delivery proceed smoothly by the influence of the universe itself, or we may say, by the will of God. If our daily lives are in harmony with the order of nature, including our dietary practices, our day to day activities and our mental attitudes, then it naturally follows that the experience of pregnancy and childbirth will be one of joy and wonder. A healthy pregnancy includes the following aspects:

1. *Freedom from Worry:*   Many people worry excessively during pregnancy. Some may fear that their baby may be born with a physical or mental defect, while others may be concerned that they or their unborn child are not receiving adequate nourishment or sufficient medical attention. Excessive worry is a sign of physical and mental disturbance caused by improper diet and way of life. For a healthy woman, pregnancy is a time of joy, hope, and boundless optimism, free from unnecessary care and anxiety.

2. *Freedom from the Fear of Childbirth:*   A woman in good health need not fear the natural experience of giving birth. If severe pain is experienced during delivery, if the labor is long and drawn-out, or if various complications require a variety of artificial procedures, we should realize that these problems are the natural outcome of a daily diet and way of life that have grown out of harmony with the surrounding environment. The natural process of giving birth is in fact one of the most fulfilling and rewarding experiences that a woman may have.

3. *Gratitude toward the Pregnancy:*   Of the countless variety of things that people attach value to, children are actually the most important and precious, even beyond their parents' own lives. Every baby is the natural manifestation of the universal creative process, and has completed a journey of billions of years to be born as a human being on the earth. Thus, each baby has an incalculable potential for growth and development and each represents the future of humanity. At the same time, children embody, and carry endlessly into the future, the spirit and dream of both parents and their ancestors extending back for countless generations. Therefore, by respecting, loving and appreciating the new life that you are creating, you are ultimately offering your respect and gratitude to the source of life itself, the infinite universe or God. Our appreciation and understanding of the great significance of pregnancy helps us to develop a universal love that embraces all beings and all phenomena.

4. *Appreciation for Related People:*   As you experience pregnancy, childbirth and then begin raising your children, you often start to remember the love and care

that you received from your parents. At this time, quite naturally, your gratitude and love goes out to them and begins to include your grandparents, great grandparents and beyond to all of your ancestors. Also, as you share more of life's experiences, the growing intimacy with your husband will develop your natural appreciation for his parents and ancestors as well. In the same way, your gratitude will often begin to be extended to friends, relatives, teachers and all the people of the world.

5.   *Gratitude toward Food and Nature:*   The creation of a new life is only possible because of food, which in turn, is a product of nature. As you begin to realize how your daily food creates and sustains your own life and that of your baby, your deep appreciation freely begins to go out to food and to all those people who made it possible for you to enjoy it. In the same spirit, your thanks will often begin to extend to the world of nature from which all food comes.

Pregnancy and Biological Evolution

During the nine months of pregnancy, the single, fertilized cell develops into a highly complex, multicelled organism, a human being. The 280 days of pregnancy correspond to the approximately 2.8-billion-year period of biological history during which life evolved in the ancient ocean. The next major biological epoch began with the emergence of land and has lasted for about the last 0.4-billion, or 400-million years. With the appearance of land, many forms of marine life, including seaweeds, algae, and fish, continued their evolution on land, initially giving rise to various types of land vegetation and primitive land animals, or amphibians.

The emergence of the continents about 400 million years ago is repeated at birth, when we leave the watery environment of the womb and continue our life on the surface of the earth. As evolution unfolded, continents formed as land gradually and repeatedly thrust upward through the surface of the oceans, giving rise to earthquakes and other geological upheavals. The contractions of birth correspond to the alternating rising and sinking of the land that occurred long ago.

The baby's development during pregnancy is influenced by the quality of the fluid environment which surrounds it and the quality of the maternal bloodstream from which the baby receives all of its nourishment. A baby's relationship to the watery environment of the womb can be readily understood when we consider how closely fish and other forms of aquatic life are dependent on their environment. When the stream, lake, or other body of water in which these creatures are living is contaminated with wastes and pollutants, they often become sick or die, or they may take on very strange, mutant forms. These creatures naturally thrive in fresh, clean water. Obviously, a similar relationship exists for the baby.

Since the 280 days of pregnancy correspond to approximately 2.8 billion years of biological evolution, each day corresponds to roughly ten million years of evolutionary history. If a woman takes aspirin or some other drug or medication during pregnancy, or if she eats some type of highly artificial or chemicalized food, the influence on her own adult condition may only last for several days. But for the developing baby, these one or two days correspond to roughly ten or twenty million years of evolutionary history. During this time, the baby must struggle to survive and develop in an unnatural, polluted environment. If the product ingested by the mother was extremely imbalanced, some type of physical or mental deformity in the child may result, especially if it was taken during the first trimester.

Therefore, the quality of the foods, beverages, and other products that you consume during pregnancy plays a decisive role in the development of your baby. Your blood, cells, tissues, organs, and amniotic fluid are continually being renewed as a result of what you eat and drink each day. The nutrients, hormones, and other substances which the baby receives are, in turn, the product of these raw materials. The quality of the nourishment which the baby receives and the environment in which it lives during pregnancy, determines the type of physical and mental constitution that the new human being will carry throughout life.

A Balanced Diet

During pregnancy a woman experiences many changes in her total condition, particularly during the first three months. Her menstruation stops, her breasts become fuller and more sensitive and her nipples harden. Increased amounts of hormones are produced that may create a wide range of emotions. A woman may have dreams about babies or about foods that she has eaten in the past. If her condition is out of balance, she may experience morning sickness.

The rapid growth of the baby during pregnancy creates a speedup in the woman's internal energy and causes her condition to become more yang and active. As a result, even if she is usually very careful about what she eats, it may be difficult for her to maintain what she considers a normal diet, especially during the first trimester. Many women crave more yin foods during this time in the natural attempt to balance their increasingly yang condition. Desires for sweets, fruits and liquids are fairly common. Moreover, the rapid acceleration in her metabolism may cause discharges that can create the desire for foods that were eaten in the past and, in some cases, women begin to want foods they have never eaten before.

Instead of being a cause for worry, these bodily and emotional changes, along with any cravings that may appear, can be a time when a woman learns to deeply appreciate the natural order of the infinite universe. Macrobiotics is the art of creating balance within ourselves and with our environment by adjusting our daily food and activity to harmonize with changing circumstances. Naturally, changes in our own condition, especially ones as profound as those experienced in pregnancy, require adjustments in our daily routine and way of eating. With just a little thought and effort, however, you will be able to find good quality alternatives in diet and activity that will help you to fully experience the joy and wonder of pregnancy.

We recommend that the standard macrobiotic diet continue to form the basis of your way of eating throughout pregnancy, with necessary modifications for which you may use the best quality foods to satisfy your needs and cravings. Needless to say, there is no one diet that is perfectly suited to everyone; each person needs to continually adapt his or her diet to suit the ever-changing conditions of their environment, with adjustments made according to season, activity, sex, age, constitution, condition, and a variety of other personal factors. In general, however, the optimum diet in a temperate, or four-season climate consists of the following foods and their approximate proportions.*

Fig. 21   The standard macrobiotic diet.

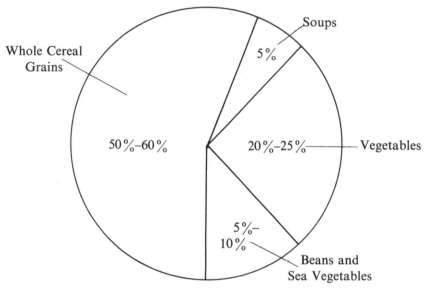

Plus occasional supplementary foods

1.   *Whole Cereal Grains:*   We recommend that cooked whole cereal grains comprise at least half (50 percent) of every meal. Cooked whole grains are preferable to flour products as they are easier to digest.

Whole grains for daily use include: Brown rice (short- or medium-grain are preferable in temperate climates, while medium- or long-grain are more suitable in warmer climates), millet, barley, corn, whole oats, wheat berries, rye, and buckwheat.

Whole grains for occasional use include: Sweet brown rice; *mochi* (pounded sweet brown rice); noodles such as whole wheat noodles (including *udon* and *somen*), buckwheat noodles (*soba*), and other whole, unrefined pasta; unleavened bread made from whole wheat, rye, or other whole grains; rice cakes; cracked wheat; bulghur; steel-cut and rolled oats; corn grits and meal; rye flakes; and cous-cous. Naturally processed whole wheat products such as *seitan* and *fu* (puffed wheat gluten) may also be used in various side dishes from time to time.

In general, whole grains should be your main dish at every meal, while flour products, such as those mentioned above, are recommended for occasional use as side dishes or in desserts.

* For a more complete explanation of the principles of macrobiotics, refer to the *Book of Macrobiotics: the Universal Way of Health and Happiness* by Michio Kushi, published by Japan Publications, Inc.

2. *Soups:* One or two cups or bowls of soup may be included daily. We recommend that your soups be moderately seasoned with *miso, tamari* soy sauce,* or sea salt so that they taste neither too salty nor too bland. Soups may be prepared with a variety of ingredients including seasonal vegetables, sea vegetables—especially *wakame* and *kombu*—and grains and beans. Barley *miso*, also known as *mugi miso*, soybean *(hatcho) miso* and brown rice *(genmai) miso* are suitable for daily use, while other types of natural quality *miso* may be used occasionally.

3. *Vegetables:* About one-quarter to one-third of each meal may include vegetables prepared in a variety of ways, including steaming, sautéing, frying, and others. In general, a smaller portion of your daily vegetable intake may be eaten in the form of unspiced natural pickles or salad. We recommend avoiding artificial chemically produced dressings and mayonnaise.

Vegetables for Regular Use Include:
  1) *Stem/root vegetables:* Burdock, carrot, *daikon* (long white radish), dandelion root, lotus root, onion, radish, rutabaga, turnip, parsnip, and others.
  2) *Ground vegetables:* Cauliflower; acorn, buttercup, butternut, and Hubbard squash; regular pumpkin and Hokkaido pumpkin; and others.
  3) *Green and white leafy vegetables:* Broccoli, brussels sprouts, bok-choy, green cabbage, carrot tops, Chinese cabbage, collard greens, *daikon* greens, dandelion greens, kale, mustard greens, parsley, scallion, chives, turnip greens, watercress, leeks, and others.

Vegetables for Occasional Use Include: Celery, cucumber, endive, escarole, mushroom, romaine lettuce, *shiitake* mushroom (a dried mushroom imported from Japan), sprouts, kohlrabi, iceberg lettuce, green peas, snow peas, summer squash, patty-pan squash, string beans, snap beans, wax or yellow beans, *jinenjo* (mountain potato), red cabbage, Swiss chard, zucchini, and others.

Vegetables to Limit or Avoid Include: Asparagus, bamboo shoots, fennel, ferns, spinach, okra, purslane, shepherd's purse, sorrel, avocado, eggplant, green and red peppers, tomato, potato, sweet potato, taro potato *(albi)*, plantain, yams, and other varieties of tropical origin.

4. *Beans, Bean Products, and Sea Vegetables:* About five to ten percent of your daily diet may include cooked beans, bean products, and sea vegetables.
  Beans for regular use include: Azuki beans, chickpeas, and lentils. Fermented bean products such as *tempeh, tofu*, dried *tofu* and *natto* may also be included on a regular basis.
  Beans for occasional use include: Black-eyed peas, black turtle beans, black soybeans, kidney beans, great northern beans, whole dried peas, split peas, pinto beans, lima beans, and navy beans.

---

* *Tamari soy sauce:* Macrobiotic quality *tamari* soy sauce is naturally fermented over two summers. It is processed from round soybeans and is made with sea salt that has not been overly refined and contains a variety of trace minerals.

We suggest that you eat sea vegetables often so that they comprise a few percent of your daily diet. Sea vegetables can be prepared in a variety of ways, for example, in soups, with beans (*kombu* is especially recommended), or as side dishes with vegetables, such as carrots or onions, or with soybean products.

Sea vegetables for regular use include: Kombu (for soup stocks, as a side dish, or in condiments), *wakame* (in soups, especially *miso* soup, as a side dish, or in condiments), *nori* (as a garnish, a condiment, or on riceballs), *hijiki* (as a side dish), *arame* (as a side dish), dulse, Irish moss, agar agar (for gelatin molds), and *mekabu* (as a side dish). Other edible sea vegetables may be used occasionally.

5. *Supplementary Foods:* Depending on your condition and desire, a small amount of white-meat fish or seafood may be eaten once or twice a week.

Suitable varieties include: Flounder, halibut, sole, carp, haddock, trout, clams, oysters, smelt, scallops, shrimp, *chirimen iriko* (tiny dried fish), and other small dried fish.

A small volume of roasted seeds, lightly seasoned with sea salt or *tamari* soy sauce, may be enjoyed as snacks.

Suitable varieties include: Sesame, sunflower, pumpkin, and squash seeds.

It is better to minimize the use of nuts and nut butters as they are high in fats and often difficult to digest. However, less oily nuts such as almonds, walnuts, and chestnuts may be enjoyed on occasion, preferably roasted and lightly seasoned with *tamari* soy sauce or sea salt.

Other snacks include rice cakes, popcorn, puffed whole grain cereals, roasted grains or beans, *sushi* (rice rolled with vegetables, pickles or fish and wrapped in *nori*), riceballs, and leftovers.

Desserts may be enjoyed now and then, on the average about two or three times per week. Unsweetened, cooked fruit desserts are preferable. However, small amounts of high quality natural grain sweeteners such as rice syrup, barley malt, or *amazake* (slightly fermented sweet brown rice) may be added occasionally. Dried and fresh local fruits in season may also be enjoyed from time to time by those in good health. The regular consumption of fruit juice is not recommended, although it may be enjoyed periodically by those in good health, especially during warm weather. Only locally grown fruits are advisable; therefore, it is better for persons living in temperate climates to avoid tropical and semi-tropical fruits and their products.

Recommended Sweets Include:
1) *Sweet vegetables:* Cabbage, carrots, *daikon*, onion, parsnip, pumpkin, and squash.
   You may be surprised by the naturally sweet taste of these vegetables.
   They can be prepared in a variety of delicious ways for use as side dishes or desserts.

2) *Concentrated sweeteners* (in small amounts): Rice syrup (often referred to as *am*é or yinnie syrup), barley malt, *amazake*, chestnuts, apple juice, raisins, apple cider, and dried temperate climate fruits.

3) *Temperate climate fruits:* Apples, strawberries, cherries, blueberries, watermelon, cantaloupe, peaches, plums, raspberries, pears, apricots, grapes, and others.

6. *Beverages:* It is recommended that spring or well water be used in the preparation of teas and other beverages.

Beverages for daily use include: *Bancha* twig tea *(Kukicha)*, *bancha* stem tea, roasted rice tea, roasted barley tea, boiled water, and spring or well water.

Beverages for occasional use include: Cereal grain coffee, dandelion tea, *kombu* tea, *umeboshi* tea, and *Mu* tea.

Beverages for use on rare occasions and in small amounts only include: *Nachi* green tea, green magma, vegetable juices, temperate climate fruit juice (apple juice or cider, unsweetened, is preferable), good quality beer, and *sake* (rice wine).
Please note that it is better to drink only when thirsty.

7. *Condiments:* Condiments may be used in moderate amounts to add a variety of flavors to foods and to provide additional nutrients. Please remember that most of these condiments contain salt so use them in moderation. Those who must restrict their salt intake during pregnancy may do so by reducing the use of condiments.
The following condiments may be used:
Tamari soy sauce: Use mostly in cooking. Please refrain from using *tamari* on rice or other grains at the table.
Sesame salt (Gomashio): Use 10 to 14 parts sesame seeds to 1 part roasted sea salt. Wash and dry-roast seeds. Grind seeds together with sea salt in a small serrated earthenware bowl called a *suribachi*, until about 2/3 of the seeds are crushed.
Roasted sea vegetable powder: Use either *wakame*, *kombu*, dulse, or kelp. Roast sea vegetable in the oven until nearly charred (approximately 350°F. for 10–15 minutes) and crush in a *suribachi*.
Sesame sea vegetable powder: Use 4 to 8 parts sesame seeds to 1 part sea vegetable (*kombu* or *wakame*). Prepare as you would sesame salt. On the average, about 1½ tea spoons of the above powders may be eaten daily.
Umeboshi plum: Plums that have been dried and pickled for over one year with sea salt are called *ume* (plum) *boshi* (dry) in Japanese. On the average, two to three plums may be eaten per week. *Umeboshi* stimulates the appetite and digestion and aids in maintaining an alkaline blood quality.
Shio (salt) kombu: Soak 1 cup of *kombu* until soft and cut into ¼-inch-square pieces. Add to ½ cup water and ½ cup *tamari*, bring to a boil and simmer until the liquid evaporates. Cool and store in a covered jar to keep as long as it remains

unspoiled. One to several pieces may be used on occasion as needed.

Nori condiment: Place five or six sheets of dried *nori* or several sheets of fresh *nori* in approximately 1 cup of water and enough *tamari* soy sauce for a moderate salty taste. Simmer until the mixture cooks down to a thick paste. A teaspoon of *nori* condiment may be eaten together with your meal on occasion.

Tekka: This condiment is made from minced burdock, lotus root, carrot, *miso*, sesame oil, and ginger. It can be made at home or bought ready made.
Use sparingly due to its strong contracting nature.

Sauerkraut: Traditional sauerkraut is made from cabbage and sea salt and is very easy to prepare at home. A small volume may be eaten occasionally with a meal.

Other condiments for occasional use include:

Takuan (dried daikon pickles):   Several pieces of this dried long pickle can occasionally be eaten with or after a meal. A variety of other macrobiotically prepared pickles may also be included as condiments on a regular basis, such as bran, *miso*, or *tamari* pickles.

Vinegar: A moderate amount of brown rice vinegar and *umeboshi* vinegar may be used from time to time. Fruit vinegars and chemically processed vinegars are best avoided.

Ginger: A small volume of fresh grated ginger root may be used occasionally as a garnish or flavoring in vegetable dishes, soups, pickled vegetables, and especially with fish and seafood.

8.   *Oil and Seasoning:*   A moderate amount of genuine, cold pressed vegetable oil can be used in cooking. It is generally advisable to enjoy sautéed vegetables and other dishes which contain oil several times per week on average and to use only a small amount of oil when preparing them. Oil may be used occasionally in deep frying grains, vegetables, fish, and seafood.

Oils for regular use include: Sesame, dark sesame, corn, mustard seed, and other traditionally used vegetable quality oils.

Naturally processed, unrefined sea salt is preferred over other varieties of seasoning. *Miso* (fermented soy paste) and *tamari* soy sauce, both of which contain sea salt, may also be used. It is recommended that only naturally processed, non-chemicalized varieties be used. Seasonings are best used moderately in your cooking. As with condiments, those who need to restrict the intake of salt may do so by reducing the amount of seasoning in cooking.

Seasonings for Regular Use Include: *Miso*, *tamari* soy sauce *(shoyu)*, white sea salt, *umeboshi* plum or paste, *umeboshi* or brown rice vinegar, or other grain vinegars. Sweeteners such as mentioned earlier in this section may also be used in desserts.

It is better to avoid chemicalized, sugared, or artificial seasonings.

9.   *Foods to Reduce or Avoid in a Temperate Climate:*

Animal Products

Red meat (beef, lamb, pork)
Poultry
Wild game
Eggs

Dairy Foods

Cheese
Butter
Milk (buttermilk, skim milk)
Yogurt
Kefir
Ice cream
Cream
Sour cream
Whipped cream
Margarine

Fish

Red meat or blueskinned fish
such as:
Tuna (though raw tuna may be served
   occasionally with *tamari* and a garnish
   of grated *daikon* or mustard)
Salmon
Swordfish
Bluefish

Processed Foods

Instant food
Canned food
Frozen food
Refined (white) flour
Polished (white) rice
Foods processed with:
   Chemicals
   Additives
   Preservatives
   Stabilizers
   Emulsifiers
   Artificial coloring
   Sprayed, dyed foods

Sweeteners

Sugar (white, raw, brown, turbinado)
Honey
Molasses
Corn syrup
Saccharin and other artificial sweeteners
Fructose
Carob
Maple syrup
Chocolate

Stimulants

Spices (cayenne, cumin, etc.)
Herbs
Vinegar
Coffee
Alcohol
Commercially dyed teas
Stimulating aromatic teas (herb, mint,
   etc.)
Ginseng

Fats

Lard or shortening
Processed vegetable oils
Soy margarines

Nuts

Brazil
Cashew
Pistachio
Hazel

Tropical Fruits-Beverages

Artificial beverages (soda, diet sodas,
   cola, etc.)
Tropical or sub-tropical fruits:

Bananas	Figs
Grapefruit	Prunes
Mangoes	Coconut
Oranges	Kiwi
Papayas	

10. *Way of Life Suggestions:* Below are additional recommendations for a healthier and more natural pregnancy:

1) Chew your food well, until it becomes liquid in your mouth.
2) Eat with good appetite.
3) Eat in a peaceful orderly manner, while sitting, and with gratitude for your food. You may eat two to three times per day, as comfortably as you want, provided your meal includes the proper proportions of food and each mouthful is thoroughly chewed.
4) It is best to leave the table feeling satisfied but not full.
5) Drink comfortably when you feel thirsty.
6) Avoid eating for approximately three hours before sleeping, as going to bed soon after eating tends to result in stagnation in the intestines and indigestion.
7) Bathe as needed, but avoid long baths or showers as they leach minerals from the body.
8) Scrub and massage every part of your body with a hot, damp towel until the skin becomes pink, every morning and/or night. At least scrub your hands and feet, including each finger and toe.
9) Wear cotton clothing directly next to the skin, especially cotton undergarments. It is best to avoid wearing synthetic, woolen, or silk clothing directly on the skin. Also refrain from wearing excessive metallic jewelry or accessories on the fingers, wrists, or neck. Try to keep such ornaments simple and graceful.
10) For the deepest and most restful sleep, go to bed before midnight and get up early in the morning.
11) Be active in your daily life. Systematic exercise programs such as yoga, *Do-In*, and sports can be helpful, provided they are not too vigorous.
12) If your condition permits, go outdoors often. Walking barefoot on the beach, grass, or soil can be enjoyable and refreshing.
13) Keep your home environment clean and orderly, especially the areas where food is prepared and served.
14) Daily living materials should ideally be of natural quality. Cotton sheets, towels, blankets, and pillowcases, incandescent as opposed to fluorescent lighting, natural wood furnishings, and cotton or wool carpets all contribute toward a more natural atmosphere.
15) It is advisable to use a gas or wood stove for daily cooking rather than electric or microwave cooking devices.
16) Avoid or minimize the use of electric objects close to the body, including electric shavers, hair dryers, blankets, heating pads, toothbrushes, and others.
17) Keep large green plants in your home to freshen and enrich the oxygen content of the air. Occasionally opening the windows permits fresh air to circulate and is refreshing even in cold weather.
18) Use earthenware, cast iron, or stainless steel cookware rather than aluminum or teflon-coated pots.

19) If you watch television, especially color TV, do so at a distance and at an angle to the set in order to minimize exposure to radiation. Avoid watching TV during meals.

20) Use naturally prepared cosmetics and body care products such as natural toothpaste, sea salt, *dentie*, or clay for tooth care.

Proper cooking is necessary for a healthy pregnancy and for a healthy life. Cooking is an essntial step in the transformation of our environment into ourselves— into our blood, cells, tissues, and organs and even into our thinking and spirituality. Women, through their ability to have children, are also able to transform these environmental factors directly into new human life. Cooking is the basis not only of our own health but also of the health and well-being of our children, our families, and our society. It is therefore important for all parents and parents-to-be to study the art of cooking as the basis for the future happiness and health of humanity.

Variety in Your Diet

To ensure that you receive all of the nutrients that your body requires during pregnancy, be sure to eat a wide variety of foods. Don't make the mistake of limiting your diet to a narrow range of products. Items like *tempeh*, *tofu*, *miso*, *tamari* soy sauce, *shiitake* mushroom, *seitan*, beans, *bancha* tea, sea vegetables, *fu*, and of course whole cereal grains and fresh local vegetables are all rich in essential nutrients, including protein, calcium, and vitamin B_{12}. We especially recommend eating sea vegetables on a daily basis, as they are rich sources of calcium, iron, protein, and minerals. They complement your grain, vegetable, and bean dishes very nicely. For those of you who are not used to eating sea vegetables, try making mild sea vegetable condiments at home. *Nori* condiment, *wakame* powder, dulse powder, *kombu* powder, or roasted sesame seed/sea vegetable powders are all fine for regular use. *Kombu* also has a very mild flavor when cooked together with grains, beans, vegetables, or in soup stocks.

The Value of Eating Well

Once a woman is married or begins intimate relations with a man, she may become pregnant at any time, unless she practices some type of birth control. If, however, she doesn't use birth control—or even if she does, although the chances are slim—a woman should be aware that conception is a very real possibility. Several weeks or more may pass following conception before a woman realizes that she is pregnant. During this time the child's fundamental constitution has already begun to form, and if she isn't eating well, her baby's basic constitution may be negatively influenced. Therefore, a woman should be cautious at all times, as she seeks, in anticipation of pregnancy, to enhance her health and biological quality by eating well and living in harmony with the order of the universe.

The growth an infant achieves after birth is less significant than the development that takes place in the womb. For example, from birth to adulthood, a child

Calcium (Ca) Content in Various Foods (per 100 grams, unit mg)

Dairy foods are known as a source of Ca, but many other foods are also rich in Ca, and often contain more than dairy foods. Following are some examples:

Dairy foods:			*Seaweeds (Sea vegetables):*	
Cow's milk	100		*Kombu* (Tangle)	800
Goat's milk	120		*Hijiki*	1,400
Cheese, various	250–850		*Wakame*	1,300
Vegetables:			*Arame*	1,170
Turnip greens	130		Agar-agar	400
Long radish greens	190		*Seeds and Nuts:*	
Mustard greens	140–160		Sesame seeds	630
Parsley	200		Sunflower seeds	140
Leaf—beet	100		Sweet almonds	282
Spinach	98		Brazil nuts	169
Watercress	90		Hazel nuts	186
Shepherd's purse	300			
Dried radish root	400			

Besides those examples, many fish and seafoods are also rich in Ca.

Beans and bean products:	
Kidney beans	130
Broad beans	100
Soybeans	190
Tofu (soybean curd)	120
Dried *tofu*	300
Congealed *tofu*	590
Natto (fermented soybeans)	92
Miso, various	70–180

Source: U.S. Department of Agriculture and Japan Nutritionist Association

Protein Content in Some Vegetable and Animal Foods (per 100 grams, unit gram)

Whole cereal grains:			*Seeds and Nuts:*	
Brown rice, various	7.4– 7.5		Various	11.0–29.7
Wheat, various	9.4–14.0		*Meat and Poultry:*	
Oats	13.0		Beef, various	13.6–21.8
Barley, various	8.2– 8.9		Pork, various	9.1–21.5
Rye, various	12.1–12.7		Chicken, various	14.5–23.4
Millet, various	9.9–12.7		Other birds and poultry	18.5–25.3
Buckwheat, various	11.0–14.5		Eggs, various	12.9–13.9
Corn, maize, various	8.2–8.9		*Dairy Foods:*	
Sorghum	11.0–12.7		Cheeses, various	13.6–27.5
Beans:			*Sea Animals:*	
Azuki beans	21.5		Fish, various	16.4–25.4
Kidney beans	20.2		Shellfish	10.6–24.8
Peas, dried, various	21.7–24.1		Seafoods	15.0–20.0
Broad beans, various	25.1–26.0			
Soybeans, various	34.1–34.3			
Mung beans, various	23.0–24.2			
Lima beans	20.4			

Source: U.S. Department of Agriculture and Japan Nutritionist Association

will increase its weight only about twenty to thirty times. Compare this to the 2.8 billion years of biological development during pregnancy in which the fertilized egg increases its weight nearly 3 billion times, and it is easy to understand why pregnancy is the period during which the child's entire destiny, including his or her capacity for health, happiness and freedom is largely determined.

If a woman is genuinely concerned about the future well-being of her child, she will naturally avoid poor quality foods, even in situations where her husband, friends or relatives are eating them. Of course husbands too must realize their responsibility by supporting and encouraging their wives. Also, husbands should remember that the quality of their sperm is largely determined by what they eat and drink.

It is of course important for a woman to pay special attention to her diet and lifestyle after she discovers that she is pregnant. But, because the quality of her egg and of her husband's sperm at the time of conception is so important to the baby's future, the ideal time to start creating a healthy baby is well before conception takes place. Then, as a couple improves their own condition, including the quality of their reproductive cells, they are at the same time establishing the health and happiness of their future children.

Living in harmony with the laws of the universe brings great rewards to ourselves and our children. By giving birth to a healthy baby with a strong constitution, we minimize any problems the child may have later in life. A healthy baby rarely cries and when he or she does, it is usually either because of hunger or the need for a diaper change. Most of the time a healthy child will be busy enjoying the wonders of his new life and will be a joy to the household.

If a mother does not take proper care of herself during pregnancy, her child may need additional care after it is born. Babies who lack a sound biological nourishment and education during pregnancy are more likely to become upset, irritable and cry for no apparent reason. These children require a much larger amount of time on the part of the parents, in the form of constant care, attention and worry. They often do not sleep well and may be suspectable to various illnesses. So please remember that a baby is strongly influenced by the degree of care the parents, and especially the mother, take in their daily eating and way of life.

Managing Cravings: The Art of Creative Substitution

Gratitude and appreciation for our food is a sign of health, as is the ability to enjoy the delicious, natural tastes of our daily meals. During pregnancy, a woman's taste for food changes, especially during the first three months. Even women who have eaten well for many years have cravings and there are many ladies who know what they should eat but still have trouble doing so. If you find yourself in this situation, try not to be conceptual; rigidly thinking that you must eat in such and such a way. Also, please don't worry. Through macrobiotics, we can create balance within ourselves and harmony in our lives whatever the circumstances.

Intuition, flexibility and a commonsense application of yin and yang, the laws of harmony and relativity, are our best guides in life, and this is especially true during pregnancy. Instead of trying to suppress cravings, it is much wiser to satisfy them by using your judgment in selecting the most wholesome foods, prepared in a variety of ways, while staying within the guidelines of the standard macrobiotic diet.

We may call this the art of creative substitution and you might be surprised to discover the variety of attractive and delicious dishes that can be prepared. For example, cravings for oily or fatty foods can often be satisfied by eating *tempura*, sautéed vegetables, fried rice, or other dishes prepared with a natural quality vegetable oil. Dishes made with a small amount of sesame or corn oil are far better that potato chips, French fries or greasy animal foods.

Finally, some women think that they are entitled to special dietary privileges because of the deep physical, mental and spiritual changes that pregnancy produces in them. As a result, they may suppose that there is nothing wrong with eating ice cream, eggs, pizza, soft drinks and other foods and beverages that they would normally avoid. Rather than forgetting about eating well, however, pregnancy is the time to be even more careful about your dietary practices. As we have seen, during pregnancy a woman is creating her baby's basic constitution and by extension, the quality of his or her future life. Extreme cravings usually diminish after the third month and it then becomes much easier for a woman to maintain her usual way of eating. Until then, please use the laws of yin and yang skillfully and creatively to harmonize yourself.

Below are suggestions for dealing with some of the more common cravings that develop during pregnancy.

1.   *Cravings for Animal Food:*   A small serving of a low-fat white-meat fish will often satisfy your craving for animal food. Also, a variety of rich tasting dishes can be made with beans, *natto*, *tempeh*, *seitan*, *fu*, and *tofu* to help satisfy any desire for animal food that might arise. These vegetable quality proteins are often more satisfying than fish and are less fatty. Root vegetable dishes, such as those made with burdock, carrots, turnips, rutabaga, and *daikon* are also helpful. Rich tasting *miso* condiments (see recipe section) may also be used occasionally in small quantities to help satisfy the craving for animal protein.

2.   *Cravings for Sweets:*   When you crave something sweet, try eating a cooked fruit dessert which can be sweetened with rice syrup, barley malt, or *amazake*. These more complex grain sweeteners are far better for your health and the health of the baby than simple sugars such as honey, maple syrup, or refined sugar. Vegetables such as onions, carrots, and squash also have a very sweet taste and can help satisfy your cravings. Fresh sweet corn is another good substitute, as are vegetable butters made from carrots or onions. Vegetable butters are very sweet if they are cooked for a long time over a low flame. A small handful of raisins or other dried northern fruit will often help satisfy sweet cravings, while desserts made with cooked apples and chestnuts are especially good for this purpose.

3. *Cravings for the Sour Taste:* The craving for foods with a sour taste is common during pregnancy. However, instead of eating highly acidic tropical fruits such as grapefruit, lemons, or oranges, these cravings can often be satisfied by eating a small volume of naturally prepared sauerkraut or sour pickles made with *umeboshi* vinegar. A small volume of brown rice or other grain vinegar can also be used as a salad dressing or in making pickles. *Umeboshi* plums, which have a strong sour taste, can also be used in salad dressings, sauces, vegetable dishes, or as condiments. If you experience some weakness during pregnancy, a small volume of *ume* extract (concentrated *umeboshi*) often helps to restore strength. Dissolve a small amount in hot *bancha* tea and drink. *Ume* extract tea can also be used on occasion to satisfy the craving for sour tasting foods. If you crave tomatoes, root vegetables cooked in *miso* or rice vinegar will often serve as a satisfying substitute, as will vegetable soups flavored with a light *umeboshi* broth.

4. *Fruit Cravings:* It is better not to eat too much fruit during pregnancy. Therefore, whenever possible, try to satisfy your craving with salads and lightly cooked vegetables. If these aren't enough, try cooking simple desserts using dried apples, raisins, apricots, pears, or other dried local fruits. It is generally better to eat cooked rather than raw fruit. During the summer, you may want to eat some watermelon, cantaloupe, honeydew, or other fresh fruit. But try not to eat them too frequently or in too large an amount. Fresh sweet corn, fresh green peas, cucumbers, celery, and fresh salads often help satisfy the craving for raw fruit. Among fruits, berries are generally more yang and are therefore better to eat. If you desire fruit juice, a small cup of hot apple or pear juice is generally preferred, while grapefruit, orange, or other citrus juices are generally not recommended. An occasional small glass of carrot juice is often better for your condition than fruit juice.

5. *Dairy Cravings:* If you experience cravings for cheese, butter, or other dairy products, try dishes made with *tempeh, natto, seitan,* dried *tofu,* or fresh *tofu.* These dishes can also help satisfy the craving for eggs. Well cooked *tempeh* with root vegetables, seasoned with *tamari* soy sauce, is often strong enough to offset these cravings. *Tempeh* can also be cooked with sauerkraut or with *umeboshi* and cabbage for the same purpose. If you crave eggs, try sautéing *tofu* with scallions and a little *tamari* soy sauce to prepare a dish similar to scrambled eggs. *Tofu* dressing or creamy sauces and dips made with *tofu* can be used to satisfy the craving for cream cheese. These sauces and dips can include things like *umeboshi,* *umeboshi* paste, onions, scallions, or chives.

Sea vegetable side dishes, which include *tempeh, tofu, seitan,* or vegetables, also help to satisfy dairy cravings, as do vegetables sautéed in a little high quality sesame oil. Roasted sesame seeds can also be used daily as a garnish or added now and then to salad dressings to satisfy the craving for dairy products.

6. *Beverages:* We do not recommend using aromatic, stimulant teas or medicinal drinks or herbs. It is far better to use your daily foods to adjust and regulate your condition. For daily use we recommend *bancha* twig tea or roasted barley tea

(*mugicha*). Any of the other beverages listed on page 75 are also fine for regular use. You can make a variety of delicious teas simply by roasting whole grains and boiling them in water. We do not recommend coffee, decaffeinated coffee, or commercial teas. These and other stimulant drinks may interfere with the development of the baby and it is best to limit or avoid them during pregnancy. Grain coffees are very delicious and are better for regular use. Mild herbal teas can be used on rare occasions, but it is better to avoid altogether the strong herbal teas.

If you crave alcohol, a small amount of high quality, natural beer or *sake* is preferred over stronger drinks (brown rice *sake* is best if you can get it). These can be enjoyed in very small quantities on occasion but are not recommended for regular consumption. It is best to stay away from stronger alcohols as they can weaken your baby's constitution and may cause problems with the baby's health.

7. *Smoking:* During pregnancy, it is better to avoid smoking. Along with other forms of tobacco, cigarettes usually contain chemicals and sugar. Tobacco smoking can cause your baby to be smaller than normal. The time when you are breastfeeding is also very important for your baby's health, and it is advisable to avoid smoking during this period as well. Smoking causes you to become dried out and thirsty. If, during pregnancy, you drink too much fluid as a result, your uterus and other bodily organs may become swollen and over-expanded. Once the uterus becomes too expanded, the baby has more room to move around in and the head may not remain in a downward position as birth approaches. The baby may therefore be born in an abnormal position.

We also recommend that pregnant women avoid chemicals, drugs, and artifical products, including vitamin tablets. It is also better to avoid exposure to radiation such as that generated by color television and fluorescent lighting.

Activity

Don't be afraid to continue with your usual physical and social activities during pregnancy. Activity tends to make pregnancy more comfortable and labor easier. It will also help you control your eating.

Light *Do-In* (self-massage) is a very good form of activity during pregnancy. Special exercises for a smooth natural birth can also be practiced if they are not too strenuous. Simple yoga exercises can also be helpful if you are careful not to injure yourself or your baby. Activities such as walking, gardening, cleaning, sewing, knitting, and crocheting are benefical during pregnancy. For those who like swimming, be careful not to let your body become too cold or to swim to the point of becoming tired.

It is a good idea to limit traveling during the first and last trimester and it is especially important to avoid long trips during the final three months. However, if you do travel, make sure that you are able to obtain the best quality food throughout your trip and that your schedule is not too active or strenuous.

Most women are able to continue working comfortably until about a month before delivery. During the final month, you may begin to prefer quieter activities around the house, together with walking and other moderate pastimes.

During pregnancy, a woman is to be treated with love, care, and respect by the people around her. However, she need not be treated as though she is suffering from some type of illness. Pregnancy is not a sickness. Pregnancy is a completely normal and natural process, and both parents are to enjoy their normal daily activities during this time.

Embryonic Education (*Tai-Kyo*)

Pregnancy is the time when a baby's basic constitution is formed and it is this constitution that primarily determines the type of life that the child will have. If a pregnant woman is very careful about her health and diet during pregnancy and puts all of her love and energy into creating a healthy and beautiful baby, then she will not have much to worry about as the child grows. As a result of this care, it will be much easier for her children to grow naturally and to develop with little artifical interference. The key to the health and happiness of the entire family lies in giving our children the proper nourishment and environment during their life in the womb.

Being happy, maintaining a sense of calm and being at ease during pregnancy all have a definite, positive influence on the developing child. Our thoughts and emotions generate vibrations in the brain that pass down along the primary channel to the abdominal energy center, located deep within the womb, where they nourish the growing baby. Therefore, the quality of our thoughts and emotions during pregnancy have a direct influence on the character of the child.

In the Orient, the traditional practice of *Tai-Kyo*, or embryonic education, was based on this relationship. This practice reflected the understanding that a baby's education starts at conception and continues throughout pregnancy. The education received in the womb was actually considered to be far more important than that received after birth. Furthermore, it was believed that a lazy, complaining or short tempered woman would give birth to children who would later become lazy, complaining and easily upset. Women were thus encouraged to remain calm and peaceful throughout pregnancy in order to produce children with similar characteristics.*

In traditional times, as soon as a woman realized that she was pregnant, she would immediately begin beautifying her home surroundings. She would remove any works of art or other objects that were sad or unpleasant and replace them with art of a religious theme or of beautiful natural scenes. Many traditional wo-

---

* *The Importance of Tai-Kyo:* When I became pregnant for the first time I started to have a big dream for my baby. I wanted my child to become like Jesus or Buddha and to be very famous and ambitious. Then, as my pregnancy went on, my dreams got smaller and smaller. I started to think, "I just hope that my baby has five fingers and not six fingers. It isn't necessary for him or her to become like Jesus or be famous or have any special talent. I will be happy as long as he or she has five fingers, two eyes, and is a normal baby."

Then, when labor started, I began to think, "Even if my baby is not normal, I don't mind. I just hope that he or she is alive and that everything goes smoothly."

So although we may have big dreams for our children, we really don't know how things will turn out; that is why *Tai-Kyo* and keeping our own condition clean and healthy is so important. In this way, we can help create a brighter future for all humanity. [*Aveline Kushi*]

men read or wrote poems, studied various spiritual or philosophical classics, and practiced meditation, chanting or prayer throughout pregnancy. At the same time, they were careful to avoid entertainment and experiences that were violent, chaotic or upsetting, choosing instead more peaceful, natural, harmonious and happy activities.

Even though the modern world is very different from the traditional one, it is still vitally important for a woman to always keep her life peaceful, orderly and harmonious, and to eat very well, not just when she is pregnant, but at all times. A husband should actively cooperate in making the experience of pregnancy as peaceful and as natural as possible for his wife because he has a strong influence on her thoughts and emotions. Also, if he is eating poorly, a husband's unhealthy quality is easily transferred to his wife through their intimate relations, even if she is eating well. This is especially true if they sleep together or continue to have sexual intercourse. Therefore husbands need to eat well, and need to be kind, supportive and affectionate to their wives*.

There are many suggestions for a smooth and healthy pregnancy which are included as a part of *Tai-Kyo*. We would like to offer several of the more important ones:

1. *Be Happy about Having a Baby:*   Today, many women conceive without having a good relationship with their husband or partner. Some women do not even want to be pregnant while others may not be completely happy about having a baby. These are not natural attitudes. If a woman is healthy, as soon as she notices the first signs of pregnancy, or if she even suspects that she might have conceived, she immediately wants to put her energy, love, and entire being into her pregnancy and into having a smooth natural birth. Remember that children are created by the order of the universe in the same way that all things are created. As parents, we are simply the means for a new human being to physicalize on the earth. If you have the spirit of genuine, natural appreciation, your pregnancy and birth will be much smoother and happier.

2. *Every Day, Pray for a Safe Pregnancy and for a Happy and Healthy Baby:*   Any style of prayer, meditation, or spiritual practice is fine, depending on your prefer-ence. However, we would like to recommend a very simple meditation to help you get started. Sit in a chair with your feet on the floor about shoulder-width apart. (You may also sit on a cushion in the lotus posture or with your feet tucked under the buttocks if this is comfortable.) Place your hands lightly together in prayer position at the level of your heart. Keep your spine straight and your shoulders and elbows relaxed.

Close your eyes and breathe normally and quietly. Keep your mind empty and free of thoughts. After sitting for a minute or so, begin to breathe more deeply,

---

* *Men Must Try Harder:* I often think that men do not really experience a challenge that compares with giving birth. So while the couple is living together and having children, the woman is getting stronger and wiser by passing through this experience many times, while the husband may not have to face such a great challenge. Especially while the mother is pregnant and preparing for birth, it is very important for the husband to be particularly busy and to make himself strong, so that he can balance well with his wife. [*Aveline Kushi*]

centering your breathing in the lower abdomen. Continue for several breaths, and then add the sound of SUU or AUM on the outbreath. Repeat several times and then return to a normal, quiet breathing, again sitting with an empty mind. After sitting for a minute or so, slowly open your eyes and dissolve the meditation. This simple practice takes only several minutes and the morning or evening are good times to practice it. During the meditation, you may also create an image of your baby, actively visualizing the child as a healthy, peaceful and spiritual person.

3. *Avoid Upsetting or Overly Stimulating Movies, Entertainment, or Books:* Ideally, a pregnant woman should take time every day to admire natural scenery, beautiful works of art, or images or paintings of various spiritual individuals.

Peaceful, natural, and inspiring images and thoughts create a more peaceful and harmonious vibration for the growing baby. Violent or unhappy thoughts produce a chaotic or disturbed vibration. During pregnancy, make an effort to see paintings depicting peaceful, natural scenery and read inspiring novels or stories about great people whom you admire. The Bible, the *Tao Teh Ching*, the *Upanishads*, the *Gospel According to Thomas*, and other religious or spiritual classics make excellent reading. Poems, fairy tales, and folk tales such as the Chinese classic, *Monkey*, stimulate the imagination and also are excellent reading material.

4. *Keep All of Your Personal Relationships Smooth and Happy:* During pregnancy, a cooperative and peaceful home atmosphere and an orderly life are important. Encourage all of your friends and family members to understand that your mental, emotional, and physical condition is changing rapidly and that pregnancy is a wonderful but tremendous responsibility. Wives, please remember that pregnancy can be difficult for husbands as well, so do your best to encourage, love, and support your husband.

5. *Wear Clothing Made from Cotton and Other Natural Vegetable Fibers:* Cotton keeps the body warm in winter and cool in summer. It is very comfortable and easy to clean and its natural, vegetable quality allows the body's energy to circulate freely. Select colors that you feel most comfortable with. Mild, pastel colors, which are soothing to the eyes, have a peaceful and harmonious effect. It is especially important to select cotton or other natural fibers for undergarments.

6. *Keep Your Home and Surroundings Clean and Orderly:* Keep your clothing, sleeping materials, kitchen, and entire house clean. Try to create a bright and cheerful atmosphere in your home. If you plan to have your baby at home, keep the delivery room thoroughly cleaned and orderly, and make sure that all of the things that you will need are ready*.

---

* *The Biggest Challenge in a Woman's Life:* As my delivery date came closer, I started to clean my room, wash out the drawers, and straighten out everything. I am sure that every mother has experienced something similar. This is different than everyday housecleaning when you may be washing dishes while your mind is far away from what you are doing. This kind of cleaning is using all of you, you are completely involved, making your surroundings and your entire life as well ordered and as clear as possible. ▶

7. *Keep Active and Busy:*   Remember that problems such as morning sickness or nausea are not really sicknesses at all but rather part of the body's adjustment to a pregnant woman's rapidly changing condition. They usually only last for a short period of time and should not keep you from being active during pregnancy. Rather than resting too much, try to keep up with your daily activities. Activity will actually help relieve morning sickness. If, as soon as you wake up, you clean house, cook, and in general keep active, you will soon notice that your morning sickness has disappeared and that you are feeling much more happy and healthy.

Please remember also that babies who have lazy or inactive mothers tend to be less healthy than those whose mothers stay busy throughout pregnancy.

When you become pregnant, it is easy to be distracted from your practice of *Tai-Kyo.* However, don't forget to eat well and to pray every day for your baby. In the morning when you wake up or at night before going to sleep, simply close your eyes and pray that your baby will come happily into this world. Also, give thanks for being the baby's mother. These simple practices, together with eating well, will make a tremendous difference for your baby.

If we could actually fashion the baby ourself, in the way that a sculptor carves stone or a painter combines color, I am sure that most women would have definite ideas as to the kind of child they would like to create. Although we can't do this directly with our hands, we can eat well, make ourselves peaceful and pray for the baby's happiness. In this way, on a fundamental level, we are shaping the child's constitution and character just as surely as the artist forms his work.

▶   Ideally, having babies should be easy, not like a trauma or sickness. But at the same time, a woman has to put her whole life into it. If you are eating well, keeping active and are in good condition, labor should not be a terrible, frightening experience. But at the same time, it is a very meaningful event to pass through and a woman has to put all of her energy and attention into it. Even if she is in good health, a mother will need to put her whole being into giving birth. Having a baby is the biggest challenge in a woman's life. [*Aveline Kushi*]

4 | Complications and Disorders

If a woman is eating properly and leading an active and busy life, her pregnancy should be an event of celebration, free from discomfort or abnormal symptoms. Today, however, most women experience a wide variety of problems during pregnancy, ranging from minor discomfort to serious and potentially life-threatening disorders. As a result, many people today think of pregnancy as a sickness or as a medical problem rather than the normal and natural event that it is.

A pregnant woman can suffer from any of the illnesses that affect the general population. Problems such as diabetes, high blood pressure, heart disease, kidney disorders, and even cancer occur during pregnancy. The macrobiotic dietary and way of life approach to these and other common sicknesses has been outlined in *Natural Healing Through Macrobiotics*, the *Book of Macrobiotics*, The *Cancer Prevention Diet*, and in other publications. In this chapter, we will discuss some of the more common disorders of pregnancy.

Anemia: Anemia is a common problem during pregnancy. It can arise when there is a reduction in the number of red blood cells or in the amount of *hemoglobin,* which contains iron, in the blood.

There are several varieties of anemia. The most common during pregnancy is *iron-deficiency anemia.* Women generally have fewer red blood cells and a lower concentration of hemoglobin in their blood than men. They experience a loss of iron due to the discharge of red blood cells every month during menstruation. Pregnancy creates an additional demand for iron since a large amount of blood is needed in the formation of the placenta and baby. In many cases, women do not get enough iron in their daily diets to make up for these losses.

The main symptoms are weakness, fatigue, and a pale white complexion. If the anemia results from the destruction of red blood cells, *jaundice* may also be present, producing a yellowish complexion and eye discoloration. Grey or white lips (healthy lips have a pinkish color), a white color in the inside of the lower eyelid (the lower eyelid should also be pink), white fingernails (pink is normal), and a decrease in sexual appetite are also symptoms of this disorder.

It is commonly believed that animal products are the best source of iron and are therefore needed in the daily diet to offset anemia. In the standard macrobiotic diet, however, grains, vegetables, beans, sea vegetables, seeds, nuts and if desired, occasional fish and seafoods, provide as much iron as the frequent consumption of meat. When compared worldwide, the average American diet is actually low in iron due primarily to its highly refined nature. Refined grains, for example, contain much less iron than do whole grains.

Oftentimes, pregnant women are told by their doctors that they are anemic or borderline anemic and are advised to take iron supplements. However, it is far better to obtain iron from whole natural foods. Sea vegetables are especially good

Iron Content in Various Foods (per 100 grams, unit mg.) Used Regularly in the Standard Macrobiotic Diet.

Whole Cereal Grains:	
Millet (whole grain)	6.8
Buckwheat (whole grain)	3.1
Soba (buckwheat noodle)	5.0
Oats (whole)	4.6
Brown rice (whole grain)	1.6
Beans:	
Azuki	4.8
Chickpea	6.9
Lentils (whole)	6.8
Soybeans	8.4
Miso:	
Hatcho	6.5
Mugi (barley and soybeans)	4.0
Vegetables (*uncooked*):	
Dandelion greens	3.1
Kale	2.2
Swiss Chard	3.2
Sea Vegetables:	
Arame	12
Dulse	6.3
Hijiki	29
Nori	12
Wakame	13
Seeds and Nuts:	
Pumpkin seeds	11.2
Sesame seeds	10.5
Sunflower seeds	7.1
English walnuts	3.1

Iron Content in Various Foods (per 100 grams, unit mg.)
(These foods are commonly found in the Average American Diet.)

Meat and Poultry:	
Beef (various)	2.5–2.7
Chicken	1.6
Chicken eggs (whole)	2.3
Lamb	1.3
Dairy Food:	
Cheddar cheese	1.0
Whole milk	trace
Condensed milk	0.1
Human milk	0.2

Source: U.S. Department of Agriculture

sources of iron and also contain plenty of calcium and other minerals. *Miso* soups made with land and sea vegetables are also rich in this element, as are foods like sesame seeds, *azuki* beans, *tempeh*, dried *tofu*, and many hard leafy green vegetables such as kale, turnip greens, and *daikon* greens.

Two practices are helpful in ensuring adequate amounts of iron with the macrobiotic diet. First, eat a wide variety of foods, and second, chew very well. Chewing makes food more digestible and easier for the body to extract the nutrients it needs. If chewing is incomplete, digestion and absorption cannot proceed smoothly and efficiently. Proper chewing also enhances the tastes of foods, thus making each meal more satisfying. Improper chewing increases the tendency to overeat and may lead to a variety of cravings.

A variety of special dishes are rich in iron, including: 1) *hijiki* or *arame* cooked with *tempeh*, carrots, and onions; and 2) *azuki* beans cooked with squash (or carrots) and *kombu*. Sesame seeds, which contain plenty of both calcium and iron, can be used frequently as a garnish. Well roasted seeds are recommended for regular use. (Sesame seeds have a high percentage of good quality oil and are preferred to using large amounts of pressed oil in cooking.) Sea vegetable condiments can also be used regularly to add iron to the diet. *Goma* (sesame)-*wakame* powder is especially good for this purpose. To prepare, crush and mix roasted *wakame* together with roasted sesame seeds (about 40 percent *wakame* and 60 percent sesame seeds).

Among the sea vegetables that are used regularly in macrobiotic cooking, dulse contains the highest amount of iron. This versatile sea vegetable, which is harvested off the coast of North America and Europe, can be included regularly in soups, salads, or in vegetable dishes. Green *nori* flakes, which are now available in many natural food stores, are also high in iron and are especially good as a condiment during pregnancy.

Be sure to include daily servings of hard leafy greens during pregnancy, as they are rich in iron, calcium, and minerals. Especially recommended are the green tops of *daikon* radishes, turnips, red radishes, and carrots. These nutrient-rich greens can be prepared in a variety of appetizing ways.

Squash and pumpkin seeds are also good sources of iron. To prepare, wash them in cold water, place on a cookie sheet, and roast until golden brown, stirring occasionally. Roasted seeds are especially good when seasoned with a little *tamari* soy sauce, and can be enjoyed from time to time as snacks.

In addition to iron, a well-balanced macrobiotic diet provides adequate amounts of vitamin B_{12}, a lack of which is associated with anemia. Vitamin B_{12} is synthesized primarily by microorganisms such as bacteria or mold. Foods that contain these organisms provide vitamin B_{12} in the diet. Products such as sea vegetables, which have microorganisms naturally attached to them, and *tempeh*, *miso*, *tamari* soy sauce, and *natto*, in which microorganisms arise through fermentation, help in providing adequate amounts of this vitamin. The occasional consumption of fish can also be of help in meeting the daily need for this vitamin, which is necessary for the production of red blood cells.

A contributing factor in many cases of nutritional anemia is the overconsumption of sugar, fruit, liquids, and other more yin foods and beverages. Nutritional anemia can also be accelerated by the overintake of flour products, dairy products, and oily and greasy foods, all of which interfere with the smooth functioning of the intestines and diminish their capacity to absorb nutrients. The lack of proper absorption naturally inhibits the formation of healthy red blood cells. In a smaller number of cases, anemia is produced by an opposite, or more yang cause. This results from using too much salt or baked foods or from not eating enough fresh green vegetables.

Women who experience more yin anemia during pregnancy can eat within the guidelines of the standard macrobiotic diet, while controlling their intake of fruit, liquid, salad, oil, and flour products. Women who experience a more yang form of anemia can also eat according to the standard macrobiotic diet, while limiting their intake of salt and baked foods and taking a larger volume of more lightly cooked vegetables, with occasional salad and a cooked fruit dessert. The special foods and dishes presented earlier can be eaten in both instances. In the case of more yin anemia, these dishes can be more strongly cooked, while lighter and less salty cooking would be more appropriate in the case of more yang anemia.

Aside from eating properly, individuals with nutritional anemia need to keep physically active. In addition, daily scrubbing of the entire body, especially the hands and fingers and feet and toes, with a wet, hot squeezed-out towel is also recommended as a way of keeping the circulation active.

Backaches: Many women experience backaches during pregnancy, ranging from mild to severe. This indicates that their daily diet and activity are out of balance with the environment. In the majority of cases, backaches are due to the overintake of more yin foods and beverages, including fruit, fruit juice, milk, tea, soft drinks, and liquid in general, plus sugar, honey, acidic vegetables, and other more expansive items. A lack of minerals and complex sugars also contributes to this condition. During pregnancy, a slight relaxation of some of the ligaments of the back is normal as a result of postural changes which occur naturally. However, if a woman consumes too many yin items and not enough minerals and complex carbohydrates, the muscles and ligaments become swollen and weak, causing additional strain.

Some backaches are caused by problems in the kidneys. During pregnancy, the kidneys must work to discharge not only the waste products produced by the mother's body but also those produced by the baby as well. Foods that weaken the functioning of the kidneys include: 1) excessive fluids, 2) cold foods or beverages, 3) dairy products, 4) fatty or oily foods, and 5) too much salt.

To help prevent backaches during pregnancy:

1) Limit your intake of more yin foods and beverages. Extreme yin foods such as sugar, tropical fruits, alcohol, coffee, highly acidic vegetables, and others are best avoided.
2) Control your liquid intake. This includes not only beverages but soups and the water used in cooking as well.
3) Keep active. Simple exercises to strengthen the back muscles can be helpful, especially for women who are physically weak.
4) Within the standard macrobiotic diet, include sea vegetables; tough fibrous vegetables such as *daikon* greens, kale, turnip greens, and others; and root

vegetables such as carrots, *daikon*, turnips, burdock, and others.

5) Beans, such as *azuki* beans, are good for strengthening the kidneys. Bean side dishes, prepared with *kombu* and vegetables, may be eaten regularly.

6) Don't overuse salt, including *miso*, *tamari* soy sauce, and various salty, mineral-rich condiments.

If pain is severe, rest until it subsides and avoid lifting, stooping, or bending. A warm compress is often helpful and can be made by running hot water from the faucet over a medium-sized towel. Squeeze and apply the hot moist towel directly to the painful region of the back. Continue for about ten minutes, changing towels as they cool. (Electric heating pads should not be used.)

In some cases, a hot ginger compress can be applied to the painful region of the back. To prepare, grate fresh ginger and place in a cheesecloth sack. Squeeze the sack so that the ginger juice drips into a pot of hot water kept just below the boiling point. Dip a towel into the ginger water, wring it out tightly, and apply hot to the painful area. Cover with a dry towel to retain heat. Replace with a fresh hot towel every two to three minutes and continue for about 15 minutes. During pregnancy, the ginger compress should not be applied to the front of the body especially to the abdomen.

Bleeding Gums: Healthy gums are pink in color. Gums that become reddish or bleed indicate the consumption of too many expansive items, including various drugs and medications. To relieve this condition, reduce the intake of more yin foods such as fruit, fruit juice, salad, liquid, and sweets. *Dentie* tooth powder, made from the tops of baked eggplants and sea salt, can be applied to the gums several times per week.

Kombu tea, which is made by boiling a strip of *kombu* and simmering it until the water turns light brown, can also be used from time to time. Sea vegetable side dishes will also help this problem.

An opposite type of gum disorder arises when too many baked foods, salt, and other more constrictive foods are consumed and when the diet is lacking in fresh vegetables and other good quality yin foods. An extreme example is *scurvy*, which is caused by the overintake of meat, eggs, or salt, and by the lack of fresh vegetables and fruit.

Constipation: There are generally two categories of constipation: more yin, in which the overintake of simple sugars, liquids, and oil causes the intestinal tissue to become swollen and loose, without enough power to move digested foodstuffs; and more yang, in which the lack of more expansive factors in the diet produces hard, compact stools and an overall constriction of the intestinal tissue. The repeated intake of fatty foods, oil, milk and dairy products, and flour products contributes to both types of chronic intestinal malfunction, as these items lead to the formation of pockets of mucus and fat in the intestines and throughout the body. A lack of proper chewing also contributes to constipation.

The standard macrobiotic diet, which is based on foods that contain plenty of fiber, will help restore the intestine to a normal degree of elasticity and regularity. The following modifications of the standard macrobiotic diet are helpful in relieving both categories of constipation:

1. It is better to eat grains in their whole form, such as pressure-cooked brown rice or boiled barley or millet, rather than as flour products. It may be necessary to limit or avoid flour products such as bread, noodles and pasta, and cracked grains until the condition improves. Sprouted grain breads may be eaten in small amounts on occasion, provided they are thoroughly chewed. A special dish of whole wheat berries, cooked together with *azuki* beans, lentils, or other grains, is also helpful in relieving constipation and may be included from time to time.

2. Nut butters, nuts, oily or greasy foods, and fruits and fruit juices may need to be avoided until the constipation disappears.

3. Fermented foods such as *miso*, *tamari* soy sauce, macrobiotically prepared pickles, and *umeboshi* plums strengthen the intestines. They may be used in moderate amounts as seasonings and in making condiments.

4. Green leafy vegetables such as kale, watercress, parsley, and celery, or *daikon*, carrot, and turnip tops may be eaten daily. These vegetables can be lightly cooked, just until they are no longer tough.

5. In cases where the intestines are very yin or expanded, avoid using oil in your cooking until the condition improves. Sesame seeds can be used as a garnish to obtain oil. *Ume-sho-kuzu* (*kuzu* tea) with a little grated ginger can be taken every day until you have a bowel movement. To make the *kuzu* (*kudzu*) drink, dilute about a teaspoon of *kuzu* in a cup of cold water, mix thoroughly and add a little *umeboshi* and grated ginger. Bring to a boil and simmer for a couple of minutes, stirring constantly. As the *kuzu* becomes clear and thickens, add several drops of *tamari* soy sauce. Drink hot.

6. When the constipation results from an overly tight or constricted condition, the *kuzu* drink can be made with a little more water and grated ginger. Oil can also be included in the diet. One or two side dishes of vegetables sautéed in a little sesame oil can be eaten daily until a bowel movement occurs. A little fresh grated ginger used as a garnish is also helpful.

7. Deep massage is helpful in stimulating the intestines. The large intestine point on the outer side of the hand (see Figure) can be used for this purpose. Massage the point by pressing deeply and rubbing with a circular motion. Massage each hand for about five minutes.

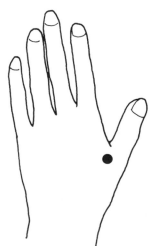

Fig. 22   The large intestine point (LI 4) on the outside of the hand.

8. For very difficult cases, an enema made with *bancha* tea and a little sea salt can be used to stimulate a bowel movement. Green salad can also be eaten for this purpose, as can a special condiment which is made by grating one tablespoon of potato with a little ginger. The condiment can be eaten in the morning before breakfast. It should not be taken too often and only for difficult cases of constipation.

9. Along with chewing properly and getting plenty of activity, persons with constipation should avoid eating for about 2½ to 3 hours before going to sleep.

10. Shoulder massage is often helpful in releasing stagnation in the intestines, since the large and small intestine meridians both run along the shoulders.* Sit in a chair or on the floor and have your husband or a friend place his or her hands on your shoulders. The person giving the massage can then knead the shoulders, beginning at the inner region near the neck and gradually working outward. Repeat several times until the shoulders become softer and more relaxed. Shoulder and neck massage is also helpful in relieving overall physical and mental tension during pregnancy.

Cramps: During pregnancy, cramps often occur in the calf muscles at night. However, cramps are simply the result of an excessive consumption of fluids, including soft drinks, fruit juice, coffee, and milk, together with the overconsumption of very yin items such as ice cream, sugary desserts, and sweets. These cramps usually occur in the region of the leg corresponding to the bladder or kidney meridian, indicating that the energy in these organs and meridians is excessive or overactive. A lack of calcium and other minerals in the diet is also a contributing factor.

When a cramp begins, flex the foot or stand up and try to walk. Activity or stretching the muscles often brings relief. To avoid cramps, cut back on your intake of liquids and other more yin foods. Temporary relief can often be obtained by drinking *tamari bancha* tea or by eating a small handful of *gomashio* or an *umeboshi* plum.

Massaging the kidney meridian, which runs from the bottom of the foot and up along the inside of the calf, is also helpful, as is massaging the kidney point (see Figure) on the bottom of the foot. If this point becomes blocked or stagnated, energy will often back up along the kidney meridian, causing a cramp. Use deep thumb pressure to release tension and stagnation in this point.

To relieve stagnation in the bladder meridian, sit in a chair and have someone massage your little toe on each foot with a pinching and rotating motion, taking a minute or so for each toe. (This can be done to release tension while a cramp is occurring, or as a general practice. All of the toes can be massaged in the same fashion to harmonize and relax your energy during pregnancy.) After massaging the toes, massage each calf with a firm but gentle motion.

---

* Complete illustrations of the energy meridians and points can be found in the *Book of Do-In: Exercise for Physical and Spiritual Development* by Michio Kushi, published by Japan Publications, Inc.

Fig. 23   The kidney meridian and kidney point (KD 1) on the bottom of the foot.

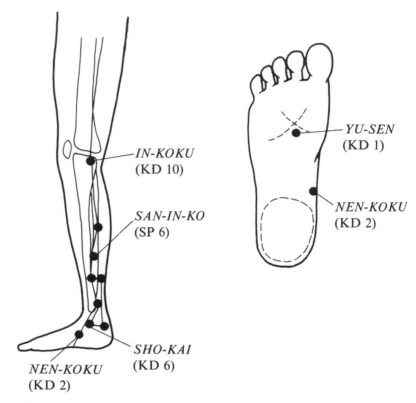

The kidney meridian on the inside of the leg shown with major points (black dots).

Depression: For a healthy woman, pregnancy is an active and happy time. However, some women experience periods of depression during pregnancy. Symptoms may include crying spells, inability to sleep, a loss of appetite for food and sex, a lack of desire to go places or do things, and feelings of discouragement or melancholy.

Physically, depression is related to problems in the lungs and large intestine and the kidneys and bladder. Depression is primarily a more yin disorder, resulting from the overintake of simple sugars, liquids, milk and other dairy products, fruit, alcohol, highly acidic vegetables, oily, greasy or sticky foods, nuts and nut butters, and flour products. Drugs and medications also contribute to emotional and mental imbalance.

Among the foods included in the standard macrobiotic diet, root vegetables are helpful in strengthening the lungs and large intestines, as are hard leafy greens. Especially good are root vegetables cooked together with their leafy tops. These include *daikon* and *daikon* greens, turnip and turnip greens, and carrot and carrot greens.

Bean dishes, such as those mentioned earlier, are helpful in strengthening the kidneys. A person who easily becomes depressed needs to minimize the intake of sweets, liquids, flour products, sticky foods, and other more yin items.

Physical activity is also helpful, as is establishing contact with nature. Walk outdoors, breathe deeply and look around you. Take time to marvel at the flowers and trees, the lakes, rivers, and ocean, the sky and stars, and other reflections of nature that help inspire and lift the spirit. A woman who feels very depressed can also try getting up early in the morning and watching the sun come up. The rising sun is symbolic of the beginning of new life.

Keeping active with friends, family, and associates is also helpful in curing depression. Social activities help to focus one's energy outward, while diminishing the preoccupation with one's own condition.

Edema (Swelling): Swelling caused by the retention of fluid is a common problem during pregnancy. Toward the end of pregnancy, many women experience some swelling in the ankles or feet especially after long periods of standing without much activity. Muscle contractions brought on by exercise help squeeze some of this fluid from the tissue spaces back into the blood vessels. A brief period of rest can also be helpful. When a woman lies flat or with her legs elevated, fluid that is accumulating in the legs or feet will be picked up again by the general circulation.

Fluid retention is related to the functioning of the kidneys. The recommendations for strengthening the kidneys presented in our discussion of backaches can also be used to relieve swelling. An excessive intake of fluids frequently contributes to the problem. In general, physical activity throughout pregnancy will help minimize swelling. In addition, the entire body can be rubbed with a hot squeezed towel every morning and every evening to keep the circulation active. It is especially important to do the extremities, the hands and fingers, feet and toes, and around the wrists and ankles.

Baked flour products such as breads, cookies, and muffins tend to make the kidneys tight and constricted. The intake of these items may be minimized by women who have the tendency to develop this problem.

If the swelling causes discomfort, a special dish can be made by boiling *daikon* with *kombu* and a little *tamari* soy sauce. This dish helps stimulate the kidneys to discharge water and salt, and can be eaten every day for several days until the problem improves. A stronger preparation, *daikon* radish tea, has been used traditionally throughout the Orient as a means of inducing urination and can be used in more severe cases of swelling. To prepare, grate *daikon* and squeeze the juice through a piece of cheesecloth. Mix two tablespoons of this juice with six tablespoons of hot water. Add a pinch of sea salt, boil and drink. (Never use without boiling.) Take only once a day, and do not use more than three times without proper supervision. This *daikon* tea can also be used in cases where swelling has developed in the hands and fingers. In some cases, it may be necessary to reduce the daily intake of salt for a short time until the condition improves. Sea vegetables and sea vegetable condiments can be used in place of salty condiments and seasonings.

Excessive Weight Gain: On the average, a woman will lose about twenty-two to twenty-six pounds in the weeks following delivery. It is usually better to keep the amount of weight gained during pregnancy to within this range. In general, the amount of weight gained during the first pregnancy tends to be less than that gained in subsequent pregnancies.

The rate of weight gain increases during the last few months as the baby grows by about an ounce per day. There is also a greater tendency to retain fluids during the latter part of pregnancy and this often contributes to an increase in weight.

If you chew your food thoroughly, keep active, and eat within the standard macrobiotic diet, the amount of weight gained during pregnancy should not be excessive. If you are overeating, you may be using too much salt, as people who overeat are frequently overly yang and seek to make balance by taking in a larger volume of food. If this is the reason for your overeating, reduce your salt intake and rely more on the natural flavor of foods. Proper chewing helps to prevent overeating as does the habit of not eating before going to sleep. Keeping your posture straight when you eat aids in digestion and makes it easier to concentrate on chewing.

Dairy products, fatty foods, and refined carbohydrates contribute to weight gain during pregnancy. It is better to avoid these items. Also, be careful not to eat too many sweets, desserts, nuts, flour products, and fruits. If you have a tendency to gain weight, it is better to keep the use of oil to a minimum and to make sure your intake of fluids, including juices, tea, and water, does not become excessive.

Daikon radish is helpful in discharging fat from the body and aiding the kidneys in the discharge of excess salt and water. It can be prepared using any of the methods described in this book and can be eaten regularly. Because of its fat dissolving properties, *daikon* can be eaten as a condiment whenever you serve fish or animal foods. Grate about a teaspoon of fresh *daikon*, add one or two drops of *tamari* soy sauce, and eat it together with your side dish of fish, similar to the way horseradish is used.

Exercise and activity help prevent overeating. Try to keep busy throughout pregnancy. Activities both in and outside the home help take your mind off of food.

Fibroids: Fibroids are fleshy growths within or on the wall of the uterus. They consist of masses of fibrous tissue and may be single or multiple, large or small. They often resemble a group of marbles.

Fibroids are widespread among women today and result from an extreme diet, especially the overconsumption of foods containing heavy saturated fat such as eggs, meat, dairy products, and poultry, in combination with extremely yin foods such as sugar, tropical fruits, oil, soft drinks, and refined flour products. When these items are eaten regularly, mucus and fat begin to deposit in the body, initially in areas connected to the outside, such as the sinuses, breasts, lungs, intestines, kidneys, and reproductive organs (for example, in a woman's ovaries, uterus, and Fallopian tubes or around the prostate gland in men).

The excess factors in the blood and lymph streams often solidify into cysts and tumors. When solidification occurs in the muscle of the uterus, the result is fibroid tumors. Fibroids often begin as small seedlings. Whether or not they enlarge depends on the quality and volume of excess that is deposited in the uterine region. Frequently, they continue growing as the result of an improper diet and begin to bulge either through the outer lining of the uterus or through the endometrium. In some cases, they bulge so far that they are pushed out on a stalk.

Fibroids may or may not produce noticeable symptoms. The most common age for symptoms to occur is between thirty-five and forty-five, although women of all ages can experience them. A common symptom is bleeding, especially in the form of heavy or prolonged periods. This happens because fibroids frequently distort the uterus so that the surface area of the endometrium is increased. A greater amount of endometrial lining is thus produced each month, thereby increasing the menstrual flow. In this case it is also more difficult for bleeding to stop since the normal spiral musculature of the uterine wall is distorted and cannot contract around the blood vessel. Fibroids may grow to become quite large, even to the size of a football, and may begin to cause pain as a result of pressing on organs such as the bladder or rectum.

In order to dissolve fibroids, it is important to avoid the extreme foods that caused them to develop. The standard macrobiotic diet, therefore, can serve as the basis for the recovery process. It is better to minimize the intake of flour products, as these can cause mucus formation, even if whole grain flours are used. It is also advisable to limit the use of oil to a few times a week. A small amount of high quality sesame or corn oil can occasionally be used in making sautéed vegetables

Fig. 24   Uterine fibroids.

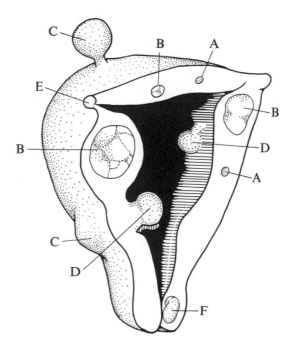

Cross section of the uterus showing numerous fibroids: A—small early fibroids in the wall of the uterus; B—larger fibroids distoring the wall of the uterus; C—fibroids bulging externally; D—internal stalked fibroids; E—fibroids blocking entrance to the Fallopian tube; F—fibroid of cervix.

or fried rice. Among vegetables, hard leafy greens can be eaten regularly. Dishes such as cooked *daikon*, *daikon* greens, and *kombu*, or shredded *daikon* cooked with *kombu* and *tamari* soy sauce are also good for this condition and can be eaten several times per week (see Recipe Guide). In general, it is better to minimize the intake of raw salad, if possible, using boiled salad to satisfy salad cravings. Among beans, it is better to use *azuki*, chickpeas, lentils, and black soy beans, and limit the use of other varieties to only rare occasions. Bean products such as *tempeh* and *tofu* may also be eaten on occasion, on an average of a few times per week.

Sea vegetable side dishes in a moderate volume are important, since minerals are needed for the smooth discharge of toxins from the body. Besides using sea vegetables in soups or with beans or vegetables, you may eat them in small side dishes on a regular basis, a few times a week. Sea vegetable condiments are also recommended for regular use.

During the healing process, it is better to minimize the use of fruit, limiting your intake to a small volume of cooked or dried temperate climate fruits only when craved. Vegetables such as squash, cabbage, *daikon*, and other sweet tasting varieties can be eaten when sweets are desired. Raw fruits and fruit juices are best avoided during the healing process, as are nuts and nut butters which contain plenty of oil and fat. It is also better to avoid animal foods or to limit your intake to a small volume of white-meat fish on occasion and preferably only when craved.

The following external applications are helpful in dissolving fibroid tumors:

1. *The ginger compress followed by the taro potato plaster:* These external remedies can be applied to the lower abdomen every day for a period of ten to fourteen days. Please note however, that they should not be used by pregnant women. The ginger compress can be applied as described on page 93. However, when treating fibroids, don't apply the ginger compress for more than five minutes and don't apply it alone without following it with a taro potato plaster. In this instance, the ginger compress is used only to prepare the body for the taro plaster.

    To make the taro plaster, remove the potatoe's skin and grate the white interior. Mix with five percent grated fresh ginger. Spread this mixture in a half-inch-thick layer onto a piece of fresh cotton linen and apply the taro side directly to the skin. Leave this on for three to four hours or overnight. If the plaster produces an unpleasant burning sensation, the grated ginger may be omitted. The ginger-taro application may be used once a day for ten days to two weeks. During the period when you are using these applications daily, it is important to eat a very clean macrobiotic diet. Following this initial period, the ginger-taro application can be used several times per week for an additional six weeks.

    Taro potato is available in most cities in North America. You can usually find it at Chinese, Armenian, or Puerto Rican grocery stores or at most natural food stores. The skin is brown and covered with "hair." Taro, sometimes known as *albi*, is grown in Hawaii and in Asia. Smaller potatoes are the most effective for use in this plaster. If you cannot find taro, a preparation using regular potato can be substituted. While not as effective as taro in collecting stagnated toxic matter and drawing it out of the body, it will still produce a beneficial result. Mix fifty to sixty percent grated potato with forty to fifty percent grated (crushed) green leafy vegetables. Crush the ingredients together in a *suribachi* and apply as above, following the ginger compress.

2. *A hot hip bath:* This is a very effective remedy for a variety of female reproductive disorders, including fibroids. Ideally, the bath water should contain dried leafy vegetables such as *daikon* or turnip greens. To prepare, hang fresh leaves so that they are not in direct sunlight. Leave them until they turn brown and brittle. (If leafy greens are not available, *arame* sea vegetable may be used.) Place about four to five bunches of dried leaves or a double handful of *arame* in a large pot. Add about four to five quarts of water and bring to a boil. Reduce the flame to medium and boil until the water turns brown. Add a handful of sea salt and stir well to dissolve.

   Then, run hot water in the bathtub and add the mixture together with another large handful of sea salt. Add only enough water to cover the body from the waist down. Sit in the tub and cover your upper body with a thick cotton towel to prevent chills and absorb perspiration. If the water begins to cool, add more hot water and stay in the bath for ten to twelve minutes.

   The hot bath will cause your lower body to become very red as a result of an increase in circulation. This along with the heat will loosen fat and mucus deposits in the pelvic region.

3. *A special douching solution:* It can be used immediately after the hip bath. To prepare, squeeze the juice from half a lemon into warm *bancha* tea or add one to two teaspoons of rice vinegar to warm *bancha* tea. Add a three-finger pinch of sea salt, stir, and use as a douche. The douching solution helps dislodge deposits of mucus and fat which have been loosened during the hip bath. The hip bath and douche can be repeated every day for up to ten days. During this time, it is important to eat very well and to avoid the foods which have contributed to this condition.

   Many women with fibroids become pregnant. Small fibroids usually do not affect the pregnancy, but larger growths may produce symptoms. During pregnancy, fibroid tumors grow, due to pregnancy hormones which, among other things, cause additional blood to gather in the uterus. If the blood contains excessive fats or other surplus factors, these accumulations are deposited in the uterine region at an accelerated rate. Women who take birth-control pills may also experience a similar growth of fibroids.

   If a fibroid enlarges to the point where it outgrows its blood supply, it degenerates in its central regions. This produces pain and tenderness which often subside after several days. This frequently occurs in the fourth or fifth month of pregnancy. Fibroids also increase the possibility of miscarriage and, in some cases, make conception less likely.

   Fibroids can reduce the elasticity of the uterine wall and prevent the baby from moving into a normal head-down position at birth, resulting in a breech or other abnormal presentation. Occasionally, they prevent the uterine muscle from properly contracting during labor, resulting in a long labor.

Fig. 25 Fibroids in pregnancy causing transverse lie.

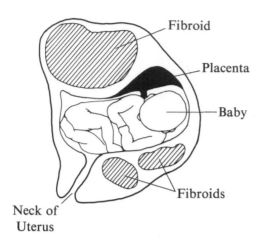

Fibroids may also produce prolonged bleeding after labor, as their presence in the uterus tends to make it contract more slowly than normal.

If you have fibroids and become pregnant, it is recommended that you eat according to the general guidelines for pregnancy, while trying to minimize or avoid the foods which contribute to this condition. However, keep in mind that during pregnancy, it is not advisable to eat too rigidly or conceptually. It is also not advisable to use the ginger compress on the abdominal region during pregnancy. The hot hip bath may be used, however, as may the special douching solution, although certain precautions need to be taken when douching during pregnancy. Therefore, consult with a qualified macrobiotic counselor, an experienced person, or a physician before using the douching solution during pregnancy.

Frequent Urination: Around the middle of pregnancy, the expanding uterus begins to press down on the bladder, causing urination to become more frequent. The ureter and kidney pelvis that carry urine from the kidney to the bladder tend to enlarge during pregnancy, and in combination with the increased activity of the kidneys, contribute to the frequency of urination.

Urination often becomes very frequent near the end of pregnancy. It is therefore a good idea to keep this in mind and try to keep yourself in situations where you have easy access to a toilet. Reducing your fluid consumption may help lessen the problem. Do not be overly conceptual about this, however, and be sure to take in a comfortable amount of fluid. It is better to avoid cold drinks during pregnancy. Hot or room temperature beverages are preferred.

For a woman who is not pregnant, the ideal number of daily urinations is three to four. If you urinate more frequently, it means that your circulatory and excretory systems are overworking due to the overintake of fluid. If you continually urinate more frequently, it is necessary to reduce your daily intake of fluids. If your daily urinations are less frequent, an increase in fluid intake is called for.

German Measles (Rubella): German measles arises when we consume too much animal fat and flour products. If we avoid the consumption of these items, or in the case of flour products, limit our intake to occasional unleavened whole grain bread or noodles, this illness normally does not arise. Foods such as cereal grains, eaten primarily in their whole form, sea vegetables, and hard fibrous vegetables, do not create the excessive condition which leads to German measles.

German measles, or rubella, produces symptoms such as fever, a light skin rash, and in some cases enlargement and tenderness in the lymph glands in the back of the neck and mild joint pains. It commonly occurs in childhood, after which a person acquires natural immunity. Forty years ago, doctors in Australia discovered that severe birth defects occurred in babies whose mothers had German measles during the first trimester of pregnancy. These deformities included brain damage and blindness. The reported incidence of deformed children following German measles in the first third of pregnancy varies from as little as 5 percent to as many as 50 percent although most texts quote the latter figure.

The medical approach to this problem is based on diagnosing whether a woman of childbearing age is immune by checking to see if rubella antibodies are present in the blood. If she is not immune, it is recommended that she take the rubella vaccine. However, in theory, the vaccine may attack the fetus and result in congenital anomalies. Therefore, it is not administered unless a woman is practicing some form of birth control which prevents her from becoming pregnant for three months after the vaccine is given.

The use of a vaccine as a preventive measure overlooks the more fundamental dietary cause of the illness and the natural immunity that can result from proper eating in a more balanced fashion.

Headaches: Headaches commonly occur during pregnancy, especially in the first and third trimesters. Even though many women experience them, however, headaches nonetheless indicate imbalance in a person's diet and physical condition. Headaches in the latter part of pregnancy may indicate toxemia of pregnancy, but in this case there are usually accompaning symptoms.

Headaches generally arise in: 1) the front of the head above the eyes, 2) the sides of the head, 3) the back of the neck and head, and 4) deep inside the head toward the back. The front is the most expanded, or yin, of these regions, while the back is more yang and compact. The sides are more yin than the back, but less yin than the front. The region deep inside the head is the most yang of all these areas.

Headaches in the front of the head result from the intake of extremely yin foods such as tropical fruits, soft drinks, fruit juices, sugar, honey, chocolate, vitamin C, and various drugs and medications. Side headaches arise more from the intake of yin foods that are less extreme, for example, oily or greasy foods, ketchup, potatoes (especially French fries and chips), dried fruits, too many fresh fruits, and various aromatic and stimulant beverages such as peppermint tea. Among alcoholic beverages, wine, which is made from fermented fruits and therefore more extreme, usually affects the front part of the head, while beer and other alcohols which are made from fermented grains more frequently affect the sides of the head.

The excessive intake of fish, poultry, eggs or more heavily salted foods can easily produce a tension headache in the back of the head. However, if you eat plenty of extremely yang foods, such as eggs, smoked salmon, bacon, liver, or caviar, a headache can easily develop deep inside the head as well.

If those who suffer from headaches avoid such extreme foods and generally eat according to macrobiotic standards, the headaches will begin to disappear. However, if you do eat some extreme food and experience a headache as a result, there are several effective treatments that can easily be done at home.

Headaches in the front and side regions are generally caused by expansion of the brain cells which results in pressure. Therefore, a cold application, such as a cold towel, will help to bring relief by causing the cells to contract. Headaches in the back of the head are generally the result of overcontraction. Therefore, a hot towel can be applied for relief. Headaches in the center of the head can be treated by wrapping a hot towel around the neck. This will help the entire area to become more relaxed.

We can also use the meridians and their corresponding toes in treating these headaches. The meridians correlate with the toes in the following manner: 1) the large toe—spleen and liver, 2) the second and third toe—stomach, 3) the fourth toe—gallbladder, 4) the fifth toe—bladder.

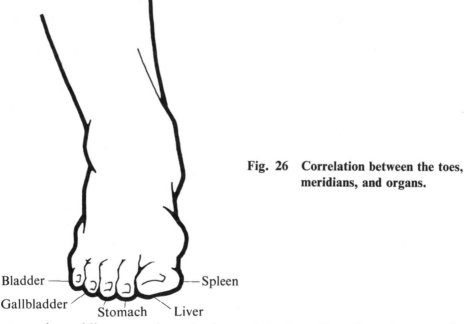

Fig. 26   Correlation between the toes, meridians, and organs.

The stomach meridian runs along the front of the face. Therefore, the stomach meridian can be stimulated when someone is experiencing front headaches.
The bladder meridian runs up along the back of the head and can be stimulated when pain arises there. The gallbladder meridian takes a very complicated course along the side of the head and can be used to treat headaches in this region.
The spleen and liver meridians can be used to treat pain deep inside the head. These treatments, summarized below, can be applied by your husband or a friend if you experience headaches during pregnancy.

1. *For pain in the front of the head:* Lie on your back, and have your friend repeatedly apply cold towels to your forehead. Then, your friend can vigorously massage the second toe, the third toe, and then both toes together. The toes should be massaged by repeatedly pulling them outward to the extent that the entire body moves when you pull. Repeat for about five minutes and then do the same thing on the opposite foot.
2. *For pain in the side of the head:* Have your friend apply cold towels to the painful region, as above, and then massage the fourth toe of each foot in the above manner.
3. *For pain in the back of the head:* Sit in a chair (lying on the front is preferable, but this position is difficult during pregnancy). Have your friend apply hot towels to the painful regions of the head. (You may need to bend forward to hold the towel in place.) After about five minutes of repeated hot towel applications, have your friend massage the fifth toe of each foot in the above manner.
4. *For pain deep inside the head:* Lie on your back and wrap a hot, squeezed towel around your neck. Replace with a fresh hot towel after the first towel cools and continue for about five minutes. Then, have your friend stimulate the first toe on each foot in the above manner.

These simple treatments, in combination with the macrobiotic diet, will help bring relief from headaches, including severe migraine headaches. During pregnancy, it is better to avoid medications such as aspirin, since they remain in your blood for several days, during which time they affect the developing baby. It is far better to use simple, natural, and effective remedies such as these which involve no artificial substances and therefore present no danger to the mother or baby.

Heartburn: Heartburn is a common complaint during the latter part of pregnancy. It occurs when the enlarging uterus pushes part of the stomach up against the diaphragm. Heartburn is often worse after meals or at night when a woman lies down to rest. Extremely yin foods and beverages, together with an excessive liquid intake, contribute to this problem as they often cause the uterus to expand abnormally. Foods that are highly acidic, such as coffee, animal proteins, and tropical fruits and vegetables, aggravate an overly-acid stomach, as do sugar and concentrated sweeteners which produce an acid reaction in the stomach. Overeating, lack of proper chewing, and eating before bed can also make the condition worse. A cup of *ume-sho-bancha* tea or an *umeboshi* plum often helps relieve heartburn.

Hemorrhoids: Hemorrhoids in pregnancy usually begin as painless swellings in the veins in and around the anus. In some cases, the swollen tissue *prolapses*, or slips outside the anus, especially when the woman strains while constipated or if she has diarrhea. Prolapse can cause the blood flow through these veins to be impeded, leading to the formation of a clot within the swollen tissue. These thrombosed external hemorrhoids bleed slightly and are very painful.

Hemorrhoids are caused by dietary imbalances. More yin hemorrhoids, which are the type that usually occur in pregnancy, result from the overconsumption of fluid, sugar, fruit, and fruit juice, salad and other more expansive items. Aside from contributing to swelling of the intestines and the development of chronic constipation and diarrhea, these items cause additional pressure to build up in the superficial veins of the pelvis and leg, causing them to become swollen and dilated. The intake of excessively yin foods and beverages can also weaken the tissues of the rectum and anus and make prolapse more likely.

In some cases, hemorrhoids result from the consumption of animal foods and salt. These more constrictive items sometimes contract the anal blood vessels too much causing them to bleed. This more yang type is far less common than that caused by the excessive consumption of yin foods, especially during pregnancy.

Herpes Simplex Infection: Every year, an estimated 10 million people develop some form of sexually contracted disease in the United States. In the past, the term "venereal disease" (named after Venus, the goddess of love) was used to describe five widespread disorders, the major ones being syphilis and gonorrhea. More recently, however, over twenty different diseases that can be spread through sexual contact have been identified. Society is now in the midst of an epidemic of these disorders.

Information about sexually transmitted diseases (STD) has become increasingly complex in recent years. A discussion of all of the known forms of sexually transmitted diseases is beyond the scope of this book. However, these disorders do occur in pregnancy and may be transmitted from mother to baby, in some cases causing serious problems with the newborn.

To illustrate the macrobiotic approach to STD, let us consider the example of *genital herpes*, a problem that now affects increasing numbers of people.

It is difficult to say with certainty just how widespread herpes has become. Estimates of the number of people in the United States with genital herpes range between 18 and 36 million. The Center for Disease Control in Atlanta estimates the number to be about 20 million, with at least ½ million new cases developing each year. As we can see, the incidence of herpes has reached epidemic proportions.

There are five main varieties of herpes viruses that affect humans. *Herpes zoster* is a widespread variety which is associated with *chicken-pox*, a disorder affecting about 75 percent of the American population by the age of fifteen. In adults, herpes zoster is associated with *shingles*, a painful blistering rash.

Herpes simplex, the virus associated with genital herpes, comes in two types: *herpes simplex virus type 1 (HSV-1)* and *herpes simplex virus type 2 (HSV-2)*. Type 1 is generally more yin and affects primarily the upper region of the body, especially the head and neck. It is associated with clusters of small red lumps around the lips that turn into painful blisters, often referred to as cold sores or fever blisters. The more yang Type 2 virus affects the lower regions of the body and is associated with painful lesions around the genitals, buttocks, and thighs. Both varieties can be transmitted through sexual contact. Not all genital herpes is the result of a Type 2 infection; an estimated 25 percent of genital infections are the result of the Type 1 virus.

Unlike other forms of STD, herpes does not respond to antibiotics. At present it is considered an incurable illness. Among women who are infected with the Type 2 virus for the first time, most show no noticeable symptoms. Among those who do have symptoms, one or more small, fluid-filled blisters usually develop on the external sex organs. The blisters are usually painful and appear within 3 to 20 days after contact with the virus. If they are located only in the vagina or on the cervix, they may be unnoticed. The blisters soon rupture, and those located externally develop into soft open sores that are very painful. The lymph glands in the groin may also become swollen and painful.

An initial outbreak usually lasts for about 10 to 12 days, after which the illness enters a latent stage. In some cases, the virus remains latent and no additional outbreaks occur. In other cases, the latent virus reactivates and the symptoms return. Recurrences may happen as often as twice a month or as rarely as once every ten years and are generally less severe than the initial outbreak.

An outbreak of genital herpes of either type can have serious consequences during pregnancy. Herpes has been associated with miscarriage, stillbirth, and infection of the baby as it passes through the birth canal. Up to 60 percent of infected babies die. The remaining babies have a 50 percent chance of brain damage or blindness. Many doctors recommend delivering a baby by cesarean section if an active infection is present at the time of labor.

The macrobiotic approach to herpes is based on reducing and preferably avoiding foods that weaken the immune system and thereby provide a fertile ground for the virus to take root. Of course, at the same time, one should begin to eat foods

Fig. 27   Regions of the body most frequently affected by HSV-1 and HSV-2.

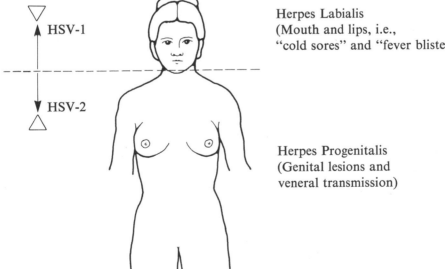

The majority of HSV-1 infections are found above the waist and the majority of HSV-2 infections occur below it. However, there is considerable crossover owing to changes in sexual practices and variations in diet: HSV-1 can infect the genitalia and HSV-2 can infect the mouth.

that strengthen the body's natural defenses. Persons with either type of herpes are advised to begin the standard macrobiotic diet with adjustments such as those presented below:

1. It is better to completely avoid all animal products, except infrequent use of non-fat white-meat fish. Historically, it is well known that the Mongols spread sexual diseases, including syphilis, throughout Asia. Their diet was rich in animal products and provided a base for these diseases to develop and persist. Among animal products, dairy fats in particular contribute to the development of herpes. Milk, cottage cheese, ice cream, and lighter, or more yin, types of dairy food contribute more to HSV-1, while heavier, solid cheeses tend to contribute more to the development of HSV-2.
2. Concentrated sweeteners are best avoided, including sugar, honey, maple syrup, and molasses, though concentrated grain sweeteners may be used from time to time.
3. Grains should be eaten in their whole form and thorough chewing is essential. Flour products, except those made from whole cereal grains are best avoided. If cravings develop, unleavened whole grain bread may be eaten. However, if it is possible to forego all flour products, the condition will improve more rapidly.
4. It is best to minimize the use of oil, even natural quality vegetable oils. A small portion of lightly sautéed vegetables may be eaten on occasion, preferably only a few times per week.
5. Among the many varieties of *miso* now available, it is better to use barley (*mugi*) *miso* and soybean (*hatcho*) *miso*.
6. It is best to eat cooked vegetables only, minimizing salads (and other uncooked foods) until the condition disappears. Among vegetable dishes, those prepared in the *nishime* style are recommended together with other styles of cooking. Vegetables such as squash, pumpkin, and cabbage may be used regularly together with other vegetables.
7. Sea vegetables such as *arame* or *hijiki*, among others, are recommended for regular use in side dishes. Beans and bean products, including *azuki* beans, chickpeas, and lentils are recommended for frequent use, together with bean products such as dried *tofu*, *tempeh*, and others.
8. Among supplemental foods, it is also better to avoid fruit, even cooked or dried temperate climate varieties. Nuts and their products are also best avoided during the recovery process. If snacks are craved, a small handful of roasted squash, pumpkin, or sunflower seeds may be eaten, preferably only on occasion.

The time needed for recovery depends on a number of factors, and particularly on the severity of the condition. Lighter or more recently acquired cases can be healed completely in as little as three weeks, while longer or more severe cases may take up to six months. During this time, it is advisable to keep the skin of the affected area clean and dry. Once recovery has been achieved, the person may eat according to the standard macrobiotic approach.

These general recommendations may also be applied in cases of gonorrhea, *chlamydia*, syphilis, and other forms of STD, although minor adjustments are of course needed in each case.

Itching: Itching results from the overintake of certain foods, especially animal fats, including dairy fats; simple sugars, including fruit sugars; oil and foods that contain plenty of oil; flour products; and other more yin foods. Itching is a mild form of skin disease and comes about when the intestines and kidneys are unable to efficiently discharge waste products. The body then attempts to discharge excess through the skin. In many cases, the problem is compounded when a thin layer of fat develops under the skin. A layer of fat interferes with the smooth discharge of various elements through the skin and makes the skin dry.

In order to clear up this problem, the following modifications of the standard macrobiotic diet are recommended:

1. Avoid all animal products, including fish.
2. Stay away from buckwheat and products that contain it.
3. Eat only cooked foods. Salad, raw fruit, and juices should be avoided.
4. Limit your intake of sweets to occasional cooked fruit desserts.
5. Avoid flour products.
6. Minimize or avoid oil, including that found in nuts and nut butters. Roasted sesame seeds can be used as a condiment during this period and other roasted seeds can be eaten as snacks.

These recommendations can be observed until the itching disappears, at which time the standard macrobiotic diet can be resumed.

A special skin wash using rice bran (*nuka*) is often helpful in relieving itching. To prepare, wrap *nuka* (this product can be obtained at most natural food stores) in cheesecloth. Place in hot water and shake. The *nuka* will melt and the water will begin to turn yellow. Wash the affected area with a towel or cloth that has been dipped in the *nuka* water.

Another external preparation, made with dried *daikon* or turnip leaves, is especially helpful in extracting excess fat and oil and in clearing up skin problems. To prepare, dry fresh *daikon* leaves away from sunlight, until they become brown and brittle. Boil 4 to 5 bunches of leaves with 4 to 5 quarts of water until the water turns brown. Add a handful of sea salt and stir well. Dip cotton linen into the liquid and lightly squeeze. Apply to the affected area, making repeated applications until the skin becomes red.

Itching is aggravated by the use of wool or synthetic fibers for clothing, especially underclothing, and for sheets, pillowcases, and blankets. Cotton or other vegetable fibers are preferred for general use. Natural, vegetable quality soaps and shampoos are also preferable to those containing chemical ingredients.

Late Delivery: Most mothers do not give birth exactly on their calculated due date. Women who menstruate on a more regular monthly basis tend to deliver closer to their due dates. Women who are generally more yang and who have shorter menstrual cycles tend to deliver a little earlier, while more yin women with longer menstrual cycles tend to deliver a little later.

The normal length for pregnancy is 280 days or 40 weeks. Most births come within the two weeks before or the two weeks after this time. Babies born before the 37th week are considered premature and those born after the 42nd week are considered postmature.

Late delivery may arise if a mother becomes too yin or if she becomes too yang. In the case of an overly yin mother, the repeated intake of too many sweets, sugars, fruits, liquids, spices, and other more yin items, weakens the muscles of the uterus and diminishes its conductivity to the forces of life vitality, especially the contracting powers.

In some cases, however, a mother becomes overly yang or constricted. When this happens, the placenta and baby are prevented from separating from the uterus. A woman in this condition literally holds on to her baby longer than necessary. In Oriental countries, however, it was considered fortunate for a baby to spend more than 280 days in the womb, as babies born several days to a week late were thought to be stronger and more developed than those born on time or early. In most cases, postmature babies seem to be no different than babies born on time. A very small percentage show some signs of malnutrition, since the placenta declines in efficiency toward the end of pregnancy and as a result provides the baby with fewer nutrients.

Miscarriage: At the present time, miscarriage is very common. Estimates of reported cases indicate that as many as one out of ten pregnancies end this way. The number of unreported cases is probably much higher as are those in which a woman is unaware that a miscarriage has taken place in the very early stage of pregnancy.

Most known miscarriages occur in the early part of pregnancy, usually between the second and third months. The expelled material frequently consists of tissue from the placenta. If an embryo or fetus is present, it is often poorly developed. These deformed embryos are referred to as *blighted ova* and result from the inability of the fertilized egg to divide properly. Blighted ova are very yin, the result of a more yin quality reproductive cell caused by the overconsumption of extremely yin foods and beverages. Such improperly formed embryos often survive for only a short period and are often discharged from the body during the first trimester of pregnancy.

In other cases, a healthy egg and sperm combine to produce a normal embryo. However, the condition of the uterus is too yin to hold the embryo inside and so miscarriage arises. This is not unlike what occurs during a nosebleed. Nosebleeds arise when we consume excessive amounts of fruit juice, water, tomatoes, fruit, soft drinks, and other strongly yin foods and beverages. When taken in excess, these items cause the capillaries in the nose to expand and burst, resulting in bleeding. Similarly, if a woman takes in too many strongly yin items, such as fruit and cold drinks, the capillaries and blood vessels that line the uterus become overexpanded and bleeding begins. If enough blood vessels rupture, the placenta and embryo separate from the lining of the uterus and are eventually discharged.

A miscarriage of this type is also more likely to occur during the first three months of pregnancy.

Factors that weaken the charge of life energy in the region of the abdominal energy center at the depths of the womb also contribute to the possibility of miscarriage. These include previous abortions, surgery in the area of the womb, and fibroid tumors.

In another type of miscarriage, the neck of the womb, or cervix, which is normally very yang or constricted during pregnancy, begins to dilate. Dilation can take place over the course of several days or weeks and can result in the onset of labor. This condition, known as *incompetent cervix*, results from the overconsumption of sugar, fruits, liquids, milk and other dairy products, cold foods and beverages, and other more extreme yin foods. It occurs most frequently between the third and sixth month of pregnancy, and can also result from previous cervical surgery.

In some cases, miscarriages arise from an overly constricted condition, caused for example when a mother eats too much salt or baked foods or eats too narrowly. The repeated intake of overly yang foods activates the more yin body of the uterus, causing it to contract. These contractions of the uterus cause the cervix to then dilate, possibly resulting in miscarriage. A miscarriage of this type is more likely to happen toward the end of pregnancy.

A sudden strong shock or an accident can trigger a similar nervous response. Therefore, a woman should try to avoid situations or activities that make her condition overly yang. Since traveling tends to make a woman more yang, it is wise to reduce travel during pregnancy and to use caution in regard to all of your vigorous activities.

The symptoms of miscarriage vary. In those involving a dilation of the cervix, a woman may be unaware of any problem until labor actually begins. In some cases, a heavy pink or brown discharge begins up to several days before labor starts. The woman may also experience a generalized aching in the back together with a sense of pressure in the lower body.

Miscarriages during the early part of pregnancy include cramps and bleeding. The bleeding often begins as a dark red or brown staining that increases after several days to a bright red flow. The flow of blood is usually heavier than that discharged at menstruation.

Bleeding or spotting do not always indicate that a miscarriage is occurring. Some women experience slight bleeding at the time of the first missed period. Often no further bleeding or problems occur. Others may experience slight bleeding later in pregnancy that subsides of itself, after which the pregnancy proceeds normally.

When a miscarriage occurs, however, the bleeding becomes heavy and is accompanied by the discharge of large blood clots together with embryonic and placental tissue. These are often grayish in color with a bluish or reddish tint. Cramps in the lower abdomen and backache usually accompany the discharge.

Whenever bleeding occurs, or if a miscarriage is suspected, it is important to eliminate all extremes from your diet. Since the majority of miscarriages result from an excess of more yin foods, and the separation of the placenta is a more yin symptom—even though the underlying condition may result from too much yang—it is important to stop the intake of all strongly yin items. This includes fruit, fruit juice, sweets, cold drinks, and even raw vegetables. Within the standard macrobiotic diet, cooked whole cereal grains can serve as the principal food. Flour products are best minimized during this time. Soup, which includes a small amount of sea vegetables and such vegetables as carrots, cabbage, onions, *daikon* or others, can be taken daily. It should be mildly seasoned with *miso*, *tamari* soy sauce, or sea salt. Among vegetables, root and fiber-rich leafy varieties are preferred, and these can frequently be prepared *nishime* style. Small amounts of cooked sea vegetable side dishes can be eaten daily, and, among beans, less oily varieties such as *azuki*, chickpeas, and lentils are to be more frequently used. (It is recommended that bean side dishes be cooked with sea vegetables such as *kombu* and land vegetables such as carrots and onions.)

It is preferable to use a lesser amount of oil at this time and to reduce eating nuts, nut butters, and other oily foods. Similarly, all fruits, except a small volume of temperate climate varieties, if craved, are better avoided, as are all animal foods, except a small volume of white-meat fish.

It is better not to season your foods strongly; a mild taste is preferred. Macrobiotic condiments can be used but in moderation.

Together with adjusting your diet, reasonable rest is also recommended.

When a miscarraige takes place, it is important to be checked by a doctor to make sure that all of the pregnancy tissue has been discharged. Therefore, save any material that is discharged for medical examination. If some material remains in the uterus, fever, headache, and pain often continue.

Warm compresses applied to the lower abdomen will often help with the discharge of any remaining material.

It is important to eat a well-balanced macrobiotic diet following a miscarriage. Within the standard macrobiotic diet, it is generally advisable to minimize the intake of animal foods and fruits for several weeks after a miscarriage. However, if you are weak after this experience, a small volume of *koi-koku* (carp and vegetable stew) can be helpful. (See Recipe Guide.)

A minority of miscarriages result from the overconsumption of salt and other more yang foods. In these cases, the diet can be adjusted to include a larger volume of lightly cooked vegetables, including some salad. Soft-cooked grains may also be used, and the intake of salt, including that in condiments and seasonings, should be reduced. The more specific suggestions presented below for yang morning sickness can also be applied in these cases.

A light *kuzu* (*kudzu*) drink, cooked with several small pieces of an *umeboshi* plum and several drops of *tamari* soy sauce, can be taken for several days following either type of miscarriage.

Caution and common sense are the best guides during pregnancy. In general, try to avoid all extreme foods and strenuous or exhausting activities. Use a very moderate amount of salt in your cooking or in the form of condiments, and also moderate your intake of more yin foods and beverages, especially during the first several months.

Morning Sickness: Although it is a common symptom during pregnancy, morning sickness is an indication that a mother's condition is out of balance. The symptoms of morning sickness include nausea, queasy feelings, or the lack of desire for certain foods or for food in general.

Some women experience these symptoms after waking up in the morning, others in the late afternoon, while some experience them throughout the day. In most cases, morning sickness results from the overintake of sugar, fruit, fruit juice, milk and other light dairy products, spices, tomatoes, and other more yin items. The standard macrobiotic diet, together with a reduction or avoidance of strongly yin foods, will help offset the more yin type of morning sickness. Stronger cooking methods are recommended in these cases.

In some cases, however, morning sickness results from the overintake of salt, baked food, animal products, and other more yang items. The overintake of these foods can cause the stomach and other organs to become overly contracted. The symptoms of the more yang morning sickness include nausea and a loss of appetite. In some cases, foods such as brown rice, cooked vegetables, and others that are normally appetizing lose their appeal.

If you experience this type of morning sickness, or if your condition becomes overly yang in general, make your diet more yin and your daily life somewhat more relaxed. Soft-cooked rice and other grains can be substituted for the usual less watery grains, and foods such as sweet rice or *mochi* (pounded sweet rice) can be eaten every day or every other day. Sweet rice is generally more fatty than regular brown rice. A condiment such as *umeboshi* plums or sour pickles can be eaten daily for a week or so. Also grated raw *daikon* may be used several times a week in a volume of a teaspoon at a time, to which are added several drops of *tamari* soy sauce together with a half sheet of toasted *nori*.

The intake of natural quality vegetable oil can also be slightly increased. Vegetables that are sautéed in a little sesame oil can be eaten more frequently. *Tempura*, or deep-fried vegetables in batter, can be eaten on occasion. Among vegetables, sweet tasting varieties such as squash, *daikon*, carrot, parsnip, and others are to be emphasized, while a small side dish of fresh salad may be taken several times a week. An overall reduction in the use of salt is recommended in restoring balance, while some fruits, especially more yang varieties such as berries, can be eaten in small quantities on occasion especially when they are cooked. A small volume of hot *amazake* (sweet fermented rice drink) or hot apple juice is also helpful, if taken occasionally. White-meat fish may be eaten on occasion by women with this condition, especially if weakness is being experienced.

In general, morning sickness is not a serious problem and often disappears after the third month. Do not become overly concerned or discouraged if you experience it. If your appetite diminishes, a small amount of *umeboshi* will often help to restore it, as will a small amount of fresh grated ginger. *Umeboshi* plum can be used with rice or soft rice, in *bancha* tea, or in *ume-shoyu-kuzu* drink. Ginger can be added to *bancha* tea (in some cases, together with *umeboshi*), *ume-shoyu-kuzu* drink, *miso* soup, cooked with fish, or used in a variety of ways as a condiment. Ginger is not often used in macrobiotic cooking, but a small amount used now and then is helpful to restore appetite.

During this time, try to discover what kinds of foods appeal to you. Among the many varieties of grains, some people prefer rice, while others may prefer barley or millet. Whole grain noodles or soft cooked grains may appeal to others. Use this opportunity to broaden the scope of your cooking and to discover the variety of tastes, textures, colors, and combinations that a well-balanced macrobiotic diet makes possible.

Multiple Pregnancy: In some cultures, it was considered unhealthy to give birth to more than one baby at a time. In modern society, twins occur once in about ninety births. Triplets occur about once every 9,000 births, while multiple births of more than three babies are more rare.

Recently, a variety of powerful new drugs, often referred to as "fertility drugs," have been recommended by the medical profession for women who are unable to conceive. Because they are extremely yin, these drugs often cause more than one egg to be released at a time, resulting in a high incidence of twin births and a relatively large number of higher multiple births of four, five, or more babies.

These multiple births are of the *fraternal* type, resulting from the separate fertilization of two or more ova. This more yin type of multiple birth can also result from the overconsumption of sugar, fruit, alcohol, spices, raw vegetables, and other more yin foods or from the use of more extreme drugs or medications.

"Identical" twins develop from a single fertilized egg. In most cases, the ovum divides soon after fertilization and each half goes on to form a baby. This can be caused by extremes of either yin or yang in the mother's diet.

Twins of both types usually develop in separate amniotic sacs. However, the placentas of identical twins are usually fused, and their blood supply is often mixed. In some cases, one of the twins receives most of the mother's blood and as a result the other grows small and poorly developed. Identical twins are not really identical; one will always develop in a slightly more active way and the other in a slightly less active way. If the mother's diet is generally balanced, the differences between them will be subtle. If her diet is extreme, however, one may be well developed while the other may be poorly developed. It is therefore very important for a woman who is carrying twins to eat a centrally balanced diet.

A well-balanced diet can also help prevent or minimize some of the other symptoms that accompany multiple pregnancy, such as more severe morning sickness, excessive weight gain, and the tendency to deliver the babies prematurely.

Nosebleeds: Many women experience nasal congestion during pregnancy arising from the intake of fats and oils, simple sugars, flour products, and too many fluids, all of which lead to the accumulation of fat, mucus, and fluid throughout the body. The sinuses are one of the most frequent sites for the accumulation of excess, as are the inner ears. As a result, many women also experience fullness of the ears during pregnancy.

This condition often becomes worse during pregnancy because the kidneys, which filter excessive factors from the blood, frequently become overworked. As a result, their efficiency may decline and fat and mucus may readily accumulate in the body.

In some cases, the overconsumption of fluids, simple sugars, fruits, fruit juices, and other more yin items causes the capillaries in the nose to expand and burst, resulting in a nosebleed. Nosebleeds can be quickly relieved by moistening a piece of tissue paper or a paper napkin with saliva, dipping it in salt or *dentie*, and placing it in the affected nostril for several minutes. Salt causes the ruptured capillaries to contract. A small amount of *gomashio* or a piece of *umeboshi* plum can be eaten every ten minutes for about one-half hour to further the process of contraction.

Ovarian Cysts and Tumors: As pointed out previously, mucus, fat, and other excessive factors frequently accumulate in the female reproductive organs. When accumulation occurs in and around the ovaries, a variety of cysts and tumors often result. There are literally dozens of varieties of ovarian growths, and each is the result of a specific excess in the woman's diet.

The most common ovarian tumor is the *simple cyst* which develops when the ovarian follicle does not rupture and release its egg but instead continues growing. These cysts are generally more yin, resulting primarily from the overconsumption of milk, butter, and other light dairy products, sugar, animal fats, and oily and greasy foods.

Another common type of ovarian growth is the *dermoid cyst*. Dermoid cysts are frequently found in younger women and often contain hair, fatty material, and sometimes "teeth." Dermoid cysts are more yang, or "hard," and arise primarily from the overconsumption of hard, saturated fat such as that in eggs, meat, poultry, and cheese.

The general dietary approach presented in the discussion of fibroids may also be applied in cases of ovarian cysts, with slight variations for each type. The external treatments introduced in that section may also be used, with the appropriate considerations for treating these problems in pregnancy.

Placenta Previa: The placenta is normally implanted at the upper end of the uterus in the general area of the abdominal energy center, or *hara chakra*. The fertilized ovum is normally attracted to the constant stream of environmental forces which converge at this point and which provide a rich supply of life energy for the growth and development of the baby.

Occasionally, however, the placenta is implanted in the lower part of the uterus. In some cases, the placenta is so far down that it completely covers the cervix, or neck of the womb. Placenta previa occurs in about one out of every hundred deliveries and usually arises when the fertilized ovum is overly yang, due to the excessive intake of eggs, meat, poultry, and other animal foods and salt. This condition is an indication that heaven's descending energy, which causes the egg to fall downward, is overly active.

Placenta previa causes bleeding in the latter part of pregnancy when the cervix begins to dilate in preparation for labor. The movements of the cervix disturb the attachment of the placenta, producing a slight show of bright red blood. Bleeding is usually intermittent and stops after several days. It may not recur for several days or weeks and when it does, it is usually much more profuse. In severe cases, hemorrhage can result.

Fig. 28   Placenta previa.

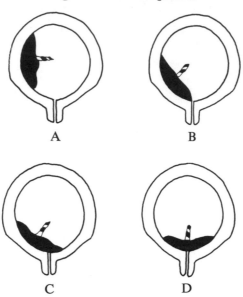

A—Normal location of placenta at upper end of uterus.
B—Marginal site approaching the neck of the uterus.
C—An incomplete placenta previa partially covering the neck of the uterus.
D—A complete cover of the neck of the uterus.

There are different degrees of placenta previa. In the marginal type, the placenta mostly covers the lower wall of the uterus and barely touches the cervix. In the incomplete type, the cervix is partially covered. In complete placenta previa, the cervix is completely covered and the baby's head is prevented from entering the pelvis during labor. With the marginal type, a normal vaginal delivery is possible, while a cesarean section is recommended for complete placenta previa. A woman with the incomplete type may be able to deliver her baby vaginally if she is in fairly good condition and if the placenta is mainly on one wall of the uterus.

Severe bleeding during the latter part of pregnancy is often due to placenta previa or to premature separation of the placenta. In either case, medical attention is necessary. Complete rest will often lessen the bleeding, as will the avoidance of extremely yin foods such as sugar, tropical fruits, soft drinks, tomatoes, and others. Eggs, meat, poultry, and dairy products are also best avoided. Strongly cooked vegetable quality foods, such as those recommended for miscarriage, are advisable in these cases.

Polyhydramnios (Excessive Amniotic Fluid): At full term, a baby is normally surrounded by about a quart of amniotic fluid. In some cases, however, up to four or five quarts of fluid accumulates. The overconsumption of liquid leads to the development of this condition, although in some cases, the overintake of salt contributes to the retention of fluid. The overintake of other more extreme yin foods, especially sugar, milk, ice cream, and soft drinks, also contributes to this condition.

Diabetic mothers frequently suffer from polyhydramnios, due to the frequent consumption of more extreme yin foods and beverages. Polyhydramnios is commonly associated with fetal anomalies such as *esophageal atresia* and fluid therefore accumulates because the fetus cannot swallow it. It is also associated with neural tube defects such as *anencephaly* and *meningomyelocele* (see Chapter 7).

Aside from reducing the excessive intake of liquids, eliminating all excessively yin items, and beginning the standard macrobiotic diet, foods that strengthen the kidneys, such as *azuki* and other bean dishes, are recommended for regular use. Dairy products and animal fats, which interfere with the smooth functioning of the kidneys, are best avoided, as is the excessive intake of salt.

Polyhydramnios often causes premature labor. Mothers with severe cases are therefore encouraged to rest and avoid strenuous physical activity. The recommendations presented earlier for edema, or swelling, can be applied in this disorder as well, with the exception of active exercise in severe cases.

Premature Birth: Like miscarriage, premature birth can arise from an excess of either yin or yang. In a small percentage of cases, a specific chronic illness or complication of pregnancy is involved. However, the vast majority of premature births, over 90 percent, are not related to specific complications but have to do more with the mother's general condition which is determined by her activity and way of eating both before and during pregnancy.

As discussed in Chapter 2, premature infants face a number of problems that full term babies do not. Aside from their size and weight, premature babies can usually be distinguished by: 1) thin skin with little underlying fat, 2) underdeveloped breast tissue, 3) a smooth scrotal sac in male babies which lacks the rough appearance found in full term babies, 4) a greater probability of undescended testes, and 5) less calcification in the long bones of the body.

The causes of premature birth are generally the same as those for miscarriage. Miscarriage is by definition a fetal loss at less than twenty weeks. All births later than twenty weeks need to be reported even though the fetus isn't considered viable until twenty-five to twenty-six weeks.

Together with eating carefully throughout pregnancy—for example, avoiding extremely yin items such as tropical fruits, sugar, and too much liquid, and staying away from more yang animal foods and dairy—it is advisable not to travel long distances, especially during the sixth and seventh months. Always keep your abdomen warm and avoid sudden movements or jolts. It is better to refrain from sexual activity during the final trimester.

If you have a premature baby, extra care must be taken during the first two years, during which time the premature infant develops more slowly than the full term baby. It is especially important not to expose the baby to strong sun, wind, or cold. Remember that the baby has entered the world of air ahead of time and therefore needs extra care in adjusting. Watch the baby very carefully. Around the age of two, however, the premature baby usually begins to develop as do other children.

The special dishes recommended in the section on recovery after birth can also be used after the delivery of a premature baby.

Premature Separation of the Placenta: In premature separation of the placenta, the placenta becomes partly or entirely separated from the lining of the womb before the baby is born. As with miscarriage, the majority of cases arise from the over-consumption of sugar, fruit, liquid, and other more yin items, all of which have the effect of depleting minerals from the body. The placenta separates prematurely in about one out of every 125 deliveries. It occurs in the latter part of pregnancy and produces vaginal bleeding.

In most cases, the placenta does not separate completely, and the baby can be delivered without complication. In severe cases, however, as much as one-third to one-half of the placenta separates. If its supply of oxygen is cut off, the baby could die. Most severe cases are accompanied by hemorrhage.

In some cases, women who have taken large quantities of extremely yin foods develop a complication in which *fibrinogen*, an element in the formation of blood clots, becomes depleted. Because the blood lacks the more yang factors needed for clotting, hemorrhaging can easily result.

Pains in the back or abdomen often accompany the vaginal bleeding. They vary in intensity, depending largely on how much of the placenta has separated. In severe cases, the pain may be strong and the abdomen becomes hard and sensitive to the touch, while in lighter cases, there may be no more than a generalized backache.

As with miscarriage, the overintake of excessive yang items, such as animal food and salt, may also cause the placenta to separate prematurely.

When severe bleeding occurs in the latter part of pregnancy, it is important to seek qualified medical advice, in order to determine whether the problem is being caused by premature separation of the placenta or placenta previa. As in cases of miscarriage or premature birth, it is important for a woman to eat very well following a case of premature separation of the placenta. The dietary recommendations presented for these problems can also be applied in this situation.

The Rh Negative Problem: The Rh factor was discovered when the blood of rhesus monkeys was injected into guinea pigs. The injections caused antibodies to form in the blood of the guinea pigs. When the antibodies were mixed with samples of the monkey's blood, the red blood cells stuck together, or *agglutinated*. When the antibody was mixed with the red blood cells of humans, agglutination took place in most, but not all, cases. The factor that was found to have caused agglutination was named the Rh factor, after the rhesus monkeys on whom the original experiments were conducted.

About 85 percent of the white population in the U.S. have this factor in their blood. When this factor is present, a person is said to have *Rh positve* blood. The remaining 15 percent in whom this factor is missing, have what is referred to as *Rh negative* blood. The percentage of people with Rh positive blood is much higher among the nonwhite population. About 95 percent of all Blacks and 99 percent of Orientals have Rh positive blood.

Some women with Rh-negative blood give birth to children with a disorder known as *erythroblastosis*. Erythroblastosis sometimes occurs when an Rh-negative woman carries an Rh-positive child. In some cases, the baby's red blood cells pass through the placenta and into the mother's bloodstream. The baby's Rh-positive cells cause antibodies to form in the mother's blood which are able to destroy Rh-positive cells. These antibodies are very small and easily pass through the placenta and into the baby's bloodstream, where they destroy the baby's red blood cells.

Erythroblastosis occurs rather infrequently. Before the advent of medical approaches to this problem, only about 10 percent of Rh-negative mothers had any problem, while 90 percent had none. Even when erythroblastosis occurred, it was usually in a mild form, with the baby recovering completely. Erythroblastosis occurs only when the mother has the specific Rh-positive antibodies in her blood. A woman with these specific antibodies is said to be "sensitized" to the Rh-positive cells. Sensitization can occur in several ways, the most common being when an Rhnegative person receives a transfusion of Rh-positive blood. It can also occur when an Rh-negative woman carries an Rh-positive baby. However, sensitization in general is relatively rare.

Erythroblastosis is far less likely when a woman is healthy and is eating a centrally balanced diet throughout pregnancy. If a woman is healthy, so is her placenta. A healthy placenta is more likely to perform its functions without mishap, for example, by completely preventing any mixing between the blood of the mother and that of her baby. A placenta that is nourished by strong, healthy blood also tends to deteriorate much more slowly, if at all, toward the end of pregnancy and is much more likely to sustain its normal functioning until the time of birth.

The sharp difference between Rh-positive and Rh-negative blood is the result of a diet which is based on the extremes of yin and yang. For example, at the present time, nearly half of the average diet in America is comprised of eggs, meat, dairy, and other animal products. These items require a large daily intake of more extreme yin items to create balance, and these are taken usually in the form of simple carbohydrates such as refined sugar, maple sugar, chocolate, corn starch, and various fruit sugars.

If, however, we consume a more moderately balanced diet, such as the standard macrobiotic diet, the Rh-factor is neither strongly positive nor strongly negative. A woman with mild Rh-negative blood is more likely to produce fewer and milder antibodies in the event that the blood of her Rh-positive baby is mixed with her own. In a case such as this, it is very unlikely that a severe erythroblastosis will occur. However, because of the possibility of complications, women with Rh-negative blood are advised to seek qualified medical advice during pregnancy.

Tingling of the Fingers: During the latter part of pregnancy, some women experience a tingling sensation in the fingers of one or both hands, especially in the first and second fingers. In some cases it becomes increasingly severe and a throbbing or burning sensation develops. This problem is caused by the overintake of fluids, including milk, soda, fruit juice, tea, coffee, and others, together with the intake of sugar, concentrated sweeteners, fruits, and other more yin items. The repeated intake of more yin foods and beverages causes the heart and circulatory systems to overwork and also produces expansion and overactivity in the lungs and large intestine. As a result, the flow of electromagnetic energy along the lung, large intestine, and heart governor meridians can easily become overactive, leading to pain, tightness, or tingling sensations. (These meridians run along the arm and connect with the thumb, index, and middle fingers.) At the same time, the over-intake of fluid causes the tissues and capillaries throughout the body to become swollen and expanded. When the tissues of the wrist become overexpanded, the nerves of the hand on the inside of the wrist can easily become compressed, result-ing in a tingling or burning sensation. Aside from reducing fluid intake, a woman with this problem can often obtain relief by raising her arm on pillows or a cush-ion. Scrubbing the arms, wrists, hands, and fingers daily with a hot moist towel will help prevent this problem and can also help bring relief.

Toxemia of Pregnancy: Most cases of toxemia occur during the last several months of pregnancy. Toxemia begins as a generalized retention of fluid which produces a rapid gain in weight. Weight gain is usually followed by noticeable swelling in the hands, feet, and face. Usually, fluid accumulates in the feet and ankles during the day when a woman is on her feet. Then, when she lies flat, it accumulates in the hands and face. A woman with this condition will often wake up with a swollen, puffy face. If the illness progresses, the blood pressure becomes elevated, protein starts to appear in the urine, and the symptoms become more severe, leading even-tually to convulsions known as *eclampsia*. (Toxemia is therefore often referred to as *pre-eclampsia*.) Eclampsia is a very serious complication of pregnancy, leading in some cases to death for both mother and baby. Once the illness has become severe, the medical approach is usually to terminate the pregnancy before convul-sions begin, after which the symptoms usually disappear.

Toxemia results primarily from the overintake of more extreme yin items such as sugar, soft drinks, refined carbohydrates, and fruits, together with the overcon-sumption of foods containing saturated fats such as milk and dairy products, eggs, and fatty animal foods. When eaten in excess, these items weaken the circulatory and excretory systems, causing both swelling and the progressive build-up of fat and mucus in the heart, kidneys, and blood vessels. The overconsumption of these items tends to weaken the intestines, so that two of the body's major organs for discharging waste products, the intestines and kidneys, often do not function as efficiently as they should. When someone in this condition becomes pregnant, the added strain imposed by the production of waste products by the fetus can become too much for these organs to handle effectively and can lead to the accumulation of fluid and other waste products in the mother's body.

Women who suffer from diseases such as high blood pressure, chronic *nephritis* (inflammation in the kidneys), or diabetes are much more likely to develop toxemia during pregnancy than those who do not have such problems. These disorders affect both the blood vessels and the kidneys.

When properly applied, the macrobiotic diet will help prevent toxemia by pro-viding an adequate balance of essential nutrients without taxing the organs which discharge excess and without causing the build-up of mucus and fat in the heart, kidneys, intestines, or other organs and areas of the body. Women with mild tox-emia can apply the specific recommendations presented earlier for backaches and edema. Bed rest is also recommended as is keeping the use of salt to a minimum both in cooking and in various condiments. The temporary restriction of salt helps to allow accumulated fluid to discharge more rapidly. In most cases, the toxemia will disappear following these adjustments.

If proper diet, including a reduction in salt intake, and bed rest do not reduce the swelling, the special *daikon* radish tea described on page 97 can be taken once a day for three days. This tea acts as a diuretic, stimulating the discharge of excessive fat, water, and salt through the kidneys.

In some cases, toxemia progresses to a more severe stage, especially when the kidneys have been chronically weakened by the previous intake of fats, sugars, and drugs and medications. The symptoms of severe toxemia include: 1) elevated blood pressure, 2) protein in the urine, 3) headaches and visual difficulties, 4) a decrease in the volume of urine, 5) a loss of clarity in thinking, and in very serious cases, 6) a severe steady pain in the upper abdomen. Because of the possibility of serious complications, a woman who suspects toxemia should seek appropriate medical advice.

Tubal Pregnancy: The condition in which the fertilized ovum implants somewhere other than in the uterus is known as *ectopic*, or misplaced, pregnancy. The most common site for implantation outside the uterus is the Fallopian tube, although implantation may occur in a variety of places (see Figure). When this happens the egg usually develops for several weeks and eventually bursts into the abdominal wall.

Tubal pregnancies result primarily from the overconsumption of extremely yin foods, especially fruits, sugar, highly acidic vegetables, and spices. Ectopic pregnancies are more prevalent in tropical regions where a larger volume of more yin foods and beverages is consumed regularly. These items weaken the egg and cause it to move too slowly through the Fallopian tube. Ectopic pregnancies can also be

Fig. 29 Abnormal implantation sites of the fertilized egg.

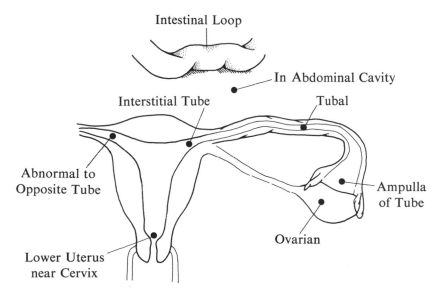

caused by mucus and fat in the ovaries and Fallopian tubes which interfere with the smooth passage of the egg. Together with the foods mentioned above, these deposits result from the repeated consumption of various animal products which contain sticky, saturated fat, along with the overconsumption of refined grains and oils. Women who have had tubal pregnancies often have histories of diminished fertility or pelvic inflammations, both of which are associated with the overconsumption of the above-mentioned foods.

When a tubal pregnancy occurs, the woman will skip a period and may experience mild symptoms of pregnancy. Soon afterward, pain develops in one side of the abdomen, frequently accompanied by slight vaginal bleeding. If you suspect a tubal pregnancy, it is important to seek medical assistance as quickly as possible, as the results of a ruptured tubal pregnancy are very serious.

The standard treatment for this condition is surgery. The dietary and way of life recommendations for care following miscarriage can be applied in this situation as well. If you experience a tubal pregnancy, it is very important to reflect on what it was in your diet and behavior that caused it to happen and to make whatever adjustments are necessary to prevent it from occurring in the future.

Urinary Tract Infections: During pregnancy, the ureter and kidney pelvis that transport urine from the kidney to the bladder tend to stretch and dilate.
The expanding uterus may also interfere with the free flow of urine through these passageways. Both conditions make it easier for infections to develop in the urinary tract, especially when a woman is eating in an unbalanced or disorderly manner. In many cases, these infections start as *cystitis*, or bladder infection, and go on to *pyelitis*, or infection of the kidney duct, and then to *pyelonephritis*, or infection of the kidney. These infections are most frequent during the third or fourth month of pregnancy.

The symptoms of urinary tract infection include pain and burning during urination (a woman with an infection of the urinary tract often desires to urinate more frequently than normal, and when she does, only a small amount usually comes out), pain in the back, and, when the kidneys become infected, chills and fever. With mild infections, the temperature often reaches 102°F., going as high as 104°F. in severe cases. The patient may also vomit and feel generally ill. In severe cases, mucus and blood are present in the urine.

In general, these infections arise when the overall condition is weakened by the overconsumption of more yin foods and beverages, including sugar, soft drinks, ice cream, tropical fruits, fruit juices, and cold liquids.

Persons with urinary tract infections can begin the standard macrobiotic diet, emphasizing dishes that are more thoroughly cooked and more strongly seasoned. Fruit and fruit juice, and animal food, including dairy foods, are best avoided during an acute attack. It is advisable to eat cooked foods only and to minimize or avoid the use of oil. The following additional recommendations are also beneficial:

1) Whole cereal grains may comprise up to 60 percent of daily meals.
2) Bean dishes may be eaten daily, limiting the intake to smaller, rounder beans such as *azuki*, chickpeas, and lentils. It is advisable to prepare beans with

kombu. Vegetables such as squash, carrots, onions, or others may also be included.

3) *Miso* and *tamari* soy sauce broth soups may be eaten daily and may have a slightly saltier flavor and thicker consistency.

4) Among vegetables, root, ground, and hard leafy green varieties may be emphasized. Longer cooking times (10 to 15 minutes) and a moderate amount of seasoning are preferred.

5) Sea vegetable side dishes may be included daily, especially those with *hijiki*, *arame*, *kombu*, and *wakame*. (A variety of vegetables may be included, in addition to *tempeh* and other bean products.) These dishes may be moderately seasoned.

6) If salads are desired, it is preferable to eat 1 to 3 minute boiled salads until the condition improves.

7) Various macrobiotic condiments may be used daily in moderate amounts. It is better to limit your intake of beverages to *bancha* stem or twig tea or cereal grain tea or coffee and to keep your daily intake of liquid moderate.

8) Seeds, such as sunflower, squash, or pumpkin, lightly roasted with a small amount of *tamari* soy sauce or sea salt, may be eaten as snacks. It is preferable to avoid nuts or nut butters until the condition improves.

During an acute attack, a *tofu* plaster can be applied to the forehead to reduce fever. To prepare, squeeze the liquid from *tofu*, mash, and add 10 percent to 20 percent pastry flour and 5 percent grated ginger. Chop either collard greens, watercress, kale, or some other leafy green vegetable very finely. Mash in a *suribachi* for several minutes. (The volume of crushed leafy greens should be equal to that of the other ingredients.) Place other ingredients in a *suribachi*, mix very well, and then spread the mixture on a piece of cheesecloth or cotton linen. Apply so that the *tofu* comes in direct contact with the skin. Change when the plaster becomes warm and continue applying a fresh plaster until the fever comes down.

A special tea made with grated raw *daikon* can also be taken to induce sweating and help reduce the fever. To prepare, mix half a cup of grated raw *daikon* with one tablespoon of *tamari* soy sauce and one-fourth teaspoon of grated ginger. Pour enough hot *bancha* tea over the mixture to cover and stir well. Drink while hot. (Do not use more than once per day for three days without the supervision of a qualified macrobiotic counselor.)

Uterine Anomalies: During the embryonic period, the paired Mullerian ducts fuse to form the uterus. If, however, the mother's diet includes an abundance of extremely yin foods such as sugar, tropical fruits, alcohol, fruit juices, and soft drinks, and does not include enough minerals and complex carbohydrates, these embryonic tubes may lack the contractive force necessary to fuse properly. The result is often some degree of a double uterus.

In the most severe forms, instead of developing as a single organ, the uterus develops as a pair of smaller tubes which are either partly or completely separated. In some cases, a septum, or dividing wall, remains and two separate cervixes and two vaginas develop. A less extreme abnormality occurs when the tubes join but the tissue of their common wall remains, leaving a septum or partition down the

Fig. 30   Types of uterine abnormalities.

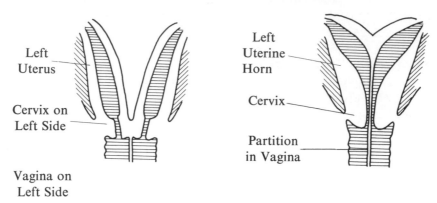

Double Uterus with two cervixes and two vaginas.

Two-Horned or Bicornate, Uterus with a partition in the vagina and cervix.

Fig. 31   Types of uterine abnormalities.

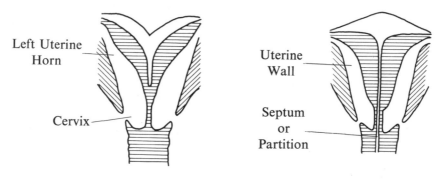

Two-Horned, or Bicornate Uterus with a single cervix.

Uterus with a Septum.

middle. In the most common form, a partial septum remains at the top of the uterus, causing the normally pear-shaped organ to become heart-shaped. This is known as a *two-horned* or *bicornuate* uterus.

Uterine anomalies are much more common in women whose mothers took DES during their pregnancies. Many women with these uterine irregularities are unaware of them. Many have normal pregnancies, but in some cases the anomaly does produce complications during pregnancy. Repeated miscarriages or premature deliveries are experienced by some women with these disorders, while breech positions and other abnormal presentations are more common in women with a double uterus. Often, the abdomen of a woman with a uterine anomaly will bulge more on one side rather than in the middle during pregnancy. Because of the increased possibility of complications, women with uterine anomalies are encouraged to eat macrobiotically throughout pregnancy.

Vaginal Infection: As explained in our discussion of fibroids and elsewhere in this book, the female sex organs are a frequent site for the discharge of excess in the blood and lymph streams which results from an excessive daily diet. Excess is commonly expelled through the vagina, producing a variety of vaginal discharges. When the localization of excess in the vagina upsets the delicate biochemical balance in this region, a variety of organisms begin to grow resulting in a vaginal infection.

Vaginal infections are common in pregnancy, especially when foods such as milk, butter, cheese, eggs, chicken, and other animal fats are eaten regularly, or when tropical fruits, sugar, soft drinks, and other extremely yin foods are consumed. Even women who eat a more naturally balanced diet can develop vaginal discharges if too many fruits, nuts, flour products, or oily foods are consumed or if they binge on items such as tomatoes, potatoes (especially French fries or potato chips), or white flour.

In the most common infection during pregnancy, a thick white discharge is produced. It is often discharged in clumps and contains a yeast or fuguslike organism known as *Monilia*. These infections often cause the labia to become red, swollen, and irritated and may cause slight pain and burning during urination.

Another common vaginal infection produces a thinner and more yellow-colored discharge which contains a microorganism known as *Trichomonas vaginalis*. It often causes an itching sensation which seems to be centered inside the vagina. This infection is, of course, sexually transmittable.

Other common discharges include: 1) a clear thin discharge which results from excessive mucus in the cervix and vaginal wall and 2) a green discharge which may contain pus as a result of an acute infection.

Clear discharges are generally the least serious, while white discharges often precede the development of a softer type of cyst. Yellowish discharges frequently accompany cysts, while greenish discharges, particularly those that are chronic, may indicate the tendency to develop cancer of the reproductive organs.

Women with vaginal infections are advised to begin the standard macrobiotic diet. The specific adjustments presented in the discussion of fibroids are also appropriate in these cases, as are the special considerations for pregnancy. The hot hip bath and *bancha* tea douching solution may also be used to bring relief, again, with the necessary considerations for their use in pregnancy.

Varicose Veins: During pregnancy, the surface veins of the genitals or legs may become swollen. They often ache and are unsightly. Varicose veins are similar to hemorroids in pregnancy. Both conditions are caused primarily by the consumption of excess fluid, including milk, fruit juices, water, tea, and coffee, together with fruit, sugar, and other more extreme yin items, and animal quality fats, especially cheese, cream, butter, and other dairy foods. The overconsumption of these items increases the fluid pressure in the veins and throughout the circulatory system and can cause the uterus and developing fetus to expand and press on the veins in the abdomen that drain the lower extremities. If a woman with this condition does not reduce or eliminate the intake of these items, the varicosities usually get worse as pregnancy progresses. After delivery, they often improve, but, without the necessary dietary changes, they may not go away completely.

Besides proper diet, varicose veins can be treated by the alternating application of hot and cold water compresses. First, hold a medium sized towel under a hot faucet, wring it out and apply hot to the affected area. Leave the towel on for about three minutes, then, run cold water over it, wring it out, and apply cold to the same area, leaving it on for about three minutes. Repeat with another hot towel, then another cold towel, and so on, for about twenty minutes.

5 | Birth and Recovery

Before she has a baby, a woman may want to become a successful businesswoman or create a large company with her husband. She may put all of her energies into endeavors such as art, music, or her career. But after her first baby is born her ideas often change. When she sees the infant smile, move around, and try to suck, and realizes that her baby is healthy and strong, she begins to feel very happy and fulfilled. Then, as her children are growing, her whole world centers on them. As a mother she gives them her greatest care and attention, even if she is active outside the home, for she is creating a new generation of humanity. She may still have great ambitions for herself and her husband, which she may go on to realize, but in the meantime, her experience of being a mother makes her whole personality and understanding so much deeper and richer.

As a woman raises her own children, she can better understand and appreciate her parents for their love and care in bringing her up. Gradually, she begins to understand love in a much broader sense, beyond sexual love or the romantic attraction between two people. Her love for her children can grow to include many other people and society as a whole.

A husband also changes after becoming a father. His care for his wife naturally grows deeper and he begins to feel more responsibility to secure his family. While he pursues his dream, he becomes more practical and realistic.

There is a great difference between people who have experienced parenthood and those who have not. People who have not had children may talk about society or about love, peace, or the future of the world. But when parents or grandparents talk about these things, they do so out of a much deeper and more practical concern. The experience of having children makes life much more full and real.

Natural Childbirth

Natural childbirth means having a baby without medication or artificial interference. It can take place at home or in a hospital. If you eat well throughout pregnancy, your chances of having a smooth delivery with no complications are better than 90 percent. Of course, you will still experience some pain, but this pain is bearable and not like a sharp knife cutting you. If a woman feels unbearable pain during birth, she has been eating improperly, especially too much fruit, sugar, or animal food. Women who chronically overeat or who are overweight also frequently experience difficulty giving birth. During labor, tissues and organs that are overexpanded frequently are forced to contract sharply, causing pain. Labor is commonly shorter for women who eat a balanced, natural diet.

If you decide to have your baby in a hospital, meet your doctor well in advance and establish good mutual understanding. Make sure he or she understands and will support your decisions regarding medication and other procedures. The following points often need to be clarified:

1. Your feelings regarding procedures such as shaving the pubic hair, routine enemas, the induction of labor, routine IV fluids, electronic fetal monitoring, the use of analgesics and anesthetics, episiotomy, forceps delivery, silver nitrate, which is put in the baby's eyes to avoid possible infection by venereal disease, vitamin K injections, which are often given to the baby immediately after birth, and the artificial hormones which are given to contract the uterus following delivery.
2. Your wish to have the baby brought to you as soon as possible for breast-feeding. State very clearly whether or not you want the baby to receive the artificial formula or glucose solution that newborns are sometimes given in the hospital. Make it clear that you are going to breast-feed the baby and do not want the medication that is given to stop the production of breast milk. (In the United States, this medication is rarely given by a doctor unless the mother asks for it.)
3. If the baby is a boy, state very clearly your wishes in regard to circumcision. (In the United States, a woman must sign a consent form to have this done.)

When a woman receives medication during labor, the quality of her milk is greatly affected. Not only is the nursing baby influenced by the quality of her milk but, prior to birth, the medications that are commonly used pass through the placenta and into the baby's bloodstream. These drugs depress the functioning of the nervous system and actually affect the baby more than they do the mother. Babies whose mothers receive medications are frequently sleepy and experience a general slowing of body functions. In rare instances, they are too sleepy to eat for several days. On the other hand, the babies of mothers who receive no medication are usually much more vigorous and alert in the first few days after birth. Some of the other problems associated with artificial delivery procedures include marks on the baby's face and head caused by the use of forceps during delivery, and swelling of the eyelids and eye discharges resulting from the application of antibiotics in the eyes. (In most hospitals, parents can sign a release form to forego use of eye medication.) In general, babies whose mothers have received medication during labor often appear to be more nervous and unstable than those who have been delivered naturally.

When a woman has her baby naturally, she is awake and fully aware of what is taking place. She is the main participant during delivery and is able to fully experience the miraculous process of childbirth. As soon as she has delivered her baby, she can hold him or her and develop further the emotional bonds that began in pregnancy and last throughout life. This experience gives a woman a very sublime feeling that is frequently missing from a medicated birth.

As far back as the early 1920's, strong criticisms started to be raised against many of the medical procedures used during labor. Encouraged by publications such as *Natural Childbirth*, a book first issued in 1933, by the British obstetrician Grantly Dick-Read, a growing movement for natural childbirth began to develop in Europe and the United States. Macrobiotics, of course, has advocated natural childbirth for more than fifty years (from its modern beginning), in Japan, Europe, and in the United States. Thousands of macrobiotic mothers around the world have experienced natural birth and, together with other individuals and groups, have helped to bring the movement for natural birth to the awareness of the general public.

Five years ago, researchers at the University of Florida discovered that medicated births can permanently damage the baby's brain and nervous system. The medicated babies who were studied were found to have I.Q.'s that were about four points lower than babies who were delivered without medication. A variety of other studies have also pointed out the detrimental effects of many hospital procedures. As a result, natural childbirth has become increasingly sought after as the preferred way of having babies. However, at the present time, we are still far from the ideal of natural childbirth. One reason is that in many cases, some type of medical intervention is still necessary mainly because the mother is not eating well. If a woman's condition is not good, she may experience a very long, painful labor, or other complications may arise. For example, the baby may be born buttocks first, as in a breech presentation, the umbilical cord may wrap around the baby's neck, diminishing the baby's supply of oxygen, or the membranes may rupture prematurely. For this reason, natural childbirth should not be approached with a rigid or fanatic attitude. Even if everything goes smoothly, it is important to be prepared in the event an emergency arises. Although for a healthy woman the chances of complications are normally very slight, precautions should nevertheless be taken. Therefore, professional guidance should be sought from an experienced midwife or doctor. Early in pregnancy, seek a doctor or midwife who can understand your wishes and who will support your approach. If you wish to have your baby at home, make sure that you have access to a nearby hospital or medical center in the event that complications arise.

Although medical treatments may be required in some cases, our long-term goal is to minimize artificial intervention in the birth process. At present, about 95 percent of the births in this country are medicated to some degree. In the future, hopefully 95 percent of all births can be done naturally, and medical treatments can be reserved for emergency cases only. As the macrobiotic way of life and proper care for delivery becomes more widely practiced, the number of women who require emergency treatment will naturally decrease.

Perhaps the ideal setting for having a baby would be a natural birth center in a comfortable, home-style facility that serves the best quality macrobiotic food. A woman could go there to have her baby and stay for a week or two with complete rest. In this way, she wouldn't have to worry about her husband, her home, or her other children if she has them. Our hope is to set up such a facility in the future.

As natural childbirth becomes more popular, husbands are increasingly participating in the birth experience. In most traditional societies, however, husbands and other men in the family customarily stayed away from direct participation in the birth experience. This was done out of deep respect for the mystery of the opposite sex, and to maintain the polarity, or attraction, between the sexes. However, in modern society the husband's participation in the delivery is sometimes considered valuable for sharing this profound life experience with the wife.

Despite their desire to cooperate, some husbands who take part in the birth process subsequently regret the experience as being too intimate. On the other hand, some couples consider the experience emotionally valuable. It is up to each couple to decide whether the husband should participate in the birth. Needless to say, however, even though the husband may decide not to be in the delivery room, it is reassuring for the wife to know that he can be easily reached if necessary.

Labor and Delivery

No two labors are the same. The type of labor that a woman has depends on her physical, emotional, and mental condition. Her condition is in turn created by her diet, activity, and way of life both before and during pregnancy. Labor can be either short or long, painful or not so painful. As mentioned previously, macrobiotic women generally have shorter, less painful labors, and experience fewer complications than average.

A number of changes in a woman's body that occur late in pregnancy indicate that labor is not too far off. These may include: 1) The baby "drops" from a more upward to a lower position in the abdomen. The downward movement of the baby is known as "lightening," and it may occur two to five weeks before birth with the first baby and usually after labor has started with subsequent births. 2) The baby becomes less active. 3) *Braxton-Hicks contractions* or *false labor* increase. 4) The mother may lose one to three pounds and experience a sudden increase in her energy level.

If you decide to have your baby at home, make sure that the birthing room is clean and that all of the supplies needed for the birth are available. Fresh flowers, plants, and a clean orderly environment help to create a calm and relaxed atmosphere. During the birth, outside distractions should be avoided as much as possible. Doors and windows of the birthing room can be adjusted to suit your needs and preferences. Once labor has started, it is important that your husband or friends be available to take care of your other children, if you have them, as well as the preparation and serving of meals for you and your family members or guests.

The Onset of Labor: When labor is starting, any of the following signs may occur:

1. *Rhythmic contractions of the uterus:* Labor begins when the rhythmic charge of heaven and earth's forces intensifies along the mother's primary channel, especially in the region of the abdominal energy center (the *hara chakra*) in the depths of the womb. The contraction and relaxation of the uterus takes place in a manner similar to the rhythmic expansion and contraction of the heart, lungs, intestines and other organs. The pattern is basic and universal: heaven's descending energy charges the organ and causes it to contract and become tighter and then earth's ascending force causes it to relax and expand. When this motion occurs in the uterus of a pregnant woman, it is referred to as *birth contractions* or *labor pains*, and these are usually felt

as mild cramps or sensations of tightness in the abdominal region. This motion normally begins in the upper portion of the uterus, in the area corresponding to the abdominal energy center, and spreads downward in the form of a wave. Contractions normally last about 15 to 20 seconds, during which time the abdomen firms and tenses. If a woman is healthy, these contractions do not cause undue discomfort. If contractions do produce an uncomfortable pain, it is generally an indication that a woman has been consuming an excess of yin foods, including fluids, or too much food in general. Painful contractions can also be caused by animal foods containing hard, saturated fat. These items harden the uterine muscle and this can cause pain when the muscle contracts.

Genuine birth contractions can be distinguished from the contractions of false labor, also known as Braxton-Hicks contractions, by their rhythm. Many women experience definite contractions for weeks before delivery, but if a steady, continuous rhythm is not established, it is usually an indication that labor is not yet beginning. Genuine contractions may start at intervals of 10, 15, or 30 minutes, but once labor actually begins, they come more rapidly and increase in intensity.

2. *Leaking of the amniotic fluid:* In some cases, amniotic fluid leaks from the membranes and is discharged from the vagina before labor begins. The membranes may also burst suddenly, causing the fluid to flow out in a gush. There is usually no pain when this happens and labor usually begins within a few hours, although in some cases, several days may go by before it begins. The *premature rupture of the membranes* occurs in about 10 percent of the births in the United States. Ideally, the amniotic sac will not rupture until late in the first stage of labor; about 10 to 15 minutes before the actual birth of the baby. The amniotic fluid moistens and lubricates the birth canal. If the sac ruptures earlier, it is often because a woman is taking too many fluids, which can cause an excess of amniotic fluid to build up and exert extra pressure on the membranes, or extremely yin foods which weaken the membranes of the amniotic sac.

As many as 10 percent of the births in the United States are initiated by the artifical induction of labor. In the past, the majority of inductions were performed for the convenience of the doctor or the pregnant mother, although elective inductions are now frowned upon by the American College of Obstetrics and Gynecology. The procedure typically begins with the insertion of a hooked instrument into the vagina which is used to tear the amniotic membranes. Following the rupture of the membranes, *Pitocin*, a synthetic version of the pituitary hormone *oxytocin*, sometimes is given to stimulate uterine contractions. In some instances, rupture of the membranes causes the umbilical cord to slip down into the vagina before the baby is delivered, resulting in *anoxia*, or lack of oxygen to the baby. Intrauterine infections, which can have serious consequences for both mother and baby, are also more likely to occur following this procedure. When administered improperly, Pitocin can produce contractions that are too strong and too long to be beneficial for the baby. Together with increasing the possible risk of brain damage, the increased intensity of contractions can cause the baby's heart rate to drop, which in some cases causes the baby to become severely distressed. Pitocin is also associated with an increased incidence of newborn jaundice. Because of these and other effects, it is recommended that the artificial induction of labor be reserved for emergencies only.

3. *A slight discharge of blood and mucus, known as "show":* This discharge may occur after the contractions of the uterus cause the cervix to dilate slightly, dislodging the mucus plug that kept the cervix sealed throughout pregnancy. The discharge resembles blood-tinged mucus.

As labor approaches, you may attend to the necessary preparations for giving birth but, as much as possible, stay calm and rested. Notify your doctor or midwife whenever any of the above signs occur. If labor begins during the daytime, you can continue with usual activities, and if it occurs at night, try to sleep or rest. You can eat or drink if you want; tea or some warmly cooked dishes are best. It is advisable to avoid cold drinks and aromatic stimulant beverages. Once labor starts, you may contact your doctor or midwife and let them know how far apart your contractions are and how long you've been in labor.

The Stages of Labor

Labor is usually divided into the following stages:

1. *The First Stage—Dilation of the Cervix:* The first, or dilation stage, lasts from the onset of true contractions until the cervix, or neck of the womb, is fully dilated. Throughout pregnancy, the cervix is maintained in a very yang condition—firm, thick, and tightly contracted. Near the end of pregnancy, it becomes more yin, softer and thinner, and may begin to open before labor starts, especially if the mother consumes too many expansive foods and beverages or if her diet is lacking in the proper balance of minerals and complex carbohydrates.

   The uterine contractions that occur during the first stage cause the baby to descend, so that the membranes and the baby's head begin to push against the cervix, causing it to open. In order for the baby to be born, the cervix must dilate to about 10 centimeters (about four inches). The dilation of the cervix proceeds more slowly during the early part of labor and then increases rapidly as contractions intensify and the first stage draws to a close.

   During the early first stage, contractions occur about every 10 to 15 minutes. Each contraction lasts about 20 to 30 seconds and is usually fairly mild. As labor progresses, the rhythmic charge of heaven and earth's forces intensifies, so that by the latter first stage, contractions usually occur every two to three minutes and last from 45 to 90 seconds. They are much stronger than those at the beginning of labor.

The length of the first stage varies. For most women having their first baby, it averages 8 to 12 hours, usually becoming shorter and easier in subsequent pregnancies. For women who eat a well-balanced, macrobiotic diet, it is often shorter.

Near the end of the first stage, when the cervix is almost completely dilated, the woman may get the urge to "bear down" or push with them. Contractions are fairly strong at this point, as it takes a powerful effort to pull the circular muscles open far enough so that the baby's head can pass through. This stage is known as *transition*. Once the force of the contractions stretch the cervix wide enough, the baby's head passes through the cervix and gradually moves into the vaginal portion of the birth canal, usually turning with a spirallic motion to the most favorable position as it descends. As the baby's head presses against the *perineum*, or tissue between the vaginal wall and anus, a feeling of numbness may be experienced as nerve endings in the area are compressed.

2. *The Second Stage—Delivery:* The second stage of labor lasts from the full dilation of the cervix to the birth of the baby. It may last an hour or two with first babies, and usually becomes much shorter with subsequent deliveries. In some cases, it can be completed after only several contractions.

Once the baby's head has passed through the cervix, a woman experiences strong urges to push or bear down. At this stage, you can push with the contractions, relaxing or easing up as the contractions cease or if you feel pain or a burning sensation.

The most favorable position for birth is for the back of the baby's head to be facing upward and the face to be looking downward. The head is the largest part of the baby and once it emerges, the rest of the body usually slips through very easily. When the head emerges and no longer slips back between contractions, what is known as *crowning* has occurred. In general, the first stage of labor is more difficult than the actual delivery of the baby. Once the cervix has dilated completely and the baby's head lies against the opening of the vagina, a few pushes are usually all that are needed to deliver successfully.

Obstetrical forceps, or specially molded steel tongs, are used routinely in some hospital births. The forceps are attached to the baby's head and the baby is then pulled out. However, if the forceps are used improperly, damage to the baby's head could result. Because they interfere with the natural process of labor and increase the risk of birth injuries, it is recommended that forceps be used only in emergency cases.

Episiotomy is a procedure in which an incision is made in the perineum, the area between the anus and vagina, in order to enlarge the birth opening. It is performed in about 85 percent of the first time deliveries in the United States. Because some women tear during delivery, episiotomy is frequently performed to prevent this and because an incision is sometimes easier to repair than an irregular tear. However, in many cases, surgical incisions are deeper and take longer to heal than natural tears.

If a mother is eating properly, delivers while in a more upright position (the supine position increases the risk of tearing), and is under the guidance of a skilled midwife or doctor, tearing is much less likely to occur. In countries where natural childbirth is more widely practiced, episiotomy is performed much less frequently. In Holland, for example, it is used in less than eight percent of deliveries and in England, in about one in seven.

3. *The Third Stage—Afterbirth:* The third stage of labor lasts from the birth of the baby until the placenta has been delivered. The placenta normally separates from the wall of the uterus within a few minutes after the baby is born. It is normally expelled completely within 10 to 15 minutes, during which time there is usually minimal discomfort for the mother. The condition of the placenta reflects the mother's diet and health as well as the condition of the baby. A mother who eats macrobiotically throughout pregnancy usually produces a clean and healthy placenta which adequately supports the baby until birth.

Birth Position

During birth, the rhythmic charge of heaven and earth's forces intensifies along the mother's primary channel. The active charging of these two energies triggers the release of oxytocin by the pituitary, producing the contractions of the uterus which push the baby downward and outward and which cause the cervix to dilate.

The charge of heaven and earth's forces in the human body is most active when we are in a vertical posture, especially when standing. An upright posture affords maximum chargeability by allowing these forces to flow vertically along the primary channel. When we sleep or lie down, these forces become less active. Our heart rate, breathing, metabolism, and other body functions become quieter when we assume a horizontal position.

It is important for both forces to charge to the maximum degree during labor. Traditionally, therefore, women would try to be active even after labor had begun and would normally give birth while in a more vertical position such as sitting or squatting. In many European countries, for example, a horseshoe-shaped *birthing stool* was used very commonly until the beginning of the 19th century, allowing a woman to deliver while maintaining a more upright position.

In early labor it is better for a woman to remain upright and vertical whenever it is comfortable. Studies have shown that being up and about during this stage results in a shorter and more efficient birth. Walking or continuing your daily routine is fine during early labor as long as it is comfortable. When walking is no longer comfortable, you can stand, sit in a chair or, sit in bed with your back supported by a stack of pillows. Changing positions when you become uncomfortable is often helpful in relieving discomfort. If labor occurs at night, you can rest or sleep. However, it is better not to lie flat on your back, as the pressure of the uterus interferes with the baby's circulation. It is also better to avoid lying flat on your back during the final trimester of pregnancy.

Examples of possible positions for giving birth include squatting, kneeling, bending forward on the hands and knees, standing, lying on the side, or semi-sitting. The *supine position*, in which a woman lies flat on her back with her knees raised is the least effective in maintaining an active charge of heaven and earth's forces. Because these forces are less active in this position, labor may be retarded and less efficient. Remaining upright during labor produces stronger, more efficient, and less painful contractions and shorter labors. The supine position causes the uterus to press on the *common iliac artery* and the *inferior vena cava* thereby reducing the amount of blood supplied to the placenta and interfering with the supply of oxygen and nutrients to the baby. Despite these disadvantages, the supine position was used in most hospital deliveries until recently. Other hospital procedures such as routine use of intravenous (I.V.) fluids and electronic fetal monitoring have tended to encourage confinement to bed and lack of movement during labor. However, conventional hospital care has begun to change; most hospitals now have birthing rooms equipped with specially designed delivery beds in which one delivers sitting up or squatting.

Fetal Monitors: Many hospitals electronically monitor the baby's heartbeat and the mother's contractions during labor. Some hospitals monitor all women in labor, while others monitor only women who have a higher than normal risk of complications. It is estimated that 50 to 75 percent of all hospital births are now electronically monitored. In 1978, the FDA estimated that electronic fetal monitors were being used on a million women a year, although the devices had not been thoroughly tested to determine their safety. Fetal monitors are attached either internally or externally. External monitors consist of two adjustable bands that are strapped around the mother's abdomen; one measures the frequency and strength of the uterine contractions, and the other uses ultrasound to monitor the condition of the baby. In internal monitoring, a wire is inserted through the vagina into the uterus, where it penetrates the amniotic sac. A tiny corkscrew at the end of the wire is then twisted into the baby's scalp. Both methods tend to restrict a woman's movements during labor and in some instances, encourage her to be flat on her back while keeping as still as possible. However, as pointed out above, this position can retard labor and interfere with the blood supply to the baby. Internal monitoring increases the risk of umbilical cord accidents, which are more common when the amniotic sac is prematurely ruptured, and denies the baby the protection of the surrounding amniotic fluid during labor. Scalp rashes occur in the majority of newborns who undergo this procedure, and on rare occasions a baby may develop a localized scalp infection similar to a boil at the site where the electrode is placed. Accidents, including placing the electrode in the baby's eye or some other part of the body, have also occurred with this procedure.

Care of the Newborn

After the baby is born, he or she will usually begin to breathe and cry within a minute after delivery. These activities help discharge mucus from the respiratory passages and prepare the baby for life in the air world. Birth contractions also help to prepare the baby for life in the more expanded environment outside the womb. In most cases, the baby will begin breathing without outside help. However, if breathing does not begin soon after birth, the baby must be shaken or spanked until it does. If these simple measures do not work expert resuscitation techniques may be needed.

When the baby starts breathing, the lungs begin to receive oxygen and the baby is no longer dependent on the placenta and umbilical cord. Usually, the umbilical cord will continue pulsating for about four or five minutes after delivery. During this time, the baby can be covered with warm towels. The baby is normally kept horizontal at about the level of the placenta until the cord stops pulsating. By keeping the baby's head higher than the level of the feet, excessive pressure is prevented from building up in the head. Once the pulsation of the cord fades, it is tied off and cut. In traditional times, the cord was cut with scissors made of bamboo and tied with a cotton thread.

As soon as the cord is tied off, the baby can be bathed in mild warm water to remove any blood and meconium, wrapped in a blanket or towels, and given to the mother to hold. Many mothers wish to put the baby immediately to breast. The sucking of the baby stimulates strong contractions and retractions of the uterus, speeding the separation of the placenta and the closing of the blood vessles to which it was attached. Not all babies begin sucking immediately, however. Some may need a little coaxing while others prefer to take their time. A more rapid separation of the placenta and the prevention of excessive bleeding following delivery are two of the more immediate benefits of breast-feeding. After the mother holds the baby for several minutes, he or she can be placed in a warm crib or a small *futon* (a cotton sleeping cushion) beside her as she prepares herself for the delivery of the after birth.

After the placenta has been discharged, the mother is cleaned and a sterile napkin is applied to receive the *lochia*, or flow of blood, from the uterus. The baby can be returned to the mother to hold or to continue nursing. When the mother returns to her bed or *futon*, the baby can be placed in a crib or small *futon* beside her. Whenever she desires, she can hold the baby to her breast.

Care of the Mother

As mentioned above, there is some bleeding from the place where the placenta was attached to the uterus. For the first several days after birth, the flow of blood is similar to that which comes out during the first several days of a menstrual period, or it may be heavier. Sanitary napkins are usually applied and may have to be changed three or four times per day for the first couple of days following delivery. Gradually, the lochia becomes lighter in color and less heavy and usually stops completely after the placental site heals, in about three to six weeks.

The contractions that follow delivery close off the uterine blood vessels and prevent excessive loss of blood at delivery and for several days afterward. The post-delivery contractions produce cramps which are like menstrual cramps or labor pains. These contractions are known as *afterpains*. Afterpains tend to be more of a problem following the birth of the second or third baby. Additional pregnancies cause the uterus to become a little more relaxed and stretched, and after delivery, it has to contract more to return to normal.

Women who breast-feed usually experience a rapid return of the uterus to its normal condition. The stimulation of the breasts brought on by the sucking of the baby causes them to become more yin or expanded, and to begin discharging liquid. As the breasts become more yin, the lower reproductive organs—in this case, the uterus—become more yang and contracted. This is facilitated hormonally by the release of oxytocin by the pituitary.

Women who eat a more naturally balanced diet heal more rapidly following delivery. Foods such as sugar, soft drinks, ice cream, tropical fruits, fruit juices, and drugs and medications tend to weaken the uterine muscle and cause the uterine tissues to become swollen during pregnancy. A swollen or weakened uterus is slower to return to normal, and its contraction frequently causes more severe pain. The intake of extremely yin foods can also slow the contraction of the uterine blood vessels, which in turn may cause the lochia to be more profuse and last longer. Saturated, fatty animal foods tend to make the uterine tissues and blood vessels harder and more rigid, thereby slowing the contracting process and causing unnecessary pain.

Following delivery, a woman can eat according to the standard macrobiotic diet, and may include a variety of special dishes which help speed recovery and aid the production of breast milk.

It is important for a mother to have a good appetite following delivery. If not, several bowls of specially prepared rice cream can be eaten with a little *umeboshi* to help stimulate it. (See the cereal grain milk recipe on page 164.)

Within the standard macrobiotic diet, special dishes made with the following foods are especially recommended during recovery:
  1) Sweet brown rice or *mochi* (pounded sweet brown rice).
  2) Light *miso* soup with land vegetables, *wakame*, and freshly pounded *mochi*.
  3) Whole wheat noodles, preferably added to *miso* soup, or served with a light *tamari* soy sauce broth.
  4) *Koi-koku* (carp miso soup). This dish can be taken once a day for several days, especially if the mother is experiencing weakness, anemia, or fatigue.
  5) Root vegetable dishes prepared *nishime* style.
  6) Vegetable stews which may include *seitan* or *tempeh*.

It is better to avoid raw fruit, fruit juice, or salad, especially during the initial recovery period, and preferably for three months afterward. The intake of more yin foods and beverages such as these can delay the normal contractions of the uterus and also tend to make the milk become more thin and watery. It is generally better to avoid iced or chilled foods or beverages following delivery, even during the summer months. Instead, only hot or warm foods and drinks should be taken.

With the exception of *koi-koku* (carp *miso* soup), which, depending on the condition of the mother, can be taken once a day for three to five days after delivery, it is better to avoid eating fish or other animal foods while breast-feeding. In the event animal food is needed, a small amount of white-meat fish cooked with a few times more leafy vegetables is recommended. Stimulants such as coffee, spices, herbal teas, and others are also best avoided while you are breast-feeding, as is alcohol. (A sip of high quality beer or *sake* can be taken on occasion.) If you crave sweets, a small volume of grain-based sweets such as rice honey or barley malt may be added occasionally to tea or breakfast cereal. If these do not satisfy your craving, simple, cooked fruit desserts such as applesauce, apples cooked in *kuzu*, and others can be eaten in small amounts. It is better to serve them warm rather than chilled.

A woman discharges a great deal of excess when she has a baby. If she eats well following delivery, she can improve her overall condition and maintain a clean, healthy state. Women were traditionally thought to be very clean and beautiful after having a baby. However, a mother can easily spoil her condition by eating sugar, oily or greasy foods and animal products, including dairy food following delivery. If a woman has experienced a smooth natural birth, both she and her baby will become very peaceful and content in the following days and weeks.

In addition to eating properly, simple external treatments can be used to make recovery from birth more comfortable. The point on the inside of both legs a few inches above the ankles (see Fig. 32) has been used for thousands of years to treat problems in the reproductive organs. It is known in Japanese as *San-In-Ko*, or "junction of three yin meridians," and is the point where three meridians—the liver, spleen-pancreas, and kidney—join together on the inside of the leg.

Oriental doctors often treat reproductive disorders by using needles, moxa, or thumb pressure massage on this point. Simple massage on this point can aid the uterus in properly contracting and help release tension. The point can be massaged every day for several days following delivery. Place your thumbs on the point, press slightly, and rub with a slow circular motion. Treat both sides in this manner.

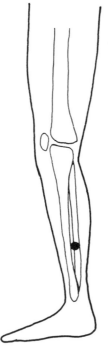

Fig. 32   The *SAN-IN-KO* (junction of three yin meridians) point on the inside of the leg.

SAN-IN-KO
(SP 6)

Another method known traditionally in Oriental countries for lessening the pain of contractions is to attach a grain of uncooked brown rice to this point (both legs can be treated). Brown rice and other whole grains continually attract electromagnetic energy, or *ki*, from the surrounding environment. The grain of rice attracts a subtle but continual charge of energy which then passes through the mother's surface meridians to the meridians of the uterus (see Chapter 2). This helps the uterus contract more smoothly. At the same time, it attracts—via the same energy pathways in the body—excessive energy that has built up in the uterine region, thereby helping to release tension in that organ. Each grain of rice can be held in place with a piece of tape and left on for about 24 hours, after which fresh grains can be put in place. The procedure can be repeated for three or four days following delivery.

Within several days, most new mothers lose four to five pounds, largely through a decrease in the volume of blood and the discharge of fluid retained in pregnancy. The total weight loss includes the weight of the baby, the placenta, and the amniotic fluid, and usually totals between 12 to 16 pounds. Most women lose additional weight in the first two weeks, depending on how much fluid was retained during pregnancy.

It is important to rest completely following delivery. It is best to rest in bed seven to nine days, during which time your husband, relatives, or friends can take care of all activities, including cooking, washing, cleaning, bringing your meals to you, preparing special dishes, and taking care of your other children if you have them. During this period, try to get out of bed only when you go to the toilet or bathe. Therefore, make sure that all of the necessary arrangements for your post-delivery recuperation are made well in advance. Resting helps you to heal more rapidly.

Following the bed rest period, we suggest that you continue to rest and take it easy for another three weeks, during which time, someone else can take care of any household chores including cooking. Try to restrict your activity to brief walks around the house and taking care of the new baby. Toward the end of this period you can begin to go outside. However, things such as long walks, climbing stairs, or carrying packages are generally not recommended.

In general, it is better to wait up to six to eight weeks before resuming intercourse. The vaginal flow should cease completely and your sexual functions should be completely recovered before resuming sex. Keep in mind that how well you eat and rest will largely determine how smoothly and rapidly you heal.

Birth Complications

The Presentations: There are a variety of positions, or presentations, in which babies are born. Babies are normally born headfirst with the chin bent down on the chest. The head, being more yang and compacted, normally takes a downward position and is the first part of the body to emerge from the birth canal. If a mother is eating well, keeping active, and in generally good condition, her baby will naturally assume the most yang position for birth. This position takes the least room and is the easiest for delivery.

When a baby is more yin, he or she may not tuck the chin down on the chest but may be born looking straight ahead, in which case, the neck is said to be *extended*. In some cases, the head is even more upward, as if the baby were looking up at the sky. This position is known as a *face presentation*, while a *brow presentation* refers to a partially uplifted chin.

Fig. 33 Positions of the fetus at birth.

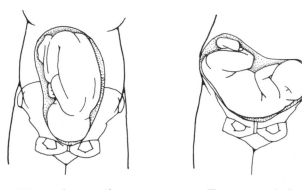 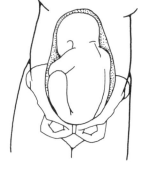

Vertex (normal)   Transverse (▽)   Breech (extreme ▽)

More yin presentations generally occur when a woman takes in sugar, soft drinks, milk, butter, too many salads, fruit and fruit juices, and other more expansive items during pregnancy. These presentations can interfere with labor but if a woman is in good condition, she will usually be able to deliver normally.

If a woman's diet during pregnancy is even more extreme, the normal balance between the baby's head and body can be disturbed, and the head may be too yin to assume a downward position. A *transverse presentation*, in which the baby lies crosswise in the mother's abdomen with neither head nor buttocks down, may result. In some cases, transverse presentations result from obstructions in the birth canal, including fibroid tumors or placentas that are situated over the cervix. Foods such as milk and other dairy products often cause the fetus to develop an enlarged bone structure, while the overconsumption of fluid can cause the baby to become expanded and swollen. When the intake of these items is excessive, the baby can become too large for the mother's pelvis and the head may be prevented from moving into a downward position.

In some cases, babies in a transverse lie in the latter part of pregnancy change positions when labor starts, and are born either head- or feet-first. If there is no obstruction of the birth canal, most obstetricians will let labor begin in hopes that the baby will change positions during labor. However, it is impossible for a baby to be delivered vaginally while in the transverse position.

In about 3 percent of the births in the United States, the baby is born feet or buttocks first, in what is known as a *breech presentation* or *breech birth*. As with transverse positions, the intake of more yin foods and beverages can cause the head to become too yin to assume its natural downward position at birth. Foods such as fruit, especially tropical fruit, fruit juices, sugar and other concentrated sweeteners, oil, coffee, spices, chocolate, and drugs and chemicals all serve to make the baby more yin and increase the likelihood of a breech presentation. Overeating and overdrinking in general also make this more of a possibility.

In some cases, a woman will consume too many yin foods and beverages because she is too tight and contracted. The overintake of salt, baked dishes, flour products, and animal foods, together with a lack of variety in the diet, especially not enough fresh or lightly cooked vegetable dishes, often cause this more yang underlying condition to develop. Cigarette smoking and an overly-active daily schedule during pregnancy can also contribute to this problem.

Breech presentations are more likely to occur when the baby is too large for the mother's pelvis or if the birth canal is blocked by the placenta, a cyst, or a tumor. Breech births are also more frequent among premature babies, especially when the mother consumes plenty of more yin foods and beverages during pregnancy. Uterine anomalies such as an intrauterine septum or a bicornuate uterus are also apt to be associated with breech presentation.

A skilled midwife or doctor can sometimes turn a baby in the breech position during the last weeks of pregnancy through external manipulation. The procedure is known as *external version* and can often cause the baby to be born headfirst. About 70 to 80 percent of breeches can be successfully turned prior to labor, and this is being done more frequently. If a mother is in good health, and if the baby is not too large, it is definitely possible for her to have a breech delivery without medications or artificial procedures. Many women have had completely natural breech deliveries. Such deliveries are usually no different than headfirst deliveries in terms of the progress of labor and in the mother's experience of it. However, delivery the of a breech carries with it a greater potential for complications than does a normal, headfirst delivery. For this reason, it is advisable for breech deliveries to be done with qualified medical assistance.

Uterine Inertia: In normal labor, the uterus will contract in waves that begin in the upper region, in the area of the abdominal energy center or *hara chakra*, and spread downward along the uterine meridians. Uterine contractions are usually strong enough to cause the tightly closed cervix to dilate and push the baby downward and outward. In some cases, however, contractions come in irregular intervals and are of weaker intensity and uneven duration and are not effective in dilating the cervix. This condition is known as *uterine inertia* and often produces a long and difficult labor.

The underlying dietary cause of uterine inertia is the consumption of extremely yin foods and beverages during pregnancy, including sugar, soft drinks, milk, yogurt, ice cream, fruit and fruit juices, coffee, and drugs and medications, together with the intake of fats and oils, especially hard, saturated fats. More yin foods weaken the uterine muscle and cause it to become loose and flabby. They also diminish the vitality of the energy center and weaken the charge along the uterine meridians. Rather than beginning in the upper region of the uterus or *hara* region, the contractions in uterine inertia often begin toward the middle of the uterus and spread upward and downward. In this case, there is a lack of the descending power of heaven's force which the highly charged abdominal energy center provides. At the same time, the intake of hard, saturated fats often causes the uterine muscle to become hard and rigid, a condition similar to hardening of the arteries. When the uterine muscle becomes harder, it loses elasticity and the ability to flexibly contract and expand. Uterine inertia is also common when the baby is too large for smooth passage through the mother's pelvis.

Umbilical Cord Accidents: At birth, the umbilical cord averages about two feet long. However, it may be much shorter or longer, depending on the foods eaten by the mother during pregnancy. In general, a diet that contains plenty of salt and other minerals, baked foods, and animal products, or not enough fresh and lightly cooked foods would tend to produce a shorter and more constricted cord. On the other hand, a diet high in simple sugars, fruit, fruit juices, refined carbohydrates, coffee, spices, and fats and oils or a diet that is lacking in minerals would tend to produce a longer and more extended cord. A more well-balanced diet would tend to produce an in-between-sized cord.

Umbilical cord accidents are not very common. Many babies are born with the cord wrapped around the neck, but in the majority of cases, no serious complication results. Accidents are more common when the cord is very short or very long. When it is very short, circulation through the cord can be impeded when the baby moves downward in labor, causing the cord to become stretched. On the other hand, a very long cord can more easily become knotted or entangled about the baby. If circulation through the cord is completely cut off for several minutes, the baby will die from a lack of oxygen. The reduction in circulation through the cord is a form of fetal distress and is a medical emergency.

Another complication involving the umbilical cord is known as *prolapse of the cord*. It occurs when the cord moves down into the birth canal before the baby does. When the cord becomes prolapsed, it may be pressed between the baby and the sides of the birth canal, causing circulation to be cut off. Prolapse of the cord occurs more frequently when the baby's head does not fill the birth canal, for example in breech or transverse positions, in premature deliveries, or when pelvic obstructions are present. It is also more common in cases where the membranes have prematurely ruptured. However, once the head or buttocks has engaged in the pelvis, prolapse is very rare.

Cesarean Section: In cesarean section, a baby is delivered by means of a surgical incision in the abdomen and wall of the uterus. Many people believe that Julius Caesar was delivered in this way. Actually, the procedure did not come into use until long after his time.

The incidence of cesarean delivery has increased dramatically in the United States. Twenty years ago, cesarean sections were used in one delivery out of twenty. By 1979, nearly one baby in six was delivered in this manner. In that same year, about 546,000 cesarean sections were performed in hospitals throughout the United States.

The most common reason for this procedure is that a woman has had a cesarean in an earlier pregnancy, usually because of *failure to progress* secondary to C.P.D. (see below). Until recently, doctors in the United States performed repeat sections routinely on all women who had had a previous cesarean in the belief that the scar from the previous operation could rupture under the force of labor. However, many physicians began to question this practice, and in 1980, the National Institutes of Health issued guidelines which held that vaginal deliveries for mothers who had previously been sectioned were as safe as, or safer than, repeat sections. (The NIH also recommended that women with uterine inertia be encouraged to move around and exercise to stimulate labor and that surgery be used only after all alternatives had been tried.) The guidelines also recommended against routine sections for breech presentations.

Cephalopelvic Disproportion (C.P.D.) is the condition in which the baby is too large for the mother's pelvis. Disproportion can exist when the pelvis is abnormally small or when the pelvis is normal but the baby is unusually large. Most mothers with small pelvises are able to deliver normally, although labor may be slower than normal. Smaller women are often more prone to disproportion, especially if they overconsume a variety of more yin foods and beverages during pregnancy, including milk and other dairy products, or if they consume excess fluid. These practices can cause the baby to become swollen and enlarged and also contribute to uterine inertia and abnormal presentations. Failure to progress can also be caused by the overconsumption of more yang items, especially animal proteins and overly salty or baked dishes. These foods can cause the cervix to remain tight and constricted and can cause a tightening of the pelvis. In most cases, cesarean sections are performed for disproportion when related complications such as uterine inertia and an abnormal position are also present.

Cesarean sections are also performed when the baby is in an unfavorable position for birth. If a baby is in a transverse position during labor, for example, vaginal delivery is impossible. However, babies who are in the transverse position prior to labor usually come into the pelvis headfirst or breech. The rate of cesarean sections is higher for breech presentations than for the normal birth position. The usual practice is to perform a cesarean when a breech baby is thought to be too large for the mother's pelvis. Cesarean sections are also performed in cases of severe fetal distress caused by twists or knots in the umbilical cord or when the mother has diabetes, some types of kidney disease, severe Rh-negative complications, or severe toxemia of pregnancy.

Because of the effects of cesarean delivery on both mother and baby, it is recommended that it be used only as a last resort in emergency cases. For example, the maternal death rate from cesarean sections is six times higher than it is with vaginal deliveries, while the rate of uterine infection following cesarean is more than fourteen times greater. About one-third of the women who have cesarean deliveries experience hemorrhaging or infection following the operation. The likelihood of this depends on the condition of the woman prior to labor. Healthier mothers do not have these complications as often.

The long-term effects of a cesarean section on the mother's physical condition are similar to those discussed in Chapter 1 for induced abortion, while the more immediate effects can include abdominal pain, temporary paralysis of the intestinal tract, severe gas pains, exhaustion, and depression. The psychological effects can include nightmares and frightening dreams following surgery—including dreams of being stabbed, cut by a knife, or strangled—together with subconscious feelings of fear. The psychological effects are generally more severe when the woman includes meat and other animal products, sugar, alcohol, spices, highly processed, artificial foods, and drugs and medications in her diet.

Babies who are delivered by cesarean do not experience the full range of the more yangizing effects of birth contractions and as a result, are generally more yin than normal babies. The contractions of birth prepare the infant for life in the more expanded environment outside the womb by helping the baby to discharge excess, especially from the lungs. Normally, excess fluid is forced from the baby's lungs by the contractions of the uterus. When the baby doesn't experience these contractions, fluid often remains in the lungs, a condition known as *transient tachypnia*. Other potential risks to the baby include those associated with the use of anesthesia and, if the baby is delivered before the actual due date, various hazards associated with prematurity.

The macrobiotic recommendations for care of the mother following birth are also suitable for women who have had a cesarean delivery.

6 | The Newborn Baby

At birth, your baby will be tiny, red, and somewhat wrinkled in appearance. Don't be disappointed if he or she doesn't fit your image of how a newborn should look. Your baby's appearance will change quickly in the weeks after birth. There are a number of things that you can check in order to assess your baby's constitution, condition, and future potential.* These include:

1. *The hair:* The skin of the newborn is covered with a fine long hair known as lanugo. The lanugo usually disappears within several weeks. Many long hairs on the head indicate that the mother took in a larger volume of more yin foods and beverages during pregnancy, including fruits, fruit juices, and raw salads. Darker colored hair results more from the consumption of vegetable-quality foods, while lighter hair results more from the intake of animal foods, including dairy products.

2. *The hair spiral:* Heaven's descending energy moves spirally and enters the body at the top of the head. The hair spiral traces this universal pattern of movement. The location of the spiral reveals much about the baby's overall constitution. A spiral located toward the center of the head shows that the mother's diet was adequately balanced during pregnancy and that the baby has a generally well balanced constitution, with the potential for a broad understanding and a well balanced mind. The child may also develop the tendency to appreciate art, literature, and other aesthetic endeavors together with the inclination towards moderation and steadiness.

A spiral on the right side of the head results when the mother's diet contains an abundance of more yang factors, such as animal food and salt, during pregnancy. A baby with a spiral on the right has the potential to become more physically or socially active. It is important for children with this characteristic to minimize or avoid the intake of meat, eggs, poultry, or other more extreme yang foods, in order to avoid becoming one-sided in their development.

A baby with a spiral on the left side has the potential to develop a more intellectually oriented personality. The hair spiral develops on the left side when a mother eats plenty of more yin items such as salad, fruit, fruit juice, simple sugars, and dairy products during pregnancy. It is important for children with this type of constitution to avoid tropical fruits, candy, ice cream, sugar, and other more extreme yin items.

Some children are born with two spirals on the head. Two spirals occur when the mother's diet during pregnancy is extremely yin. The normal condition is for

---

* Many of these points are outlined in more detail in the books, *How to See Your Health*, *The Book of Do-In* and *Your Face Never Lies* by Michio Kushi. —ed.

heaven and earth's forces to flow along one main channel. However, children with two spirals have two channels, one of which conducts heaven's force and another which conducts earth's force. Their character has a tendency to alternate between extremes. When the channel conducting heaven's force is more active, they can become more masculine or aggressive, and during periods when the channel of earth's force predominates, they can suddenly change and become more quiet and passive. The spiral that conducts heaven's force is activated by the intake of meat, eggs, or other more yang foods, while the opposite channel becomes more actively charged when sugar, spices, and other more extreme yin foods are consumed.

It is important for someone with this characteristic to eat a more centrally balanced diet in which whole grain cereals are the principal foods in order to help stabilize the tendency toward extremes. If your baby has two head spirals, it is recommended that you eat a slightly larger volume of whole grains and cooked vegetables during the time you are breast-feeding.

3.   *The head:* A newborn's head will often have a somewhat unbalanced shape, due to some molding which occurs during passage through the birth canal. The bones of the baby's skull are not yet fixed in their positions as they are in adults, and there is a slight separation between them. The head usually develops a more normal shape within the first month after birth.

Toward the front of the head in the middle is an opening known as the major *fontanel* or *soft spot*. The fontanel is covered by a tough layer of skin and normally closes within six months to one-and-a-half years as the bones of the skull fuse. The fontanel often pulsates in rhythm with the heartbeat and may appear slightly depressed when the baby is sitting. It often tenses up when the baby cries. Many babies also have a smaller soft spot toward the back of the head. It is usually barely noticeable and closes soon after birth.

No one's head is perfectly symmetrical. If the left side is more developed than the right, the baby has a greater potential to develop a more intellectual or idealistic character. If the right side is more developed, the baby can easily become a more practical minded person.

If the back part of the head is prominent, the small brain is well developed. A baby with this characteristic has the tendency to be somewhat more active or aggressive throughout life and must be careful to minimize animal products, especially meat, eggs, or poultry, as well as refined sugar and products that contain it. These foods could promote a tendency toward wild behavior.

4.   *The eyebrows:* By seeing the angle of the eyebrows, we can understand the baby's physical and mental constitution and know the quality of foods eaten by the mother during pregnancy. Downward slanting eyebrows indicate that a larger volume of vegetable-quality foods were consumed during pregnancy and that the consumption of animal food was less. In general, babies with downward slanting eyebrows will usually have a more gentle and understanding character. They tend, however, to have a disposition for disorders of the hollow organs such as the stomach and intestines.

Upward slanting eyebrows are caused by the opposite or more yang quality of

Fig. 34 Angle of the eyebrows.

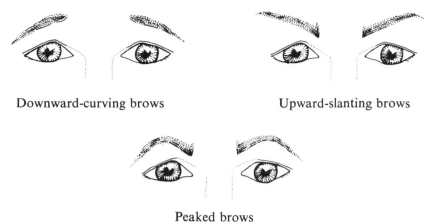

Downward-curving brows   Upward-slanting brows

Peaked brows

food during pregnancy. Babies with this characteristic can easily develop a more aggressive or offensive character as they grow, especially if animal foods are part of their regular diet. They are also more susceptible to future problems in the more compact organs such as the heart and liver.

Eyebrows that slant upward toward the middle, peak, and then curve downward show that the mother's diet contained plenty of animal foods during the first part of pregnancy, and then changed to include a larger volume of vegetable foods toward the end of pregnancy. A baby with this type of eyebrow tends to be more active and aggressive during the first half of life, and then more quiet and retiring during the latter part.

Smooth, curving eyebrows, which have an orderly and balanced angle, are the result of a well balanced diet during pregnancy. A baby with eyebrows such as these has a more balanced constitution and has a potential ability to adapt to various conflicting experiences.

5.   *The eyes:* If the baby is a boy, small eyes indicate that he has a strong constitution and the tendency to develop determination and self-discipline. It is preferable for a baby girl to have larger and more widely opened eyes. Large eyes indicate that a girl has a healthy womb and ovaries and can naturally develop into a very loving and tender-hearted person.

In the Orient, the word *sanpaku* describes a condition in the eye in which three sections of white are showing. The term *sanpaku* means literally "three whites," and there are two types of *sanpaku. Upper sanpaku* means that white is showing above the iris and indicates that a person has a more yang condition. In *lower sanpaku,* white is showing beneath the iris. Lower *sanpaku* shows that a person's condition has become overly yin and is a sign of physical and mental deterioration due to overexpansion of the brain and other tissues. It is caused by the chronic consumption of extreme yin foods and beverages.

A slightly more yang *sanpaku*—the iris is more down—is normal in babies and young children. As the child grows, the iris will normally move upward so that no

Fig. 35   Types of *Sanpaku* (three whites).

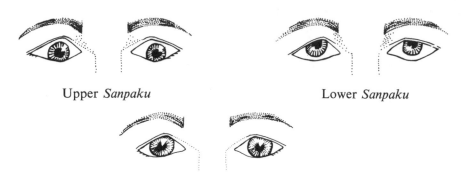

Upper *Sanpaku*   Lower *Sanpaku*

Normal adult eyes

white is showing above or below it. In babies, upper *sanpaku* shows a strong constitution and good vitality, as does infrequent blinking. If the eyes do not show this condition, or if the baby blinks more than one time per minute, he or she is somewhat yin as a result of the mother's consumption of more extreme yin foods, including liquids, fruits, and juices, either during pregnancy or while breast-feeding. In adults, the normal position of the iris is directly in the center, with no white showing above or below it. In adults, upper or lower *sanpaku* is an abnormal condition and indicates physical and mental imbalance.

Some newborn babies have a tiny spot of bleeding on the white of the eye. The eruption of blood vessels in the eye-white of a newborn baby is the result of the mother's consumption of more extreme yin foods such as sugar, fruit, fruit juice, soft drinks, and drugs and medications during pregnancy. If your baby has this characteristic, be careful not to consume extreme yin foods or beverages following delivery and at least as long as you are breast-feeding.

Many babies have mucus discharge from the eyes. *Eye discharges* are often caused by the medication that is put in the baby's eyes shortly after birth. They are also caused by the mother's intake of fatty or oily foods, sugar, fruits, milk, and other more yin items during pregnancy or while she is nursing. These items lead to the development of mucus and fat in the mother's body and in her milk, and this quality is passed to the baby and often discharged through the eyes. Babies who consume cow's milk, which contains plenty of fat, or artificial infant formula frequently develop this condition.

If your baby develops an eye discharge while you are nursing, eliminate fatty or oily foods from your diet, including items like nuts, nut butters, and fried foods. Fruit and fruit juices can also be avoided until the baby's condition improves. The eyes can be wiped clean with a clean cotton cloth or piece of sterilized cotton dipped in warm bancha tea.

6.   *The nose:* If the baby's nose points upward at the tip, the mother ate plenty of animal foods, especially fish and seafood, during the middle part of pregnancy. A baby with an upward pointing nose can easily develop a certain sharpness in thinking later in life but may become narrow-minded, if a large volume of animal

products are part of the daily diet. A nose which droops is caused by the excessive consumption of more yin items such as fruit, salad, and fluid. It shows the tendency to develop a more gentle or timid character and there is an increased likelihood of heart, kidney, and bladder troubles, if a large volume of more yin foods and beverages are consumed throughout life.

Larger nostrils indicate that a person has a more masculine character. It is therefore better for a boy to have larger and more well developed nostrils. Smaller nostrils indicate a more feminine character and are more natural for girls. Boys with smaller nostrils may develop feminine characteristics later in life, especially if fruit, sugar, milk, and other more yin foods are eaten, while girls with larger nostrils can easily become more masculine if they eat a large volume of animal foods.

A baby should not have a runny nose. A runny nose indicates that the baby's condition has become overly yin. It can easily occur if the mother consumes too much fruit, fruit juice, oil, liquid, salad, sugar, soft drinks, concentrated sweeteners, or other more yin items while nursing. These items can cause her milk to become overly thin and watery and can result in the discharge of mucus and liquid from the baby's nose.

7. *The ears:* The baby's entire constitution is reflected in the ears. A sound, healthy constitution is reflected in ears that begin at eye level and have lobes extending down to the level of the mouth, with the lower part of the ear attached to the head at the level of the nose. Ears of this type indicate that a mother had the proper balance of minerals, proteins, and carbohydrates in her diet during pregnancy. Thick ears also indicate that the baby has a strong native constitution which is produced by a properly balanced diet.

Ears that are smaller, pointed at the top, and positioned higher on the head indicate that excessive animal food was consumed during pregnancy. Those with little or no lobe show that the mother's diet was not properly balanced as a result of an insufficient intake of minerals. Ears such as this show less constitutional vitality and a possible tendency toward narrowness in thinking and attitude.

The angle of the ears is also important. Ears which lie flat and close to the head indicate that the mother ate a generally well balanced diet during pregnancy. They show that the baby's constitution is more harmoniously balanced and indicate the child's potential to become active in society.

Ears that stick out from the head, especially beyond a 30-degree angle, show that more yin foods were consumed during pregnancy, including salad, fruits, and fruit juices, and in more extreme cases, sugar, soft drinks, chemicals, and drugs. If the ears protrude but to less than 30 degrees, the baby has a tendency to be more active mentally than physically. Ears that extend beyond 30 degrees show a possible tendency toward skepticism, suspicion, and narrowness in thinking and behavior.

In some babies, the skin behind the ears begins to take on a dry, cracked appearance. As discussed in Chapter 2, the ears are related to the kidneys. Cracking behind the ears is an indication that mucus, fat and liquid have built up in the baby's kidneys as a result of the mother's intake of fatty, oily, and overly watery foods, including nuts, deep-fried vegetables, nut butters, dairy products and other animal foods, together with sugar, fruit, fruit juice, and flour products. If this problem occurs while you are nursing, we recommend that you avoid these excesses and make your diet as clean as possible. As the baby begins to receive less fatty, sticky milk, the problem should begin to clear up.

8.   *The mouth:* As pointed out in Chapter 2, the mouth reflects the development and condition of the digestive system as a whole. A smaller mouth indicates that the digestive system—and overall physical and mental vitality—is natively strong. Ideally, the mouth should be of the same width or narrower than the nostrils. Smaller mouths were generally more common until several generations ago. The increase in the average size of mouths in recent times is an indication that people have largely lost the constitutional strength and vitality of their ancestors.

If the mouth is much wider than the nose, the baby's overall constitution is more yin, meaning that the function of the digestive system and other organs and systems is generally weaker than normal. This results from the overconsumption of more extreme yin foods and beverages during pregnancy, including items such as potatoes, tomatoes, sugar and other sweeteners, soft drinks, milk, fruit and fruit juices, oil and fat, and coffee, herbal teas, and other stimulants. These foods and beverages deplete minerals from the mother's body. The intake of a larger proportion of protein in relation to carbohydrates, especially complex carbohydrates, also contributes to the formation of a larger mouth. Minerals and complex carbohydrates produce a more contractive effect in the body.

9.   *The hands and fingers:* When babies are born, their fists are clenched and their arms and legs take the form of tightly wound spirals as a result of consuming more yang, animal quality food—mother's blood—during the period in the womb. These spirals begin to relax and unwind after the baby begins consuming more yin forms of nourishment, especially mother's milk.

The hand grasp should be strong and tight. The strength of the grasp reflex corresponds to the contracting power of the heart. If the grasp reflex is not strong and tight, the heart is generally weaker as a result of the mother's overconsumption of more yin foods and beverages during pregnancy.

The fingers generally show the baby's capacity for mental and artistic development, while the palm reflects the physical constitution. Longer fingers indicate the tendency to become more artistic or intellectual, while shorter fingers, indicate the tendency to become more physically or socially active.

As pointed out in Chapter 2, the lines of the palm correspond to the major systems of the body. (Refer to the Fig. on page 000). If the three major lines of the palm are generally long, deep, and clear, the baby has a sound native constitution. The life line, which corresponds to the digestive and respiratory systems, should be the longest of the three, ideally extending to the wrist. The nervous system line should be the shortest, while the length of the circulatory-excretory line should be in between the other two. The lines of the right hand correspond to the influence received from the mother, while those of the left correspond to the influence received from the father.

10.   *The neck:* Some babies are born with cysts on the neck which appear as lumps or masses. Neck growths result from the consumption of fatty, oily, and greasy foods during pregnancy, together with the intake of sugar, soft drinks, fruit and fruit juices, and other more expansive items. Animal fats in particular contribute to the development of these growths. It is recommended that nursing mothers avoid consuming these items until the cyst disappears. Within the standard macrobiotic diet, limit the intake of oil, flour, nuts and their products, animal food, including fish, and fruit and fruit juices until the condition improves.

If a mother consumes too many yin foods while nursing, the baby's neck may become red and moist. This is a sign that her milk has become overly yin. To recover from this problem, avoid extreme yin foods and beverages and slightly emphasize more yang factors in your diet. The problem should clear up within a week or so.

11.   *The skin:* A healthy newborn has a deep red color. In Japan, babies are called *Akanbo.* (*Aka* means "red" and *bo* means "small child.") Once the baby starts to take mother's milk, he or she will begin to change from red to light pink.

The skin of a healthy newborn is clear and free of markings. In some cases, however, the skin of the head becomes swollen, especially the scalp region, as a result of the excessive consumption of fluid and other more yin items during the latter part of pregnancy. In some cases, the head becomes swollen and cannot pass smoothly through the birth canal. The pressure of the contractions may then cause one of the small blood vessels in the inner tissue lining next to the skull to burst. This in turn causes a soft round bulge to develop at the side of the head, a condition known as *cephalohematoma.* The swelling often lasts for several weeks and can also result from the use of forceps during delivery. If either condition develops, it is important for the nursing mother to avoid extreme yin foods or beverages during the first several weeks following delivery.

At birth, the baby's skin is covered with blood and an oily coating known as vernix caseosa. During the baby's first bath only the blood and meconium are washed off. The vernix caseosa is best left on as it serves to protect the baby's skin from infection. The vernix is eventually absorbed into the baby's skin.

Small yellow or white dots are often present on the newborn's nose, chin, or cheeks. These spots result from the overintake of oily or fatty foods during the latter part of pregnancy. Foods such as nuts, nut butters, chips, fried foods, and dairy products contribute to this condition. These items cause excess oil and fat to build up in the baby's bloodstream, and cause the *sebaceous glands* to secrete excessive amounts of oil and fat. These secretions often become trapped in the pores of the skin, causing tiny yellow or white spots to develop.

The consumption of sugar, fruit, fruit juice, coffee, and drugs and medications during pregnancy often produces *skin markings.* Small, faint red spots or blotches on the upper eyelids, on the back of the neck, or on the bridge of the nose and forehead are one of the more common varieties. The overconsumption of more yin foods and beverages, including sugar, coffee, fruit and fruit juice, and soft drinks, causes blood capillaries to expand toward the surface of the skin. These markings are similar to the reddish coloration that often appears on the nose or cheeks in adults who consume too many yin foods and beverages.

Another type of skin marking is the *strawberry mark* or *strawberry nervus*. It occurs in about 10 percent of the babies born in America. The mark is bright red and looks as if a strawberry had been cut in half and attached to the skin. It usually appears on the face or neck. These markings are usually small at birth and enlarge and reach a peak size after about six months. The majority of them disappear during childhood. If your child has a strawberry mark it is important not to eat an overly yin diet while nursing or to feed the child too many foods such as fruit and fruit juice, sugar and other sweets, stimulants or spices. The standard macrobiotic diet will help cause the expanded blood vessels to contract and the mark to disappear.

Another type of birthmark is known as the *port wine stain*. It appears as a red discoloration, often taking the form of a diamond on the forehead which extends to the bridge of the nose. It is caused by the overconsumption of sugar, chemicals, drugs, medications or other extreme yin items during the third or fourth month of pregnancy. The standard macrobiotic diet during pregnancy will prevent marks such as these from developing and can help cause them to fade as the child grows older.

Of the primary colors, purple is the most yin. Birthmarks that have a purple color indicate that the mother took in some type of drug, medication, or other extreme yin item during pregnancy.

Skin rashes can easily occur if the nursing mother is eating in an excessive or unbalanced manner. One type of skin rash, known as *erythematoxicum*, results from the overconsumption of simple sugars, such as those in fruit, refined sugar, corn syrup, and honey, in combination with fats and oils such as those in milk, butter, nuts, and vegetable oils. In erythematoxicum, a red blotch develops with a small white raised center. The rash usually appears on the face, neck, and trunk.

Prickly heat, or *heat rash*, is also common in newborns. It is caused by the types of foods mentioned above. The excessive consumption of fats and oils causes them to build up in the sweat glands near the surface of the skin. If the sweat glands become blocked, toxins that are normally discharged through the sweat glands accumlate under the skin, resulting in inflammation. Prickly heat is made up of many small, red spots with slightly raised whitish centers. The best way to prevent it is to avoid excessively yin foods plus oily or fatty foods including all dairy foods, while you are nursing.

If your baby develops a rash while you are nursing, we recommend that you eat within the guidelines of the standard macrobiotic diet, while reducing or avoiding the intake of fruit, fruit juice, concentrated sweeteners, oil and oily foods such as nuts and nut butters, flour products, raw salads, and fish. The standard macrobiotic diet can be resumed once the condition improves.

12. *The first cry:* When your baby is first born, he or she will normally utter a loud cry. Someone with experience can tell whether the baby is a boy or a girl just by hearing the first cry. Boys usually have a louder and more penetrating cry, while girls tend to make a softer and more gentle sound. In both cases, if the baby is healthy, he or she will have a strong and clear cry.

If the first cry is weak or if the baby does not cry, it may be the result of some type of physical problem or may indicate a future tendency toward physical weakness and a decreased resistance to illness. Traditional cultures attached great importance to the first cry of a newborn. In Japan, for example, it was referred to as the "first word." People would listen for this first word with great anticipation, hoping that it would be loud and strong.

Early Care

Bathing: During the first three weeks, a baby undergoes many rapid changes. Babies can normally be given warm water baths once a day during this period, as bathing will help make the process of change smoother and easier.

Babies were traditionally washed in warm water in which rice bran, or *nuka*, was dissolved. The liquid from the rice bran contains natural oil that helps keep the skin smooth and healthy. To prepare a *nuka* bath, put about 2 to 3 tablespoons of rice bran into a sack made of thin cotton cloth or cheesecloth. Sew or tie the sack tightly to keep the *nuka* from falling out. Place the sack in the bath water and squeeze it. A milky liquid will come out. Mix the liquid in the bath water, and use the mild milky water to wash the baby. Rice bran can also be used by women instead of soap to keep their skin smooth and beautiful.

If rice bran is not available, rolled oats can be substituted. Use about ¼ cup of oats in place of rice bran.

After the bath water has been prepared, use a light terrycloth or smooth cotton facecloth to wash the baby. Gently washing the baby activates the circulation and the flow of energy throughout the body. It is important that the circulation be active in the hands and fingers, feet and toes, and in the peripheral parts of the body. Bathing has an effect similar to *shiatsu* massage. The flow of energy in the major organs and along the meridians becomes more active and harmonized.

When washing the baby, support the head and neck with one hand, leaving the other hand free for washing. As mentioned earlier, don't try to scrub off the vernix caseosa, because it protects the baby's skin from infection. If you wash the baby in a porcelain or stainless steel sink, place a cotton towel or facecloth on the bottom to prevent the baby from slipping.

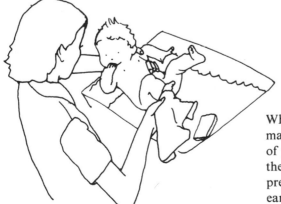

Fig. 36 Position for bathing.

When washing the baby's head, you may use the thumb and middle finger of your supporting hand to gently fold the earlobes over the ear openings to prevent water from entering the inner ears.

Circumcision: At birth, the head of the penis is covered by a retractable sleeve of skin known as the foreskin. It is something like the bud of a flower. When the baby has to urinate, the opening at the tip of the foreskin, which is normally closed tightly, opens slightly and allows the urine to flow out.

Gradually, the adhesions which attach the underside of the foreskin to the head of the penis dissolve and the foreskin becomes loose. This natural unfolding is like the blossoming of a flower from a small, compact bud. Once the foreskin has become completely retractable, the boy is naturally capable of having intercourse.

When a baby is circumcised, this natural process is artificially accelerated. In this procedure, soon after birth, the sleeve of skin is surgically cut away. The operation itself is very painful, and the baby will experience pain and sensitivity for several days after the operation, especially when the newly exposed part of the penis comes in contact with a diaper.

When the head of the penis is artificially exposed through circumcision, the flow of heaven and earth's forces along the primary channel is stimulated. This in turn activates the adrenal glands and the pituitary gland, together with the endocrine system as a whole. As a result, the boy physically matures more rapidly than normal.

In many traditional cultures, however, later maturity was preferred over earlier maturity. Later maturity was especially preferred in Japan, China, and other Oriental countries, and it was symbolized in the expression, *Tai-Ki-Ban-Sei. Tai* is translated as "large" or "great"; *Ki* as "human capacity"; *Ban* as "late" and *Sei* as "maturity" or "accomplishment." This expression refers to the Oriental belief that a great person often takes a longer time to develop and mature.

Circumcision is completely unnecessary as a means of preventing infection. Infections on the head of the penis develop as a result of eating greasy, oily, or fatty foods, including dairy products. A similar process causes women to develop ovarian cysts, vaginal discharges, and fibroid tumors. If the mother and baby eat a clean, naturally balanced diet, infections will not develop in this area. One of the problems experienced by uncircumcised babies is that many doctors tell the mothers to retract the foreskin to clean the penis. This is painful for the baby and can promote infection. It is important for mothers to understand that they don't have to and should not attempt to retract the foreskin.

Clothing, Blankets and Sleeping Materials: Baby clothes made of 100 percent cotton are recommended for daily use, as are cotton blankets, sheets, and pillowcases. It is also preferable to make or purchase a 100 percent cotton *futon* (sleeping cushion) or mattress for your baby to sleep on. Synthetic fabrics are not recommended. Wash the baby's clothing and accessories with a mild, high-quality natural soap. If the weather permits, hang them outside in the sun to dry.

Care of the Navel: Until recently, bellybands made of cotton were tied around the baby's abdomen to allow the navel to heal properly and to prevent clothing or diapers from rubbing against, irritating, or pulling off the remaining section of umbilical cord. These bands were made of light, soft cotton and were similar to the Japanese *hara-maki*, or *hara* warmer, the cotton belt traditionally worn around the abdomen. Unfortunately, these special belts are only rarely used in the United States now.

When giving the baby a bath, try not to touch the remaining part of the umbilical cord. The remaining cord begins to shrivel within a few hours after birth and becomes drier and smaller until it drops off, usually within the first or second week after birth.

After the cord has fallen off, the navel can be cleaned daily, although for the first few days, it is better to very lightly pat the navel clean with sterile cotton.

As pointed out in Chapter 2, the wall of the baby's abdomen below the navel is open during part of the embryonic period. It normally closes before birth. In some cases, however, the opening does not close properly—a condition known as *umbilical hernia*. Failure of the abdominal wall to close properly results when sugar, fruit, soft drinks, spices, stimulants, juices, medications and other more yin items are consumed during pregnancy. These items deplete minerals in the mother's body and slow the contraction of the abdominal wall. In many babies with this disorder, complete closure does not occur until after the first year of life and, in some cases, not until the age of four or five. Since umbilical hernia is the result of an excess of more yin factors in the diet, if your baby has this condition, it is important to avoid the intake of extreme yin foods or beverages while you are nursing and to avoid feeding these items to your baby once he or she begins taking solids and liquids. Within the standard macrobiotic diet, vegetables such as *daikon*, carrot, turnip greens, and other tough, fibrous greens can be included daily. Sea vegetables, which are rich in minerals, can be used daily in soups, with vegetables, and on a regular basis as side dishes. Small side dishes of *hijiki* and *arame* are especially recommended and can be eaten several times a week.

Skin Care: Other than bathing, a healthy baby's skin requires no special care. Chemicalized soaps, oils, lotions, and powders are best avoided.

One problem experienced by many babies is *cradle cap*. Cradle cap is caused by the buildup of dried oil and excess protein on the scalp and resembles dried, scaly skin. The accumulation of dried oil is caused by the mother's intake of oily or fatty foods during pregnancy or while breast-feeding, including nuts, nut butter, fried or sautéed foods, dairy products, and animal fats. The consumption of salt and baked flour products causes oil in the body to become drier and harder, and can also contribute to cradle cap. The overintake of beans and bean products, which contain plenty of fat and protein, can also lead to this condition.

Cradle cap can be kept to a minimum through proper washing with rice bran, rolled oats, or a high-quality natural soap, in addition to eating properly. Wash the scalp gently with *nuka* or oat water and lightly scrub with your fingers to loosen any cradle cap.

Diaper rash is another common skin problem. It is caused by the mother's overintake of fruit, fruit juice, sugar, maple syrup, grain sweeteners, and other more yin items, or by the consumption of fats and oils. Diaper rash will clear up quickly if you reduce or avoid these foods while nursing.

Arrowroot flour can be applied to help keep the affected area dry and make the baby more comfortable. Chemicalized preparations, including ointments made with zinc oxide, are best avoided for skin conditions.

Skin rashes can be aggravated by the chemicals used in the preparation of disposable diapers or by the detergents and bleaches used by commercial diaper services. Rubber pants, which hold in heat and keep air from entering, can also aggravate rashes. Ideally, diapers should be washed at home with a natural detergent and hung outside in the sun to dry. If your baby develops a rash, we recommend that you use this method until it improves. Similarly, rubber pants are best used only when really needed and preferably not until the baby is three to four weeks old. Traditionally, diaper covers were made of thick quilted or layered cotton. Cotton allows air to enter and does not lock in heat.

Sleeping Position: The most natural position for sleeping is on the back. Sleeping on the back is unique to human beings. No other animal sleeps in this position. Sleeping on the stomach is an indication of chronic weakness in the digestive system. Digestive weakness can result from overeating on the part of the baby or from the intake of dairy and animal products, sugar, fruit, and fats and oils by the mother or baby.

Babies often sleep with their heads to one side. If your baby does this, periodically turn the head to the opposite side so that the baby sleeps an equal amount of time facing in both directions. If you don't alternate the position of the head, the side that the baby most often sleeps on will tend to become flatter and the other side will become more well developed.

Babies can use a very low, almost flat pillow for sleeping. A cotton receiving blanket can also be folded over and placed under the baby's head to serve as a pillow. High, large pillows are not recommended for infants.

In general, it is better for the baby to sleep with the head pointing north or, if you live in the Southern Hemisphere, pointing south. By facing the poles when we sleep, our billions of brain cells become especially charged with the vibrational energy generated by the heavens.

If you eat well during pregnancy and while nursing, your baby should enjoy peaceful and undisturbed sleep. If a baby wakes up often during the night, crying and fussing, it is often due to an imbalance in the daily diet. Too much fruit, juice, sweetener, flour products, oil, or overeating can easily create an unbalanced quality in a mother's milk, which can cause the baby to frequently wake up crying during the night. Overconsumption of animal food can also cause the baby's sleep to be disturbed.

Keeping Warm: Babies often kick their blankets off, especially during the summer. Therefore, always make sure that your baby's abdominal region is covered, either with a blanket or a loose fitting cotton wrap such as the *hara-maki*, or *hara* warmer, worn by the Japanese. It is important to keep the baby's abdominal region warm even if the hands and feet are uncovered. During the first several months, be especially careful to keep the baby away from cold drafts or wind. If your baby is exposed to cold, for example, in an air conditioned room, he or she may become very fussy or irritable. If you are in a cold area, make sure that the baby is well covered and protected.

Going Outside: In general, it is better to wait three to four weeks before going outside with your baby. This is especially important if you live in a cold climate and the baby is born in a cold season. Of course, if your baby is born in a hospital, going outside is unavoidable when you leave the hospital.

Make sure that your baby is properly dressed in cold weather, especially until he or she is about six months old. It is also important to keep a newborn from being exposed to too much direct sunlight, especially during the warmer months or at the beach. Make sure to properly cover your baby on these occasions.

Nursing Your Baby

As we have seen, a newborn baby is very yang from being nourished by a diet of 100 percent animal food in the womb. Babies are small and red, have high body temperatures, and very active pulse rates.

Because they are so yang, newborns instinctively seek yin, which nature provides in the form of mother's milk. Breast milk is simply mother's blood that has risen in the body and been converted in the breasts into a sweeter and less salty liquid. The formation of breast milk is similar to the rising and separation that occurs in fermentation. Mother's milk is therefore very similar in quality to *amazake*, a fermented sweet rice drink. Since breast milk is so yin and fragile, it should not be exposed to air, as its quality changes easily. The baby's quality also begins to change as a result of taking mother's milk, on the whole becoming more yin.

As the baby starts drinking mother's milk, the fats, proteins, and other more yin components that it contains are attracted toward the upper part of the child's body, while the more yang minerals are attracted downward toward the legs and feet. At birth, the head is more yang, so the most natural position for delivery is for the head to be downward. However, as the baby begins taking mother's milk, the legs become more yang and the head becomes more yin. The baby's position then begins reversing; he or she gradually begins to crawl and finally stands upright.

Colostrum: When a baby first begins to nurse, the breasts secrete a thick yellowish liquid called colostrum. Colostrum is an intermediary food—we can consider it to be in between mother's blood and mother's milk. Biochemically, colostrum is more like blood than milk. Like blood, it contains numerous living cells such as *lymphocytes* and *macrophages* which protect the body from disease organisms and foreign substances. Because it contains antibodies, colostrum helps convey a natural immunity to the baby. It is especially rich in viral disease antibodies, which are present in colostrum in much higher concentrations than in mother's blood.

While mother's milk is more yin and provides the basis for growth, colostrum serves to make the baby more yang. Therefore a newborn will usually lose a small amount of weight for the first several days until he or she begins receiving mother's milk. Colostrum is also believed to promote constriction of the microscopic openings in the wall of the intestine through which digested food particles are absorbed. The inner lining of the baby's intestine thus becomes impermeable to large molecules, including many disease organisms. The reduction of intestinal permeability also promotes more complete digestion of large protein molecules and may help prevent the absorption of whole proteins, a factor believed to be associated with a variety of allergies.

When a baby receives colostrum created by the mother's well balanced, natural diet, and is nourished by a healthy quality of breast milk, and later by a properly balanced natural diet, artificial immunizations are usually unnecessary. Babies who do not receive colostrum, or who are nourished by a poor quality of breast milk or an unnatural substitute for it, are often susceptible to disease organisms. Because of this, artificial immunizations are thought to be necessary. It is far safer to let the baby suck at his or her mother's breast immediately after birth as a way of providing immunity against illness. Colostrum also acts as a natural laxative which cleanses the baby's intestine of meconium.

The Need to Suck: It is very important for a baby to learn to suck as soon as possible after birth. Most new mothers are surprised at how hard healthy newborns suck. Sucking may be difficult for some babies, and it may take several attempts before nourishment is received from the breast.

Many of the newborn's movements are governed by a variety of automatic reflexes, with rudimentary consciousness. These include the *rooting response*, in which a baby will turn his or her mouth toward any object that comes in contact with a cheek, be it a finger or the mother's nipple. Rooting helps the baby to locate the nipple. Sucking and swallowing are another example. Anything that touches the baby's lips will normally produce sucking movements. Grasping is also a reflex action; the pressure of a finger on the palms or soles of the feet will automatically cause the fingers or toes to curl in to grasp the pressing object. As with rooting and sucking, it is better for the grasping reflex to be strong and well developed at birth. The baby's reflexes are examples of the well developed mechanical consciousness that human beings possess at birth. The senses gradually develop and begin to come under conscious control as the baby grows. At this time, a baby will begin to reach for and grasp at objects which are first seen, or will visually search for the mother's breast. The grasping and rooting reflexes decrease once sensorial consciousness becomes stronger.

Advantages of Breast-Feeding: Breast-feeding is the most natural way for babies to eat. It has a number of distinct advantages over artificial methods of feeding. These include:

1) *Availability and convenience:* Breast milk is always available, sterile, and at the right temperature for the baby. No special equipment is necessary to prepare food for the baby. Breast-feeding is very economical; it requires no special investment of time or money.

2) *Better health for the baby:* As we have seen, colostrum provides the baby with natural immunity against many illnesses. Breast milk also contains antibodies, and breast-fed babies have a much lower incidence of upper respiratory infections and a variety of other disorders. In one study conducted at the Northwestern University School of Medicine, bottle-fed children were found to have four times as many ear infections, four times as many colds, eleven times as many tonsillectomies, and twenty times as many

diarrheal infections than children who had been breast-fed for six months or longer. The study was based on the rates of illness in a group of 178 children between birth and age ten. A similar result was obtained in a study conducted in Great Britain in which *ulcerative colitis* was found to be 100 percent more common in adults who were weaned from breast milk before two weeks than in those who breast-fed for longer periods.

It is now widely known that babies fed only breast milk develop far fewer allergies than babies fed artificially. In the Northwestern study mentioned above, artificially fed children were found to have had from eight to twenty-seven times as many reported allergies than their breast-fed counterparts.

3) *Nutritional compatibility:* The quality and proportion of nutrients in human milk are perfectly compatible with a baby's digestive and excretory systems. No other form of nourishment is so well suited to a baby's physiology. The composition of milk changes throughout the period of lactation to adapt to the baby's changing condition and needs. Let us consider how breast milk supplies the essential macronutrients:

Human & Cow's Milk Nutrients

Substance	Human Milk	Cow's Milk
	(Percent)	
Water	88.3	87.3
Inorganic salts	0.2	0.7
Protein	1.5	3.8
Fat	4.0	4.0
Sugars	6.0	4.5
Reaction	Alkaline	Acid

From *Anatomy and Physiology, Volume* 2 by Steen & Montagu; p. 253

- *Minerals:* As we can see in the above table, breast milk contains a smaller percentage of minerals than does cow's milk. For example, breast milk contains about a fourth as much calcium as does cow's milk. However, the proportion of minerals in human milk is ideally suited to the development of a healthy body structure. Babies fed cow's milk formulas tend to develop larger, heavier bone structures which are not necessarily compatible with overall health, adaptability, and endurance. The high mineral content of cow's milk also puts an additional burden on the excretory system, which must continually work harder to discharge much unused calcium and phosphorus.

  Some people believe that breast milk is lacking in iron. In actuality, it contains more iron than cow's milk. The iron in healthy breast milk, together with the release of stored iron from the baby's liver, is generally adequate to sustain the baby until solid foods are introduced.

- *Protein:* Cow's milk contains more protein than human milk, however, the protein in cow's milk must be diluted before the human body can tolerate it. In its natural state, cow's milk forms a large, tough curd when mixed with digestive juices. Even after being diluted and heated, the curds of cow's milk stagnate in the baby's stomach, often leading to a variety of digestive disorders.

The curds in human milk are produced from a more suitable balance of proteins and are soft and delicate, with an almost fluid consistency. The stomach of a breast-fed baby therefore empties more quickly and easily. A breast-fed baby wants to eat more frequently, usually every two or three hours. Frequent nursing helps stimulate the production of breast milk.

The protein in human milk is mostly soluble *lactalbumin*, which is easily digested. Cow's milk contains mostly *casein*, which is relatively insoluble in the digestive tract. Human milk contains a large proportion of essential amino acids, which are absorbed and utilized by the baby just as they are. Colostrum is especially rich in amino acids.

The protein in breast milk is utilized with almost 100 percent efficiency. Nearly all of the protein in breast milk is used by the baby; little or none is excreted. The proteins in cow's milk, however, are utilized with only about 50 percent efficiency. About half of the protein in cow's milk is wasted; some passes through the system and is discharged in the feces, while some is digested but cannot be utilized by the baby's cells and is excreted in the urine. Therefore, bottle-fed babies must take in a much larger volume of milk in order to obtain enough usable protein.

The elimination of unusable protein and mineral salts puts additional strain on the formula-fed baby's kidneys, which are not fully mature in infants. Babies fed cow's milk need additional water, not only for their metabolism, but also to allow the kidneys to eliminate excess salts and proteins. Breast-fed babies get enough water for their metabolic needs from mother's milk and do not need to take in water beyond what they receive in milk.

● *Fat:* Breast milk contains about the same amount of fat as undiluted cow's milk. However, breast milk contains much less saturated fat and is easier to digest. The long term excess of saturated fat in the diet has been associated with a wide range of disorders, most notably heart disease and a variety of cancers.

● *Carbohydrate:* Mother's milk contains far more carbohydrate (in some cases, about twice as much) than whole cow's milk. Therefore, some type of sugar is generally added to cow's milk formulas to provide enough calories. However, highly refined and processed sugars, such as cane sugar, brown sugar, corn syrup, and others are usually added, all of which create harmful effects.

The carbohydrates in breast milk are mostly in the form of *lactose*, while cow's milk includes *galactose*, *glucose*, and other carbohydrates. Lactose is more easily digested; it also facilitates a more efficient utilization of proteins and calcium.

In the digestive tract, the secretion of digestive juices alternates between alkaline and acid: for example, the saliva secreted in the mouth is alkaline while the digestive juices of the stomach are primarily acid; the digestive secretions of the pancreas and duodenum are primarily alkaline, while those of the small intestine are more acidic. The digestion of the lactose in breast milk helps the small intestine maintain a normal acid medium. However, the sugars present in cow's milk cause an opposite, or alkaline medium to develop in the intestines. An alkaline medium furthers the development of harmful and putrefactive bacteria, while an acid medium prevents those bacteria from developing. Breast milk contains a carbohydrate compound known as the *bifidus factor*, which furthers the growth of a beneficial organism known as *Lactobacillus bifidus*. This compound, not present in cow's milk, helps make the baby's intestinal tract resistant to harmful bacteria.

- *Vitamins:* In general, breast milk contains from two to ten times more of the essential vitamins than cow's milk. The vitamin content of breast milk varies according to the type of diet eaten. If the mother is eating a well balanced macrobiotic diet, and if she and her baby are both getting sufficient activity, including exposure to sunlight, nursing will provide the baby with all of the necessary vitamins. Because the vitamin content of cow's milk is less, bottle-fed babies usually require vitamin supplements and the early introduction of various types of artificially formulated baby foods.

4) *A strong bond between mother and child:* Nursing creates a strong emotional and physiological bond between mother and baby. Both experience a natural sense of oneness that continues throughout life. Breast-fed babies tend to develop natural love and respect for their mothers, and a woman who breast-feeds enjoys the satisfaction of early and prolonged contact with her baby. Nursing has a calming and relaxing effect on both mother and baby.

5) *Rapid healing after delivery:* As mentioned previously, nursing releases a hormone known as oxytocin, which causes the uterus to contract following delivery. Frequent nursing of the newborn lessens the mother's risk of hemorrhaging and causes the uterus to return to its normal size quickly and naturally.

6) *Normal development of the baby's teeth and jaws:* Sucking on the mother's nipple leads to a more natural and adequate development of the baby's teeth, palate, and jaws. Bottle-feeding frequently distorts the development of the teeth and jaws and is a major factor in problems with dental and facial development in children.

Breast-feeding allows some of the excess in a woman's diet to be discharged from the body, thus helping to prevent or minimize the accumulation of toxic substances, especially in the breast region. This could be a factor in the prevention of breast and other types of cancer. Breast-feeding also helps a woman return to a more normal and healthy weight following delivery. Some of the weight gained during pregnancy is in the form of calcium and other nutrients which are stored for future use during lactation. If the woman does not breast-feed, some of these nutrients remain in the body as added weight. This happens after each pregnancy in which the mother does not breast-feed, and the continual storage of excess can lead to a variety of disorders, including cancer.

In summary, mother's milk is the perfectly suited form of nourishment for human babies. Just as a mother's diet during pregnancy plays a decisive role in the development of her baby, how she feeds her newborn during the first part of the baby's life is also vitally important for the child's future health and happiness. Always remember that your baby has passed through the equivalent of billions of years of evolution in order to physicalize upon the earth as a human being. After having passed through this long journey, it is indeed unfortunate when parents allow their baby to become the foster child of a cow or of an infant formula factory, instead of providing the proper nourishment for human health and happiness.

The Process of Breast-Feeding

As pointed out earlier, the breasts have a complementary relationship to the reproductive organs in the lower part of the body. Before and during pregnancy, blood and energy tend to gather in the lower reproductive organs during the monthly maturation of ova and during the development and growth of the fertilized egg. At full term, for example, the blood supply to the uterus is substantial; as much as one-fourth of the output of the heart goes to this organ.

Following delivery, the focus of bodily activity shifts upward toward the breasts. Blood and energy now gather there as the function of lactation begins. The output of estrogen and progesterone, the two principal ovarian hormones, declines, while the output of *prolactin*, the pituitary hormone which stimulates lactation, rises.

The mammary glands begin secreting milk within 24 to 96 hours after delivery. The appearance of milk in the breasts is known as the "coming in" of milk, and many women experience this as the sensation of fullness in the breasts.

Milk is secreted in the mammary glands and temporarily stored in the aveoli, which are tiny sacs surrounded by special cells which contract like muscles. When the baby suckles, nerve endings in the nipples are stimulated and the impulses signal the brain to produce two hormones, prolactin and oxytocin. The more yin prolactin stimulates the breasts to produce milk while the more yang oxytocin causes the cells that surround the aveoli to contract and squeeze the milk out of the aveoli into large ducts leading to the nipple. The discharge of milk from the alveoli is known as the "letdown reflex."

The breasts will continue to produce milk as long as they are stimulated by the baby's sucking. The more stimulation that the breasts receive, the more milk is produced.

During pregnancy, the breasts ready themselves for nursing by becoming larger. The nipples are kept free of harmful bacteria through the antibacterial action of sweat and oil secreted by the nipple, together with the antibacterial action of newly secreted milk. The nipples are therefore ready for sucking whenever the baby wants.

When milk comes in, the breasts often become firm, full, and tender. Any discomfort that is experienced at this time, however, will normally disappear after several days of nursing. At the same time, the nipples may become tender during the first week of nursing. In most cases, this too disappears after several days. Simple massage of the nipples is often helpful in relieving tenderness.

When nursing, allow one breast to empty completely before changing to the other. Since earth's expanding force is stronger in the right side of the body, the milk from the right breast has the effect of actively stimulating the baby's growth. Heaven's descending force is generally more active on the left side of the body, and milk from the left breast has a strengthening or stabilizing effect on the baby. These differences are in the subtle electromagnetic effects of the milk and would not show up in chemical analysis. The ideal method of nursing is to feed the baby completely from one breast and then switch to the other, alternating continually so as to balance the baby's mix of these energy forces.

The most reliable guide to the length of each feeding is the behavior of your baby. Nursing can be stopped once the baby slows down and appears to be full and satisfied. In general, babies can be nursed whenever they appear to be hungry. Remember that breast milk is easily and rapidly digested and will not upset the baby. Nursing according to a schedule determined by the clock disturbs the natural development of the baby and is not recommended.

Problems with Nursing

In some cases, milk does not come in properly. A lack of breast milk is often a sign that a woman's condition has become overly yin, especially if she is eating a large volume of sugar, fruits, salad, honey, maple syrup, spices, tomatoes, and potatoes, or if she received medication during delivery or is presently consuming various types of drugs or medications. This condition can be offset by emphasizing more variety and combinations within the standard macrobiotic diet and by avoiding extreme yin foods and beverages.

In some cases, however, a lack of breast milk is the result of an overly yang condition. A woman needs to be strong and in good health in order to produce enough high quality milk. If, however, her condition becomes overly tight as a result of eating too many heavily salted or baked foods, or if she does not have enough variety in her diet or in the method of preparation, there may not be enough rising or expanding energy in her body to produce sufficient amounts of breast milk. Mothers who experience this problem should: 1) make their diets somewhat wider, for example, by including grains such as sweet brown rice or *mochi*, which contain more protein and fat than regular brown rice or other frequently used grains; 2) reduce the intake of salty seasonings and condiments; 3) include more lightly cooked green vegetable dishes; 4) use lighter cooking methods; 5) eat products such as *tempeh, tofu*, and other vegetable products that contain plenty of protein. A small volume of *amazake* or high quality beer can also be taken on occasion by women with this condition to help stimulate the production of breast milk.

If, however, a mother is still unable to produce milk, there are several alternatives to be considered:

1. A wet nurse can be found to provide breast milk for the baby. Traditionally, a mother who could not nurse would make arrangements with a healthy new mother who had an ample supply of milk and who had given birth within two to three months of her delivery date. Ideally, a mother should be sought who is eating a macrobiotically balanced, natural diet.
2. The baby can be given artificial formula, in which case he or she becomes the child of an infant formula factory.
3. The baby can be given formulas made with goat's or cow's milk, in which case he or she begins to develop as a kid or calf rather than naturally as a human baby.
4. The baby can be fed primarily with a milk substitute made from whole grain cereals and other natural food ingredients, in which case he or she can develop naturally as a human being.

With the last alternative, cereal grains and other whole natural foods are used to imitate the natural bodily processes in which mother's milk is produced from the cereal grains and other foods that she eats. *Cereal grain milk* is prepared at home in the kitchen using the basic food materials that produce ideal breast milk.

Brown rice is the principal ingredient in cereal grain milk, since in terms of the proportion of macronutrients, it comes very close to mother's milk. In order to simulate the sweet taste of mother's milk and provide enough protein and fat for the baby's growth, more yin sweet rice, which contains more of these factors, can be included, as can barley or other whole grains.

When making grain milk, use approximately four parts brown rice (short grain), three parts sweet brown rice, and one part barley. Millet and oats may be included from time to time. Buckwheat, wheat, and rye are not recommended for use in grain milk. To prepare grain milk:

1. Soak the cereals overnight, or for 24 hours if the weather is very cold. Pressure cook with a small piece of *kombu* (the *kombu* does not always have to be eaten) and five times more water (use the soaking water to cook the grain). Cook for about one and a half hours. Use a medium-low flame after the grain comes to pressure, or
2. Soak the cereals as above and boil with ten times more water and a small piece of *kombu* until half the original amount of water is left. When the cereal comes to a boil, turn the flame to medium low and simmer.

When preparing grain milk for a newborn or very small baby, place the cooked mixture into a cheesecloth sack and strain it to remove the bran. Then, it can be sweetened by adding one teaspoon of barley malt or high quality traditionally processed rice syrup to one cup of grain milk. Heat the sweetened mixture and simmer for several minutes before use.

When preparing the grain milk for an older baby, after the mixture has finished cooking, put it into a *suribachi* (a clay grinding bowl with a wooden pestle), or into a hand food mill, and mash it very thoroughly. Do not use a blender or electric device for grinding. After mashing the mixture, add a small amount of barley malt or rice syrup. Just enough concentrated grain sweetener should be added to give the mixture a sweetness similar to that of mother's milk.

Once it has been prepared with the proper taste and consistency, heat the cereal grain milk to about body temperature and put it into a baby bottle. Cereal grain milk can be stored in a glass jar and reheated before subsequent feedings.

If either of the above cereal grain milks do not flow smoothly through the nipple, they can be further diluted with water and strained several times through cheesecloth. You may also enlarge the opening of the nipple with a large darning needle. Sterilize the tip of the needle by holding it over a flame before using it to enlarge the opening. Among nipples, special orthodontic nipples are preferred as these tend to foster the natural development of the teeth and jaws.

The ingredients and proportions presented above can be varied slightly, depending on the age and needs of the baby. Grain-milk can also be used as one of the first soft foods that a baby is given once foods other than breast milk are introduced. In general, a more watery grain milk is recommended for younger babies, while older infants can receive a firmer mixture; the proportion of water to cereal can be 10: 1, 7: 1, 3: 1, etc., depending on the age of the baby.

Sesame seeds may be added to either of the cereal grain milk recipes. The seeds should be well toasted and thoroughly crushed in a *suribachi* before being added. About 5 to 10 percent crushed seeds can be cooked along with the cereals.

The baby can also receive naturally processed *soy milk* as a supplement to cereal grain milk. To prepare, soak about 3 cups of soybeans overnight, strain, and discard the soaking water. Grind the beans in an electric blender (this is one of the rare instances in which electric devices are used in macrobiotic cooking). Or, if you have time and patience, a Foley hand food mill can be used. Add about 6 quarts of water and a 1-inch piece of *kombu* to the bean mash and bring to a boil. Reduce flame to low and simmer for about five minutes. Stir continuously to prevent burning. Sprinkle cold water on the mash to stop bubbling and bring gently to a boil again. Sprinkle cold water once more on the mash and again bring to a boil. (Don't cover the mash as it will bubble over the top of the pot.) Place a cotton cloth or cheesecloth in a strainer and pour the liquid—called soy milk—through the strainer and into a bowl. Fold the corners of the cloth together to form a sack and squeeze out the remaining liquid. (The pulp, known as *okara*, can be saved and used in other dishes.)

Put the soy milk in a bottle and feed to the baby. If the soy milk does not flow smoothly, dilute it with water and strain through a cheesecloth until the desired consistency is achieved. Soy milk is usually very sweet, but if additional sweetener is desired, barley malt or rice syrup can be added as in the grain milk recipe. Soy milk can be stored and reheated to body temperature prior to use.

In Oriental countries, babies who were unable to nurse were also given the heavy liquid which rises to the top of the pot when grains are cooked with plenty of water, for example 5 to 10 parts water to 1 part grain. A small volume of grain-based sweetener was usually added to provide a taste approaching that of mother's milk.

In addition to the foods mentioned above, babies can also be given *special rice cream* from time to time. To prepare, pressure cook brown rice with 3 to 6 parts water and a 1-inch piece of *kombu* for at least two hours. (Do not add salt.) Squeeze the cooked rice and liquid through a piece of sanitized cheesecloth into a bowl. Put this thick liquid into a baby bottle, diluting and straining again if necessary. On occasion, the rice can be roasted prior to pressure cooking.

Babies can also be given the juice from cooked vegetables. Bring vegetables such as carrots, squash, cabbage, broccoli, corn, or others to a boil. A small, 1-inch piece of soaked *kombu* may be added. Simmer the ingredients over a low flame for 30 to 45 minutes. Strain the liquid from cooking the vegetables through sanitized cheesecloth. Place in a bottle and give to the baby.

If, during the time that you are feeding your baby in the above manner, you notice that he or she fails to gain weight or seems to be not developing properly, seek advice from mothers who have had experience in feeding their children macrobiotically or from a qualified macrobiotic counselor. It is also advisable to work along with a pediatrician who supports your desire to feed your baby naturally, in formulating an appropriate feeding plan.

One problem experienced by some women during lactation is a breast infection known as *mastitis*. Mastitis most frequently results from stagnation in the breast caused by the clogging of a duct. Milk backs up, and the affected area tends to become overfull. The area may become tender and slightly reddish and infection may appear. A slight fever may develop, together with a general feeling of being ill.

The most common dietary cause of blockage in the ducts is the consumption of fatty, oily, or greasy foods, especially animal quality fats, together with sugar, fruits, fruit juice, spices, stimulant beverages, and other more yin items. These latter items contribute especially to the development of infection.

In a smaller number of cases, the flow of milk is temporarily impeded as a result of an overly constricted condition resulting from the intake of too many salty foods and baked items. However, infection is not likely to develop unless more extreme yin items such as those mentioned above are also being consumed.

In the past, doctors frequently advised women with mastitis to wean their babies; however, this approach is now being questioned, as taking the baby off the breast results in an increased backup of milk and can make a breast abscess more likely to develop.

A less drastic approach to mastitis is to continue nursing and to try to establish an active flow of milk in the affected area. Frequent nursings from the affected breast are therefore recommended, as there is nothing in the milk that will harm the baby. A hot ginger compress can also be applied to the affected area to stimulate the blood circulation and help relieve stagnation. The compress can be applied twice daily until the condition improves. It is also advisable to avoid the intake of fatty, oily, or greasy foods, together with sugar, fruit, fruit juices, spices, stimulant beverages, and other more extreme yin items. The standard macrobiotic diet is recommended as the basis for recovery from this condition. It is advisable to limit or avoid the use of oil or the intake of nuts and nut butters until the condition improves. Similarly, all animal products, including white-meat fish, are best avoided. Among grains, barley can be included regularly as a principal grain together with rice, while flour products, which can lead to stagnation, are not recommended. Hard, leafy green vegetables such as kale, *daikon* greens, and turnip and carrot tops can be lightly steamed and eaten daily, as can root vegetables such as *daikon* and carrots. Cooked *daikon* is especially effective in helping dissolve fat and mucus accumulations. It can be prepared with *kombu* and other vegetables or can be used in the dried and shredded form. *Miso* soup, made with *wakame*, *daikon*, and *shii-take* (dried mushrooms), is especially good for this purpose and can be eaten daily until the condition improves.

It is recommended that sea vegetables be included daily, while it is better to limit the intake of beans and use only varieties that are low in fat. Bean products such as *tempeh* may be eaten but in small amounts and not on a daily basis. It is better to avoid raw *tofu* until the condition improves; dried *tofu* can be used in place of raw *tofu* in a variety of dishes.

In general, the taste of your daily meals should not be overly salty. Lighter cooking methods are preferable to longer methods of cooking. If the condition is accompanied by fever, a raw *tofu* plaster can be applied to the forehead while the special *daikon* tea described in Chapter 4 can be taken for a few days.

In cases where mastitis leads to the development of a breast abscess, either a *taro potato* or *lotus root plaster* can be applied to the affected breast following a five minute ginger compress. To prepare the taro plaster, peel one large or several small taro potatoes and grate the white interior. Mix with about 5 percent grated ginger and spread the mixture in a half-inch layer on a piece of cotton linen. Apply the potato side directly to the skin of the affected breast. The plaster can be tied in place with a cotton cloth or bandage and left for about four hours.

To prepare the lotus root plaster, grate fresh lotus root and mix with about 10 percent whole wheat pastry flour or unbleached white flour. Add 5 to 10 percent grated ginger and spread the mixture on a piece of cotton linen and apply as above. The ginger compress can be applied for five minutes before either of these applications to warm the body and increase circulation in the affected area. This procedure can be repeated daily until the condition improves.

If itching is experienced when the plaster is applied, the grated ginger can be omitted.

Your Baby's Daily Condition

While you are nursing, it is important to continually observe your baby's changing condition. Remember that problems are most often caused by the foods you eat which the baby receives indirectly through your milk.

The most basic things to check when monitoring your baby's day to day condition are:

Bowel Movements: For the first day or so after birth, a baby's bowel movements are normally greenish black with a smooth sticky consistency. Once the meconium has been discharged, the bowel movement should become a light, golden yellow. A breast-fed baby usually has several movements per day during the first several weeks. Bowel movements tend to become less frequent as the baby gets older; however, at least one movement per day indicates that the baby is in a normal, healthy condition.

A baby's bowel movements are not as firm as an adult's but have a softer consistency. If the bowel movement becomes too soft and watery, very sticky, or has a greenish color, however, the baby's intestines are becoming too loose. An overly expanded condition in the bowels is normally the result of the mother's intake of such yin foods as potatoes, fruit, tomatoes, honey, or the overconsumption of flour products and a lack of vegetables. These foods frequently cause the baby's bowels to become expanded and sluggish. At the same time, animal fats, oils, and animal proteins frequently cause breast milk to putrefy in the baby's intestines and contribute to the formation of toxic bacteria. Intestinal putrefaction also contributes to greenish bowel movements. Dark brown or hard bowel movements indicate that a nursing mother is eating too much salt, baked flour products, or overly cooked dishes.

A breast-fed baby's bowel movements should not have an unpleasant odor. Strong, sour-smelling bowel movements often indicate that a nursing mother is eating too many fruits and other strong yin items. It is better, therefore, to minimize or avoid the intake of fruit while you are breast-feeding. In hot summer weather, foods such as corn on the cob and fresh leafy green vegetables are better than eating a large volume of fruit.

Always check your baby's bowel movements on a daily basis. If you find that they have become abnormal, make the appropriate adjustments in your daily diet to restore proper balance. Whenever your baby has a problem, first check his or her bowel movement. The underlying cause can often be discovered through this basic observation.

Urination: A healthy baby's urine has a light yellow color which is almost clear. It does not have an overly strong smell. If the urine becomes darker, the mother's diet has become too high in salt or minerals. If the urine begins to have a strong, ammonia-like odor, it may indicate that the mother has eaten too much animal food or sea vegetables.

Sleeping: During the first several months, a newborn will sleep from feeding to feeding, waking up only to take milk and soon going back to sleep. Healthy babies sleep peacefully and soundly. Continual sleeping furthers the process of growth. Some babies are unusually wakeful right from the beginning or have difficulty in sleeping deeply and soundly. The inability to sleep well is frequently a sign that the baby's condition is overly yang or tight as a result of the mother's overintake of animal foods, salt, and baked flour products without enough fresh or lightly cooked grain and vegetable dishes. If your baby has trouble sleeping, these items can be reduced and more fresh, lightly cooked grain and vegetable dishes can be eaten. In this case, a small volume of natural quality beer or *amazake* can be taken from time to time, as can occasional cooked fruit desserts, to help the mother and baby relax and to make the quality of her milk slightly more yin. However, more extreme yin items such as coffee, stimulant teas, spices, and simple sugars can easily make the baby hyperactive and unable to sleep well and are therefore best avoided.

A baby will gradually sleep less and less as he or she gets older. Each baby develops his or her own pattern of sleeping and waking. If older children continue to sleep for extended periods, however, the cause is frequently an excess of more yin factors in the diet.

Crying: Healthy babies generally cry for three reasons: 1) Because they are hungry, 2) because they need a diaper change, or 3) because they are too hot, too cold, in a noisy or disruptive environment, or if they are being bothered by insects. If mosquitoes or other insects are attracted to the baby, it is a sign that the mother's milk has become overly yin, usually as the result of eating too many fruits, juices, or sweets.

If a baby cries for any reason other than the above, it is an indication that there is some imbalance in his or her diet or surroundings.

A common cause of upset in babies is sharp pains in the intestines, or *colic.* Colic is related to problems in the lungs and large intestines and occurs most often between the hours of 6 and 10 P.M. Babies with colic frequently experience swelling in the abdomen, caused by the retention of gas, and often pull up or stiffen their legs, scream, and pass gas via the rectum.

Colic is caused by an improper diet. The most common dietary cause is a reaction to artificial cow's milk formula, which, as has been pointed out, is not properly suited to the delicate digestive system of the newborn. The degree of intolerance to these formulas varies from what is considered a "normal" degree of crankiness to convulsions and progressive emaciation. Symptoms such as frequent and painful gas, vomiting, periodic irritable crying, and crying during bowel movements are far less common in breast-fed babies, as are problems such as continually watery stools and diaper rash.

When colic does occur in the breast-fed baby, it is the result of an imbalance in the mother's way of eating. Some babies are unusually tense and restless during the first several weeks. Their bodies can't relax well, and they frequently startle easily at slight noises or sudden changes of position. Infants with this problem are referred to as *hypertonic* babies. The inability to relax is usually an indication that the baby's condition is overly yang, as a result of the mother's intake of salt, animal products, baked foods, or overly cooked dishes throughout pregnancy and while nursing. The overconsumption of ice cream, candy, and other highly sugared foods, and iced beverages—especially sugared soft drinks—can also cause this condition.

The type of colic described above, in which the infant's abdomen becomes distended and gas develops, results from an expanded condition in the intestines, which in turn results from the intake of sugar, fruit, fruit juice, milk, carbonated soft drinks, honey, and other more yin items. These items frequently combine with animal fats, excess oil, and flour products to produce a more undigestible quality of milk which causes the baby to develop indigestion and gas.

Common Problems

Below are several common problems that may arise with newborns, together with the macrobiotic approach to restoring balance.

The Overuse of Salt: The correct use of salt is very important for babies and children. Although the breast-fed baby does not receive salt directly, the mother's intake does affect the quality of her milk. Too much salt can inhibit the natural process of growth. A baby will begin to crawl and stand as a result of taking mother's milk followed by vegetable-quality foods. If the baby receives too much salt, the natural process of growth is disrupted, and the baby may not be able to stand up or, after having begun to stand, may return to all fours. The excessive intake of salt can cause the baby's thinking ability to degenerate as well. When you begin introducing grains and vegetables to the baby, therefore, no salt should be included for about the first year after birth and sometimes longer. Creamy cereals made from roasted flour are also too yang for the baby, as are baked flour products.

Since a baby can't tell you how he or she feels, you may not know whether you are taking in too much salt or giving the baby too much. However, there are a number of symptoms which you can recognize, including:

1. Excessive hunger.
2. Excessive screaming. There are generally two main varieties of crying, 1) screaming, which usually means that the baby is too yang, and 2) whining, which often means that the baby has become too yin.
3. Tightness or lack of flexibility in motion or lack of motion.
4. Loss of the ability to crawl or walk.
5. The development of bowed legs, as in rickets.
6. The failure to grow. If a baby is small at birth, for example, five to six pounds, there is no reason to worry; since they are more yang, smaller babies often have more vitality and capacity for growth than over-sized babies. Following birth, however, a baby should actively begin to yinnize (expand) and should grow rapidly. Salt can prevent this from occurring and cause the baby to remain small.
7. Sluggish circulation, resulting from constriction of the peripheral capillaries.
8. Abnormal weight. There is no set rate at which a baby will gain weight. Some babies gain weight more rapidly, others more slowly, while others gain at a medium rate. Babies who are smaller at birth tend to gain weight more rapidly, while babies who are larger tend to gain weight more slowly. As a baby grows and becomes more yin, the rate at which weight is gained slows down.

   As long as your baby has a good appetite, you needn't be overly concerned about his or her weight, for example, to the point of weighing the baby every week or every month. However, if the baby becomes unusually thin or unusually heavy, it may be a sign of too much salt. Excess salt causes an unusually thin baby to contract and tighten, while in the opposite case, it causes the baby to retain water, fat, and other more yin substances.
9. Dry skin. A baby's skin is normally soft and smooth.
10. A change in the baby's bowel movement toward dark or hard stools. (See the previous discussion.)
11. In some cases, a high fever. Salt-induced fevers are less common than the other symptoms presented here. Fevers can be caused by a variety of other dietary imbalances in addition to salt.
12. Irregular appetite. As mentioned above, salt can cause a baby's appetite to become excessive. However, the baby's appetite may soon diminish as the

digestive tract becomes overly tight and constricted.

If your baby has any of these symptoms, or if you suspect an overly yang condition, the first step toward restoring balance is to reduce or avoid the excessively yang factors in your diet. (If the baby is older and is eating grains and vegetables, review his or her diet and make the appropriate adjustments.)

When adjusting your diet, reduce or avoid using salt or salty condiments and seasonings in your cooking or on your food. In general, the naturally sweet taste can be emphasized more. Grains such as sweet rice or oats, which are higher in fat and protein, can be served more often, and grains can be cooked with a little more water than usual in order to create a softer consistency. Sweet-tasting vegetables such as squash, carrots, or onions can also be served more frequently, and lighter, shorter cooking methods can be emphasized. *Shiitake* (dried Japanese mushrooms) can also be cooked with your vegetable dishes or used in soups on a regular basis. Sea vegetable condiments, such as green *nori* flakes or roasted *kombu* or *wakame* powder, may be used in place of *gomasio* or other condiments containing salt.

Be careful, however, not to take foods that are overly yin in your attempt to restore balance. Taking an excessive volume of fruits, liquids, concentrated sweeteners, or other more yin items will make you and the baby weaker and, unless the excessive yang factors in the diet are reduced, will not help solve the problem. A small volume of cooked applesauce, apple juice, or fruit compote can be eaten on occasion to relieve excessive tightness caused by salt, but again the volume and frequency should be moderate. If possible, it is better to adjust your cooking methods and types of grains and vegetables that you are using in order to balance an overly salty condition. Time, patience, and flexibility are especially important when making adjustments in your baby's condition.

Adjusting the baby's environment is also helpful in balancing this condition. Warm baths help discharge salt and other minerals and can be given to the baby on a daily basis. Keeping the baby in a quiet room, with few visitors or distractions, handling him or her with slow movements, and making sure that the baby is always lying on a soft cushion or blanket can also help relax an overly tight and irritable condition.

Digestive Problems

1. *Diarrhea:* When a baby develops diarrhea, the color of the stools usually changes to green and remains so over some period. A baby who has an occasional green bowel movement does not necessarily have diarrhea. Together with a color change, the stools of an infant with diarrhea are very watery and expansive. Babies with diarrhea frequently pass many stools. Mucus in the bowel movement is also a common symptom.

As mentioned above, diarrhea is usually an indication that the mother and baby's nourishment is overly yin, including the intake of cold, icy foods and drinks. However, diarrhea can also arise from the intake of eggs, poultry, meat, or other unbalanced items that cause an immediate toxic effect. If your baby develops diarrhea while you are breast-feeding, avoid eating excessively yin foods such as fruit, fruit juice, carob, honey, maple syrup, and other concentrated sweeteners, and highly acidic vegetables. Raw salad is also best avoided until the baby's condition improves, as are flour products, oily, greasy, or sticky foods, including nuts and nut butters, and animal products. In general, it is better to cook with less water than usual so that your foods have a slightly drier consistency. It is also important to eat only hot foods during the period in which the diarrhea is active.

If the condition causes discomfort in the baby, simple *palm healing* is very effective in bringing relief. Several methods of palm healing are discussed in the following section.

2.   *Constipation:* There are several varieties of constipation seen in newborn babies, ranging from mild to severe. Constipation can arise from an excess of either more yin or more yang items in the mother's diet.

After the first several months, a breast-fed baby's bowel movements normally become less frequent. Once a day is normal; however, some babies have them only every other day or even further apart. In some cases, when the baby does have a bowel movement, it is of normal color and consistency. In others, it is very watery.

In the case of irregular bowel movements with a normal appearance, the cause could be an excess of either more yin or more yang factors in the mother's diet. An excess of more yin factors causes the intestines to become swollen and loose and lacking in the contracting power necessary to move digested foodstuffs with the normal frequency. An excess of more yang factors causes the intestines to become overly contracted and lacking in the flexibility to create the rhythmic expanding and contracting movement needed to move digested foodstuffs properly. Flour products, an excess of more sticky foods, and baked or overly salted dishes can contribute to this condition.

In the case of watery and irregular bowel movements, the cause is an excess of more yin factors in the mother's diet, which makes her milk too thin and watery. The intestines then become overly loose and expanded, and the baby must strain through muscular exertion to try to force the bowel movement out.

Another type of constipation is caused by an overly yang condition, and the main symptom is hard, dark stools which are often difficult to pass. More yang constipation can arise when the mother is eating too much salt, flour products, animal foods, too many baked or overly cooked dishes, or not enough fresh or lightly cooked dishes. This type of constipation is far more common in babies fed cow's milk formula.

In most cases, constipation can be relieved by making adjustments in your diet or, in the case of older children, in the child's diet. For example, soft, lightly cooked foods are often helpful for more yang constipation, and occasional special dishes such as cooked applesauce or lightly sweetened *kuzu* can also be eaten. Supplementary treatments are usually unnecessary. However, if the baby develops a high fever as a result of, or together with, constipation, or goes several days beyond his or her usual schedule without having a bowel movement, then an enema can be given.

The enema solution can consist of warm water (about body temperature) or warm *bancha* tea in which a pinch of sea salt has been added. A small infant can receive about four ounces of solution and a one-year-old can receive about eight ounces.

It is recommended that a rubber ear syringe with a soft tip be used when giving an enema to an infant or small child. Fill the bulb completely so that air will not be introduced into the intestines. The tip can be lubricated with a small amount of sesame oil. Gently insert it about an inch or two and squeeze the bulb slowly and gently. As you insert the tip, rotate it in a slow spiral motion; the more slowly you insert it, the less liable it is to make the baby feel uncomfortable and expel it.

The large intestine expands and contracts in waves, and if you feel a strong resistance, wait until it relaxes before pushing again. Slowly squeeze the bulb until it is empty. As you withdraw the tip, press the buttocks together in order to hold the solution in for several minutes and allow it to begin softening the stools. If the water does not come out after 15 or 20 minutes or if it comes out without much stool, the enema can be repeated. There is generally no danger from the solution staying in.

It is usually not advisable to give enemas too often for the problem of constipation. The most effective method for relief of constipation is to review your diet and make the appropriate adjustments. However, various supplemental treatments can also be helpful. Babies who have become constipated due to the tension caused from the overintake of salt will often relax following a warm bath. Palm healing, which will be discussed in the next section, is also effective in bringing relief.

3. *Spitting Up and Vomiting:* Babies frequently swallow air while nursing which causes an air bubble to develop in the stomach. Holding the baby face down on the shoulder and lightly patting the back will help bring up any air that has been swallowed. This procedure is known commonly as "burping" the baby. Burping can be done after each feeding, during any long pauses in the course of a feeding, or if the baby shows some sign of discomfort following a feeding.

Babies sometimes spit up small quantities of milk while burping. Spitting up can occur if the baby takes more milk than the stomach can hold comfortably or if the baby is shaken or held too tightly. If the breast milk becomes too thick and sticky, it may not flow rapidly enough from the breast. It can also lead to swallowing air and frequent spitting up and burping. Foods that create a thick, sticky quality of breast milk include oil, flour products, concentrated sweeteners such as maple syrup, rice honey, or barley malt, dried fruits, nuts, various types of hard candies, including those made from grain sugars, mushy oatmeal, and other items with a thick or sticky consistency.

An opposite or more watery quality of milk can cause the same symptom. If taken in excess, items such as raw fruits, salads, fruit juices, carbonated beverages, and beer and other fluids make a woman's milk too thin and watery. Watery milk tends to flow more quickly through the nipple and can lead to the frequent swallowing of air and to the baby's taking an overly large volume at each feeding.

Vomiting is different from the type of spitting up described above. Vomiting means that the contents of the stomach are ejected forcibly, so that they are propelled several inches from the mouth. Frequent vomiting usually means that the baby is having stomach trouble, probably including the presence of mucus. Foods that make the milk thick and sticky contribute to the formation of excessive mucus, as do animal fats, including dairy products, fruits, and refined sugars. If a breast-fed baby vomits frequently, it is important for the mother to avoid these items and to eat a very clean, macrobiotically balanced diet. Cow's milk formula also leads to the formation of excess mucus and to frequent spitting up or vomiting.

Sneezing and Coughing

Babies sometimes sneeze when their noses have not been cleaned properly. Sneezing is one of the natural processes through which excessive mucus is discharged. There are generally two types of sneezing which babies experience, and these are dependent upon the quality of nourishment being received. A sticky quality of milk frequently causes hard, dry mucus to form in the nostrils. When the mucus causes irritation, the baby will sneeze in an attempt to discharge it. A thin, watery quality of milk frequently causes the tissues which line the nostrils and nasal cavities to become swollen and easily irritated. If a particle of dust or lint enters the nasal passages, irritation can trigger a sneeze. Similarly, dust or lint are more likely to accumulate or cause irritation if the nasal passages are sticky and filled with dried mucus.

Today, the majority of people suffer from chronic blockage of the sinuses. Many of these cases begin in infancy and are caused originally by the quality of nourishment received at that time.

If your baby sneezes frequently while you are nursing, review your diet so as to determine the factors that are causing excess to develop and then make the necessary adjustments. Cotton swabs or a nasal syringe can also be used to help keep the nostrils clean and free of mucus.

Along with accumulating in the sinuses, mucus frequently builds up in the lungs. Coughing is the natural mechanism that helps the baby to discharge these excessive factors. It is caused by the foods listed above and, in most cases, will disappear once these excesses are reduced or avoided in the mother's diet. If a baby coughs frequently, it is important for the mother to be very careful about her diet until it improves. Flour products, concentrated sweeteners, fruits, and fruit juices are best avoided during the recovery process. If more yin items are craved during this time, it is preferable to eat lightly cooked vegetables, sweet tasting vegetables, sweet tasting grain dishes, and boiled salads.

In some cases, the buildup of mucus and other excessive factors in the baby's boby triggers a variety of discharge mechanisms, sometimes all at once. The most common symptoms include a runny nose, sneezing, and coughing, and, in some cases, fever. These symptoms are generally referred to as the "common cold" and result from excesses in the mother's diet which are transferred to the baby. In most cases, the symptoms of a cold are usually mild in infants under one year of age. However, if the underlying dietary imbalance which causes the buildup of mucus and other excessive factors continues, the child faces a greater possibility of experiencing more severe symptoms in the future, including high fever, inner ear infection, tonsillitis, vomiting, diarrhea, bronchitis, and other complications. These symptoms are generally more common after the first year.

In some cases, the accumulation of mucus in the nose makes it difficult for the baby to breathe while nursing. Nasal obstruction can usually be relieved by sucking the mucus out with a nasal syringe. To do this, squeeze the bulb, insert the tip into the nostril, and then slowly release the bulb.

Measles

If a baby is nourished macrobiotically and is in good general health, there is only one sickness that can be considered normal and necessary. That sickness is measles. Every baby should have the measles, and the sooner it appears, the better; ideally within three years after birth.

Measles is actually not a true sickness. True sicknesses are caused by excesses in the diet. Suppose, for example, that a person consumes an excessive amount of fruit or cold liquids during the summer. As the weather begins to cool during the fall, the more yin elements contained in these foods become excessive, and in order to balance the environment, they are discharged through symptoms such as fever, coughing, or diarrhea in what is commonly referred to as a "cold." Conversely, items such as salt, and oily, heavy foods such as fish and *tempura* are frequently consumed during the winter. As the season changes to spring, often the body cannot tolerate this excess and various symptoms of discharge begin. This discharge of excessive yang factors is often referred to as "spring fever."

Measles is also caused by the discharge of excess but, unlike other sicknesses, it is not the result of excessive dietary factors or seasonal changes. Rather, it occurs as a baby enters a new period of growth and is similar to a snake shedding its skin. During the embryonic period, a baby is nourished by a diet of concentrated animal food in liquid form, the mother's blood. After birth, a baby must become more yin in order to grow, and for growth to proceed smoothly, the excessive yang quality accumulated during life in the womb must be discharged. Measles is nothing but the discharge of these excessive yang factors.

A baby cannot grow smoothly without having the measles. A healthy baby will normally have the measles within the first three years and preferably before he or she is a year old. However, if a mother consumes more yin items like sugar, milk, orange juice, and others throughout pregnancy, or while she is nursing, her baby's more yang quality will often be weakened and the onset of measles may be delayed until the child is much older.

At the present time, measles is often viewed as an abnormal process and as something that should be prevented through injection with a vaccine. However, as with the removal of the tonsils and adenoids, this approach overlooks the underlying cause and the fundamental importance of this natural discharge process.

When a child develops the measles, he or she must be attended to very carefully. Inexperienced parents may make mistakes and not handle the situation properly.

Measles normally begins with a fever and other symptoms resembling a cold, such as red, watery eyes, a slight loss of appetite, fatigue or tiredness, and a hard, dry cough. The temperature usually rises as each day passes; children under the age of two generally have lower temperatures, while older children frequently have higher ones. The rash usually appears within three or four days, beginning as indefinite pink spots behind the ears. The spots gradually spread over the face and body, and become larger and darker colored. The day before the rash begins, tiny white spots surrounded by redness appear on the inside of the cheeks next to the lower molars. These are known as *Koplik's spots*, and they normally go unnoticed.

Usually, several days go by before the rash comes in fully, during which time the fever may remain high and the coughing continue. The fever and other symptoms normally begin to go away once the rash has reached its peak.

The best way of approaching the measles is to encourage the rash to come in as completely as possible. The rash and fever are signs that the more yang quality accumulated in the womb is now coming out. Since this more yang quality is unnecessary for life in the air world, it is important that the baby discharge as much of it as possible.

In general, external treatments or special dishes are not needed when treating the measles. If the condition occurs while you are breast-feeding, the best approach is to make your diet as clean and simple as possible, avoiding extremes that could cause complications such as ear abscesses, bronchitis, or pneumonia.

It is important not to apply *tofu* plasters or any of the other external treatments or special dishes for reducing fevers. Instead, we recommend encouraging the baby to discharge his or her excess. Discharge will occur more smoothly if you make the baby's surroundings as yin as possible. To do this, you can:

1) Keep the baby in a somewhat darkened, quiet room. Pull all of the shades down, close the curtains.

2) Keep the air slightly moist by placing a pot or two of steaming water in a corner of the room. Electric steam vaporizers can also be used, but they are generally less efficient than humidifiers. Care is also needed because a small child may touch the vaporizer or knock it over. An electric hot plate can also be used to heat a pot of water in the baby's room, or wet towels can be placed on a radiator.

3) Keep the baby warm, but not hot. Keep the windows closed and the child properly dressed and covered. However, occasionally allow fresh air to come in the room by opening the window slightly. The room should be kept comfortably warm.

Many parents do not understand the importance of allowing the measles to discharge. A common mistake is to try to stop the fever. Some parents try to do this by applying cold towels, *tofu* plasters, or ice packs to the baby's head, or by putting a fan in the room or leaving the windows open to let cool fresh air in. These methods prevent the measles from discharging fully. As a result, the discharge is directed inside toward the lungs, intestines, stomach, or other organs. The suppression of the discharge and the internalization of the measles weaken the internal organs. If it occurs together with an excessive or unbalanced diet, more serious complications are likely to occur. Complications are generally more frequent and more severe in children over the age of three or four, as older children have had more time to accumulate excessive factors from their diets. If parents take a baby outside in the fresh air and sunshine as soon as the measles appear to be over, some portion of the discharge will also go toward the inside. Accordingly, a baby should be kept at home for about a week after the measles have been completely discharged and have disappeared.

If the measles are not handled properly, the discharge of excess will probably take another form. A high fever may arise after a week, a month, or several months, at which time a more serious complication may develop.

Meningitis is one of the complications that can result from handling the measles improperly. Meningitis is the medical term for inflammation of the membranes surrounding the brain and spinal cord. It is accompanied by a very high fever and, if not treated properly, can cause death or extensive brain damage.

A breast-fed baby receives antibodies which convey protection from a variety of illnesses. Meningitis is one of the illnesses that breast milk helps protect the baby against, and the incidence of meningitis is far lower among breast-fed babies than it is among babies who are fed by other means. However, it can arise among breast-fed babies if the quality of milk becomes overly yin from the intake of sugar, sugared drinks, milk, yogurt, other dairy foods, tropical fruits, alcohol, drugs, spices, stimulants, and other more expansive items. It can also arise if a child eats too many of these foods.

If meningitis is suspected, there are several traditional remedies that can be applied as a part of home care. First, a *tofu* plaster can be placed on the head—preferably all over the head—in order to reduce the fever. The *tofu* plaster can be prepared by squeezing the water from *tofu*, mashing it, and adding 10 to 20 percent pastry flour and about 5 percent grated ginger. The mixture can then be spread onto a piece of cheesecloth or cotton towel and applied so that the *tofu* comes in contact with the skin. The plaster can be changed as soon as the *tofu* becomes hot and used in this way until the fever begins to come down.

With the *tofu* plaster in place, hot towels can be repeatedly applied to the base of the spine for 10 to 15 minutes in order to activate the circulation and reduce the probability of the infection becoming lodged in or around the spine. A third application—a mustard plaster—can be applied to the back of the neck and spine following the *tofu* plaster and hot towel application. Either yellow mustard or mustard powder can be used. To prepare, dilute mustard (or mix dry mustard with water and stir into a paste) with 30 to 40 percent whole wheat pastry flour, spread onto a paper towel, sandwich it between two thick cotton towels, and apply this "sandwich" so that it covers the back of the neck and the back of the head behind and between the ears. It is here that the infection of meningitis frequently lodges and causes damage to the brain and nerve membranes, or *meninges*. The mustard plaster can be left on for about 10 to 20 minutes during which time the skin will become red and warm. However, do not allow the skin to become too hot, for example to the point where blisters start to form. Clean off any remaining juice with a warm towel after removing the plaster. If, after the plaster has been removed, the skin remains hot and causes obvious discomfort, cool cabbage leaves, Chinese cabbage leaves, or other leafy greens may be applied to the hot area for several minutes to absorb the remaining heat. The mustard plaster helps prevent the infection from penetrating into and lodging itself in the deeper tissues of the brain and spinal cord. The possibility of brain damage can therefore be minimized through this procedure.

Meanwhile, a nursing mother must be very careful with her diet during this period, taking care to avoid all excessive or extreme foods. At the same time, in order to minimize the spread of infection, she can make the quality of her milk more balanced by taking *ume-sho-kuzu* drink once each day for several days. (If the child is no longer breast-feeding, a very mild *ume-sho-kuzu* drink can be given directly.)

A high fever does not always mean that meningitis has developed. As mentioned above, the measles usually require no additional home treatments other than changing the baby's environment. However, if the temperature rises to 103°F., or over, there may be danger of some harm to the brain. When a very high fever arises, a plaster made of finely chopped, raw green vegetables, known as a *chlorophyll plaster*, can be applied. To prepare it, chop fresh greens such as collards, bok-choy, or Swiss chard very finely. Mash the chopped leaves thoroughly in a *suribachi* for about two or three minutes. Spread the mashed leaves about a quarter-of-an-inch thick onto a piece of cheesecloth or small cotton towel. Apply to the forehead so that the mashed greens come into direct contact with the skin. The plaster can be applied for a short while until the temperature drops slightly.

If your baby develops a temperature above 103°F., you need to consider the possibility that meningitis, pneumonia, or some other complication is developing. With meningitis, the temperature can reach 105°F. or higher. However, other symptoms are usually present when more serious disorders develop. Pneumonia can be suspected when the temperature climbs rapidly, the breathing becomes rapid, and there is a cough. In addition to a high fever, the symptoms of meningitis include vomiting, stiffness of the neck with a tendency of the head to be pulled backwards on the shoulders, twitching, spasms or stiffness in the arms or legs, convulsions, restlessness, irritability, dilation of the pupils, and frequent squinting caused by increased sensitivity to light. If any of these symptoms appear, the home care treatments described above can be started immediately. Medical assistance should also be sought immediately, due to the possibility of serious complications.

Fever

Because of the complications that sometimes result from improper handling of the measles, if your baby has not had them, it is better to treat a fever as you would the measles. In this way, there is less danger of driving the discharge inside as a result of suppressing the fever.

A baby's body temperature doesn't stay fixed at 98.6°F., but fluctuates slightly depending on the time of day and on the baby's activity. It is normally lowest in the early morning and highest in the later afternoon. The body temperature is also frequently higher following activity than it is after a period of rest. The temperature following activity may go as high as 100°F., without necessarily indicating a fever. In order to tell whether or not the baby has a fever due to illness, the temperature can be taken after a period of rest or minimal activity.

The average temperature taken by mouth is 98.6°F. Rectal temperatures normally average 99.6°F., since the area where the temperature is taken is more inside the body. The temperature of the armpit, which can be used when taking the temperature of an older child, is generally in between. A well cleaned rectal thermometer can be used in the mouth, and a mouth thermometer in the rectum, provided it is inserted slowly and gently.

It takes from one to two minutes for the thermometer to register in the rectum, slightly longer in the mouth, and up to four minutes for an accurate reading from the armpit. Shake the thermometer down before using it. Hold the upper end firmly between the thumb and finger and shake with a sharp, snapping motion. Shake the thermometer until the mercury goes down to about 97°F. When taking the rectal temperature, dip the bulb of the thermometer into sesame oil. Place the baby on his or her stomach across your knees, and insert the thermometer gently into the rectum. Push it in with a gentle twisting motion, and allow it to find its own direction. Don't hold the thermometer rigidly but allow it to move slightly as the baby moves. Once it has been inserted, lay the palm of your hand across the buttocks and hold the thermometer lightly between two of your fingers in a manner similar to the holding of a cigarette.

To take the temperature in the armpit, place the bulb of the thermometer in the armpit and then hold the arm flat against the chest. Either type of thermometer can be used. It is usually necessary to wait until a child is five or six before taking the temperature by mouth. It is recommended that thermometers be used only when necessary and not excessively.

Fevers can be caused by the excessive intake of more yang items such as meat, fish, shellfish, poultry, eggs, or salt; by the excessive intake of more yin items like sugar, ice cream, fruit, fruit juice, and concentrated sweeteners; or by the combination of both extremes. When a fever arises, it is important to check to see whether other symptoms are present which would indicate that measles or some other specific disorder is developing. By taking the baby's overall condition into account, the underlying cause of the problem can be determined together with the proper dietary adjustments and home care.

If your baby develops a fever without additional complications, a variety of medicinal foods or external applications can be used to reduce it. Fevers that represent the simple discharge of excess are often the result of constipation. If the baby turns out to be constipated, an enema will frequently bring relief and help lower the fever. In many cases, this treatment is sufficient; no other special treatments are necessary and the fever will often come down by itself.

It is better for the baby not to have a bath during a fever, and the baby should be kept warm.

In some cases, the baby can be given the juice from a sour, or Pippin, apple. Cut an apple in half, grate it, and squeeze the juice into a saucepan. Add one or two grains of salt, bring to a boil, reduce the flame and simmer for about a minute. Let it cool to body temperature and feed to the baby on a teaspoon. A teaspoon or so should be sufficient.

The apple juice helps to quiet any disturbance in the stomach, while applesauce helps to reduce fever in the intestines. Although sour apples are preferable, if you cannot locate one, a regular apple can be used.

To keep the baby from becoming dehydrated, keep the temperature of the room warm and the air moist. Any of the methods described previously can be used. The baby can also drink a small amount of rice or barley tea.

A baby will normally begin to perspire after drinking juice or tea. Keep the baby well dressed in cotton clothing and wrapped in cotton blankets. Change the cloth-

ing or blankets if they become wet with perspiration. If the hands or feet become
cold while the fever is discharging, they can be gently scrubbed with a facecloth
that has been dipped in mild warm water. Remember that it is important to keep
the baby from developing a chill during a fever. If the fever is localized in the head,
keep the chest and abdomen warm. If the baby shows signs of chilling, a warm
roasted salt pack can be applied to the abdomen. To prepare, roast salt in a dry
pan until hot and then wrap in a thick cotton linen or towel. Allow the salt to
cool slightly and then apply to the abdomen.

Children over the age of one can be given a slightly stronger medicinal bever-
age to reduce fever. Either *shiitake* mushroom tea or a tea made from dried shredded *daikon* and *shiitake* can be used. To prepare *shiitake* tea, place one dried *shiitake* mushroom in a saucepan and add a cup of water. Bring to a boil and simmer
for several minutes as you would when preparing other teas. To prepare the dried
daikon and *shiitake* tea, place one *shiitake* mushroom and one tablespoon of dried
daikon in two cups of water. Bring to a boil, reduce flame to medium low, and
simmer until one cup of liquid remains in the saucepan. Babies should receive no
more than one or two teaspoons of the liquid. Small children may have up to half
a cup. The usual grated *daikon* teas which are recommended to reduce fever in
older children and adults are too strong for small children or infants.

If the temperature goes above 103°F., the chlorophyll plaster described previously can be used to help lower the temperature, especially in the head. If the
chlorophyll plaster does not cause the temperature to drop sufficiently, a *tofu*
plaster can then be used. However, remember that *tofu* is very cold and, except
for specific emergencies, is best left on for no more than 10 minutes.

Bronchitis and Pneumonia

Bronchitis and pneumonia, while similar in that they both affect the lungs, are
actually opposite in nature, and should be treated quite differently. Bronchitis is
a disease of the more peripheral part of the lungs—the trachea and bronchi. It is
a more yin disorder, lingering for a longer time, while pneumonia is usually more
sudden and acute. Pneumonia is a much deeper condition, affecting the alveoli, or
compact air sacs deep within the lungs. People with more frail constitutions are
usually afflicted with bronchitis, while stronger, more hardy types often get pneumonia, especially if their diet includes a large volume of meat and animal products.

1. *Bronchitis:* There are many degrees of bronchitis, from very mild with no
fever, to severe with high fever, chest pain, loss of appetite, and frequent coughing.
A child with bronchitis may make a squeaky noise while breathing, and mucus
can often be felt vibrating when a hand is placed on the chest.

Bronchitis is caused by the consumption of strong yin foods including sugar,
cold drinks, fruit, and soft dairy fat. The severity of the symptoms depends upon
the type and volume of the items consumed. Extreme yin items such as sugar, ice
cream, and tropical fruits tend to produce more severe cases of bronchitis, while
less extreme items such as locally grown fruits and juices, concentrated sweeteners
such as maple syrup or grain malts, herbal teas, or too much liquid would tend to

produce a milder case. The consumption of excessive yin items during pregnancy helps create a more frail or weakened constitution with an increased susceptibility toward bronchitis.

The fever and coughing of bronchitis are nothing but the body's attempt to burn off and expel accumulated excess. If possible, it is better to let the fever run its course. If it becomes dangerously high, a chlorophyll plaster can be applied as described previously. If the green vegetables do not bring down the fever to a suitable level, the short time *tofu* plaster described above can be used.

If the bronchi are tight and filled with mucus, so that the baby is obviously experiencing discomfort, a mustard plaster can be applied to the upper chest or upper back. (The preparation of the mustard plaster is described in the discussion of *meningitis*.) However, when a mustard plaster is used on an infant or small child, do not use mustard or mustard plaster only, as this is too strong. Dilute the mustard or powder with 30 to 40 percent whole wheat pastry flour. Apply the mustard plaster for a short time only—just until the skin becomes slightly red—and clean off any remaining juice with a warm towel after removing the plaster.

Since the underlying cause of bronchitis is the overconsumption of excessive yin foods and beverages, these items are best avoided until the condition improves. If you are breast-feeding, even the consumption of fruit or foods cooked with too much water can delay the baby's recovery. If a mother's diet contains too much fruit, oil, liquid, or flour products, her baby can easily develop a chronic cough that periodically erupts into bronchitis.

2. *Pneumonia:* Pneumonia frequently comes on after a child has the symptoms of a cold for several days, although, in contrast to bronchitis, it may arise suddenly. It can result in serious complications or even in death if not treated properly. Pneumonia occurs frequently in the spring or summer, while bronchitis is more common in the autumn and winter. The underlying dietary cause of pneumonia is the repeated consumption of more yang foods, such as animal food, heavily salted dishes, or strongly cooked dishes including fried and deep-fried items, in combination with extreme yin foods like sugar, ice cream, or iced drinks. Pneumonia can be suspected when the temperature climbs to 103°F. or 104°F., the breathing becomes rapid, and the baby develops a cough. The cough is often less frequent than with bronchitis. Although drugs are usually effective in relieving the acute symptoms of the disease, the underlying cause is not addressed.

Aside from the more common pneumonia described above, a variety of "atypical" pneumonias also occur. Many of these unusual varieties are more yin than the acute variety. The symptoms are often less severe, although the illness tends to last for a longer time.

Pneumonia often comes on when someone whose overall condition is overly yang suddenly takes in strong yin. It often results from an attempt to balance extremes in the diet, for example, taking cold, sugared drinks in an attempt to neutralize the effects of eating eggs or meat. Therefore, if your child develops pneumonia while you are nursing, immediately simplify your diet by eating soft-cooked grains and very mild vegetable dishes.

Then, in order to reduce the activity of the inflammation, a cold application can be applied to the lungs. The most effective application for reducing the fever of pneumonia is a plaster made from carp. Carp is a very yin, slow moving fish. Carp meat is therefore very effective in neutralizing the more yang condition which underlies pneumonia.

If you can obtain a live or freshly killed carp, then you can first give a little of the carp's blood to the baby. Giving a small volume of carp's blood is only recommended if the fish has been very recently killed; otherwise the blood becomes too toxic to use safely. Carp's blood can be taken in a small cup, about the size of a *sake* cup. An infant can be given about one-eighth of a cup and an older child about one-quarter of a cup.

Then, wrap the carp in a towel and crush it with a hammer as you would crush ice. Apply the crushed carp to the baby's chest and check the temperature frequently, as it will probably drop very quickly, most probably within 30 minutes. Remove the application when the temperature has dropped to about 97°F.

If you are unable to get a live or freshly killed carp, you can apply high-fat, chopped raw hamburger, cold, directly to the chest and the back. Replace with new hamburger when the application becomes hot. Continue applying raw hamburger until the fever drops, usually within a few hours.

The home treatments for bronchitis and pneumonia produce opposite effects in the body. With bronchitis, a hot compress to the chest increases circulation and helps break up tightness and congestion, while, in order to subdue the chest inflammation of pneumonia, a cold compress is required. Although the symptoms of these sicknesses often seem similar, it is important to carefully determine which illness the baby has before treatment is applied. If the wrong treatment is applied in either case, the result could be very serious.

Ear Infections

The ears are a common site for the accumulation of fat, mucus, and other excessive factors in the body, as are the lungs, bronchi, and sinuses. The cause of accumulation is excess in the diet, especially more yin items such as fruit, sugar, milk and other dairy foods, concentrated sweeteners, fruit juice, and sugared drinks, together with animal fats and oily or greasy foods. In the case of nursing infants, a mother's intake of these items affects the quality of her milk and can also cause the buildup of excess. Coughing, a runny nose, fever, and ear infections represent the body's attempt to localize and discharge accumulated excess.

Ear inflammations frequently accompany colds during the first several years of life, especially if a mother consumes an excessive volume of more yin foods and beverages while she is nursing or if the child consumes them on his or her own. It is difficult to tell whether an infant has a painful ear inflammation since he or she can't tell you what is wrong. However, a baby with a pain in the inner ear may continually rub the ear or may cry steadily for several hours. A fever may or may not accompany ear infection.

If your baby develops an ear infection while you are nursing, stop the intake of excessive yin foods, including fruits, fruit juice, milk and other dairy foods, concentrated sweeteners, including grain sweeteners, salad, and reduce the intake of fluids. A cool chlorophyll plaster can be applied to the painful ear, while several drops of heated and strained sesame oil can be put in the ear with an eye-dropper. To prepare, warm several tablespoons of sesame oil in a saucepan, until it just reaches the boiling point. Strain through sanitized cheesecloth or sterile cotton and store in a small jar. Before applying the oil, place the jar in a saucepan of water and heat until lukewarm. Put several drops in the ear with an eye-dropper. If the ear is discharging thin watery pus, it is better not to use the sesame oil drops. In this case, the chlorophyll plaster described in this chapter can be applied, and a piece of sterile absorbent cotton can be placed in the ear opening to collect the discharge. A *tofu*/green vegetable plaster, applied directly behind the ear, can also be helpful. Mix an equal amount of *tofu* and mashed leafy greens in a *suribachi*. Add 10 to 20 percent whole wheat pastry flour and spread on cheesecloth or cotton linen. Apply to the region of the head directly behind the painful ear. Replace with a fresh plaster when the application becomes warm.

Palm healing is also effective in relieving inner ear pain. Please see the following section for a description of the methods for use in these cases.

Jaundice

Jaundice is the yellow discoloration of the skin and whites of the eyes resulting from an elevated level of *bilirubin* in the blood. Bilirubin, a more yang chemical, results from the breakdown of hemoglobin. Red blood cells, which have an average lifespan of 120 days, are broken down in the lymph system. The bilirubin which results from the breakdown of red blood cells is carried to the liver where it is chemically processed and secreted into the bile. Most of it passes into the small intestine and is discharged with the feces. A small amount is excreted by the liver into the bloodstream. The accumulation of bilirubin in the bloodstream indicates that a person's condition is overly yang.

A large percentage of newborns experience what is referred to as *physiologic jaundice*. On the second or third day, the skin and whites of the eyes begin to take on a yellowish color. In many instances, the discoloration begins to fade by the end of the first week.

If a mother consumes too much salty food, hard baked flour products such as hard, "brick type" bread, cookies, muffins and similar items, and not enough fresh, lightly cooked vegetables, her condition, as well as that of the baby, can easily become overly yang or contracted. In many cases, the internal organs, especially the more compacted organs like the heart, liver, spleen, and kidneys, become small, tight, and unable to function normally. Any disturbance in the functioning of the liver can interfere with its ability to process bilirubin. In many cases, the liver cannot produce enough of the more yin enzyme that causes the bilirubin to dissolve in the bile.

The injection of synthetic oxytocin to induce or stimulate labor can also cause jaundice in the newborn. Oxytocin is the more yang pituitary hormone that causes the uterus to contract during and after labor.

To offset jaundice, a nursing mother can change her style of cooking and choice of foods to emphasize more lightly prepared dishes. More soft cooked grains, lightly steamed green vegetables, and dishes with a very light taste would be suitable for this purpose. Salads, with a small amount of *umeboshi* or brown rice vinegar dressing may be included in the diet, together with a small volume of cooked fruit such as applesauce or apples cooked in *kuzu*. A small amount of barley malt may be added during the preparation of these desserts. In general, the salty taste should be reduced. In many cases, simple dietary changes such as these can help the baby recover from jaundice within several days.

Palm Healing

Of the many natural treatments available for the recovery of health, simple palm healing is one of the most effective and easy to use. Because it is based on the subtle adjustment of the body's electromagnetic energy, and requires nothing other than our two hands, it is very safe and carries no risk of harmful side effects. It is an ideally safe method for helping babies recover from sickness.

In Japan, palm healing is referred to as *Te-Ate*, or "hand application." It was widely used in the past as a method of restoring health together with dietary adjustment. (The term *Te-Ate* is still used in Japan to describe medical treatment in general.) References to palm healing can also be found throughout history. In the Bible, for example, there are many recorded instances of its use, especially among Jesus and his disciples.

Palm healing is derived from the intuitive use of our native healing abilities. People often use it without realizing it. When someone has a headache, for example, or a stomachache, they often place a hand on the afflicted area for relief. Or, when a child falls, a mother will often comfort the child by placing her hand on the hurt area or by gently stroking the forehead. It is from intuitive practices such as these that palm healing developed into a highly refined art.

To activate your healing power before practicing palm healing, sit with your spine straight and shoulders and elbows relaxed. Place your hands together, lightly touching. Extend your thumbs outward, and place them on either side of the vocal cords in the region of the throat *chakra*, or energy center. Keep your elbows raised slightly, close your eyes, and breathe normally and quietly. Sit in this position for about a minute and then begin breathing more deeply, allowing your abdomen to expand during the in-breath and contract with the out-breath. After several deep, slow breaths, add the sound of SU on the out-breath, continuing five or six times. Then return to normal, quiet breathing and slowly detach your thumbs from the throat energy center and gradually separate your hands. Slowly open your eyes and relax your posture. You are now ready to apply your palms for healing.

This practice helps to increase your conductivity to heaven and earth's forces while activating the flow of healing energy in the palms and fingertips.

Below are examples of palm healing in the treatment of common problems in infants and children.

1. *Digestive problems:* To treat diarrhea, constipation, gas, or other intestinal problems, place the baby on his or her back, sit close by with a straight but relaxed posture, and breathe in a normal quiet way. Place one hand lightly

nter of the palm covers the navel or
your eyes and breathe with a quiet
keeping your hand lightly on the
also add the sound of SU on the
after 15 to 20 minutes.

If the baby is experiencing problems in the stomach, place your hand further up on the abdomen in the area just below the ribcage. The breathing can be done as above. This method is especially good for calming a baby who is colicky or hyperactive as a result of indigestion or gas pains. Palm healing can be given several times a day until the condition improves.

2. *Eye problems:* To treat problems with the eyes, including mucus discharges, watery or bloodshot eyes, and others, place your palm across the bridge of the nose so that it covers both eyes. (An alternative method is to treat each eye separately by placing the center of your palm directly over the eye.) Breathe as described above.

3. *Nasal blockage:* To treat blocked sinuses and/or nasal passages, place your hand across the bridge of the nose. Treat as described above.

4. *Ear problems:* To treat inner ear infections, dry, cracked skin behind the ear, or other ear disorders, place your hand over each ear and treat as above. To treat the related organs, the kidneys, place your hand across the middle of the back and treat as above.

5. *Skin problems:* To treat lumps or masses on the neck, place your hand lightly on the neck so that the center of your palm is directly above the cyst. Treat as above. For swelling in the head or scalp, place your hand over the swollen area and treat as above. You may also place your hand on the side of the head so that the center of the palm covers the temple. Treat one side at a time. Skin markings, such as those described earlier in the chapter, can also be treated with palm healing. Apply your hand to the affected area so that the center of the palm is directly above the skin marking. Skin rashes or discharges can be helped by treating the intestines and kidneys. When treating skin rashes directly over the affected area, however, do not actually touch the skin. Treat by holding your palm slightly above the skin.

6. *Difficulty with sleeping:* If your baby has difficulty sleeping, apply your palm to the forehead and treat as above. Then move your hand to the side of the head and treat each of the temples as described in number 5 above. It is also advisable to treat the abdominal area as described above.

7. *Crying and nervousness:* To help quiet a nervous or hysterical baby, apply your palm to the forehead and treat as above. Then, apply your palm to the base of the spine and treat as above. Following this, you can also apply your palm to the top of the head and slowly slide it down the back of the head and down the spine to the buttocks. Repeat several times, using a slow gentle motion. These treatments are also effective in calming hyperactive children.

As mentioned earlier, crying and nervousness are often related to indigestion and problems in the intestines. Treating the intestines is recommended in these cases.

8. *Lung or bronchial troubles:* To treat lung mucus, coughing, bronchitis, or other respiratory problems, place your hand across the chest region and treat as above. You may also treat each lung separately. The lungs can also be treated by placing your hand on the upper back in the region of the shoulder blades.

9. *Fever:* Apply your palm to the baby's forehead and treat as above. You may also apply the treatment to the back or sides of the head or back of the neck. Since fevers are often related to blockage or stagnation in the intestines, it is recommended that they be treated as well. In some cases, fevers are localized in particular organs. Treat the affected organ in these instances.

10. *Jaundice:* Treating the liver and gallbladder is often helpful in cases of jaundice. Place your palm on the right side of the abdomen just below the ribcage and treat as above. (You may also treat the liver or gallbladder from the back or sides.)

Caring for Your Baby

When your baby becomes sick, it is important to remember that he or she cannot tell you what is wrong. Unlike adults, children do not know what to do for their condition. It is usually much easier for adults to judge their own condition and when problems arise to apply their understanding to determine whether it is serious and what treatments are needed.

However, a baby's symptoms are often a great deal more difficult to understand. Since a baby's metabolism is much more active than an adult's, problems may develop, change, and produce new symptoms at a much faster rate than in adults. Babies are also more sensitive to strong foods than adults are. If we give them some special food or drink, or if a nursing mother changes her diet, it will affect them much more strongly.

When caring for your baby, it is important to keep your condition clean and your judgment as sharp and quick as possible, in order to adapt to the speed and sensitivity of the baby's condition. It is also wise in many cases to seek the advice of experienced macrobiotic parents or doctors who understand your way of life.

However, remember that such situations also arise for your benefit, to make your judgment sharper and clearer. Learning to solve problems with your children's health is part of your responsibility as a parent and part of gaining a deeper and more practical understanding of life, health, sickness, and the laws of nature.

In one sense, caring for your children is simply an extension of caring for your own health. But in a larger sense, caring for your family also develops your understanding of society and ability to care for all of humanity.

Baby Food

When a baby is six to eight months old and the teeth start to grow, and he or she begins to half-stand, you may begin giving the baby soups and lightly cooked green and root vegetables, together with softly cooked whole cereal grains. You can also begin introducing a small amount of sea vegetables in the baby's diet.

Since babies are very yang and are growing quickly, their food should be very light and soft—more yin than the usual adult food. If you give your baby plenty of raw vegetables, however, the result is a weakening of the baby's digestive tract. Baby food needs to be cooked with plenty of water over a low flame. It can then be mashed in a *suribachi* or baby food grinder. (Electric blenders are not recommended.) The baby's cereals can be made a little more yin—as mother's milk is more yin—by adding a small amount of sweetener such as barley malt or rice honey. Of course, salt or salty tasting foods are not recommended while the child is still small.

The baby can receive only breast milk until teeth start to come in. You can then decrease the amount of milk and begin introducing other foods. Babies often show interest in what you are eating at the table. They often begin to reach for food and try to put it into their mouths. However, do not give the baby the same foods that you are eating. You should begin preparing special food for their stage of growth, food which is milder and lighter than that which you are eating.

For the next four months you can continue decreasing the amount of breast milk while increasing the amount of semi-solid foods. In the beginning, the baby's main foods, whole grains, should be very soft and sweet tasting, with the flavor and consistency of mother's milk. You can gradually make the grains harder and firmer by cooking them with less water. You also can increase the amount of vegetables, which in the beginning are thoroughly cooked and mashed, and begin to introduce beans, sea vegetables, and other side dishes. However, it is recommended that the majority of the foods that you prepare—at least 50 percent—be in the form of cereal grains of different varieties.

You can begin to stop nursing about four months after the baby's teeth start to come in. A slightly salty taste can be added between the ages of 14 and 18 months, but it should be *very* mild, not at all like adult food. At that time you can begin using a very small amount of sea salt, *miso*, and *tamari* soy sauce. Then, by the time the child is about four years old, he or she can generally eat the same types of foods that adults do, however, with a much milder taste. You can usually give the child normal adult food after he or she is about six years old, while still being careful with foods that are especially salty or strong.

Throughout childhood, always observe your child's condition and be flexible in your selection of foods and in how you prepare them. If you notice that the child is always thirsty, for example, modify the diet by making it less yang. Also, some babies like brown rice so much that they eat too much of it and do not eat enough vegetables or other side dishes. As a result, they may become overly yang and contracted; their legs may become tight and fail to develop in a straight, strong, and flexible way. As you can see, parents must watch their children carefully to make sure that enough vegetables, beans, and other side dishes are eaten and that the child has enough variety.

Below are specific suggestions for introducing foods to your baby:

- *Whole cereal grain milk* can be introduced after eight months to one year as the main food. (The recipes for preparing grain milk are presented on page 164.) The main ingredients are brown rice, sweet brown rice, and barley. Millet and oats can be included from time to time, while buckwheat, wheat, and rye are usually not recommended. If you introduce grain milk at an early age, for example, at less than five months, it is best digested if it is very thoroughly mashed in a *suribachi* or food mill. For babies under the age of one, a small volume of rice honey or barley malt may be added as a sweetener. The proportion of water to grains can vary, depending upon the age of the baby. Younger babies generally require more water in their preparation. Grain milk which is made from flour products or creamy grain cereals which are made from flour are best avoided.

- *Soups* may be introduced after five months. They may include vegetables, together with *wakame* or *kombu*, that have been thoroughly cooked and mashed so that they have a creamy consistency. It is recommended that sea salt, *miso*, or *tamari* soy sauce not be added before the baby is ten months old.
- *Vegetables* can be introduced when teeth start to come in and usually after the baby has been eating grains for about a month. It is better to begin by introducing sweeter tasting vegetables such as carrots, cabbage, squash, onions, *daikon*, and Chinese cabbage which have been thoroughly boiled or steamed and then mashed into a creamy form. Because babies often have difficulty with green leafy vegetables which are tough and fibrous, special efforts are often necessary to make sure that they eat them. Children often prefer more sweet tasting greens like kale and broccoli over more bitter tasting ones like watercress and mustard greens. Very mild seasonings may be added after the baby is ten months old.
- *Beans* can be introduced after eight months. It is better to use only small amounts of *azuki* beans, chickpeas, lentils and other beans which are cooked with *kombu* or vegetables. Beans can also be well cooked and thoroughly mashed.
- *Sea vegetable* dishes can be introduced as part of daily consumption after one and a half to two years, although from the beginning grains, beans, vegetables, and soups can be cooked with sea vegetables, even though the sea vegetables themselves need not be eaten.
- *Fruit and fish* are generally not needed as a part of daily consumption. However, for occasional use, locally grown, temperate climate fruits can be cooked or mashed after one and a half to two years of age and introduced to the baby in small amounts. A moderate volume of white-meat, non-fatty fish may also be introduced at this time.
- *Quick, light pickles* may be introduced after two to three years of age.
- *Beverages* may include spring or well water that has been boiled and cooled; *bancha* twig tea, cereal grain teas, apple juice (warmed or hot), and *amazake* which has been boiled with twice as much water and cooled.

By the age of four, children can eat according to the standard macrobiotic diet with a very moderate use of salty seasonings or condiments. Fish is generally unnecessary as a part of daily consumption, although older children may have a small amount of it on occasion. It is generally recommended to avoid giving fish or ginger to babies or infants. Among the possible tastes, the naturally sweet taste is used most frequently in preparing baby foods.

7 | Birth Defects

It is vitally important for every woman to guard her own health and that of her baby during pregnancy. If through the intake of improper foods or other substances a woman damages or destroys the condition of her blood, the quality of her offspring could be permanently damaged. Women are the biological guardians of the human race. If they disregard their natural biological superiority, as many women are now doing, the biological foundation of humanity will collapse, and the quality of the human species as a whole will rapidly decline. Therefore, the correct practice of macrobiotics, especially during pregnancy, is particularly relevant in our modern age. The practice of macrobiotics is crucial to the future health and development of the human race as a whole.

Heredity or Diet? A Discussion of Birth Defects

The memory of biological evolution is stored within the *deoxyribonucleic acid*, or DNA, in each cell. Although DNA is composed of only six basic substances, it can store about three billion genetic messages or "memories."

DNA is constructed like a spiral staircase; a pair of coils wind around each other, one charged more with heaven's force or contracting effects and the other with earth's force or expanding effects. The spirally twisted coils are linked by rungs composed of four different chemical bases. The sequence of bases differs with every species, and it is this sequence, together with the vibrational quality of the DNA as a whole, that determines the type of baby that is born.

Although the combination of the bases may vary almost to an infinite degree, all human babies have the same basic structure. The memory of the evolutionary process, therefore, must be generally the same for all people. Individual differences must be the result of differences in the quality of each person's DNA in combination with differences in the types of nourishment that each of us receives during pregnancy and throughout life. Individual differences also vary almost infinitely.

If DNA is somehow damaged, the memory that it contains becomes incomplete. If this occurs in the DNA contained within an egg or sperm that combine at conception, the baby that develops may "forget" how to create two eyes, a nose, or a fully-developed brain. The baby may be born with one eye or with three eyes, or with some other structural defect. What is the origin of these defects? They must originate prior to conception when the quality of the parental reproductive cells is being determined. Since the quality of the reproductive cells is already established at the time of conception, what the mother does after that has little or no effect in this respect.

Usually, babies with such fundamental deformities are capable of living in the watery environment of the womb, since all of their essential functions are taken care of by the placenta. However, most of them are unable to survive outside the womb—where they must assume their own vital functions independently—and die soon after birth. The number of such deformed births is higher than most people realize. According to some estimates, the incidence of major congenital deformities is about 2 percent of all live births in the highly industrialized countries. When combined with minor defects, the incidence may be as high as 10 percent.

The quality of the DNA in the reproductive cells is not fixed or static but changes in response to variations in the quality of the blood which continually nourishes these cells. Our daily food is the most important factor in determining the quality of our blood and therefore is crucial in determining the quality of the reproductive cells and the DNA which they contain. In the female reproductive system, for example, the egg must pass through the ovarian follicle during the process of maturation. The follicle cells are continually nourished by blood, the quality of which changes from day to day as a result of the foods that are eaten.

The father's diet also affects the health and well-being of his children. His eating habits change the quality of his sperm cells and the DNA they contain. The quality of his reproductive cells, in turn, is transmitted to each child he and his wife produce.

If the reproductive cells, and the DNA that they contain, are normal when they combine at conception, the baby will in most cases develop a complete human form. The fertilized ovum has but one goal, to develop into a complete human being. To accomplish that goal, the baby must be continually nourished by a clean and healthy quality of blood. The highest quality of blood is created by eating whole cereal grains and other foods that are suited to human development. However, if a pregnant woman takes in foods or other extreme substances that upset her blood quality, or if she is exposed to some extreme environmental stimulus, such as radiation, her baby may not develop properly, even if there is no defect in the DNA. Some types of mental retardation, for example, arise as a result of what a woman takes in following conception. In other types, including many cases of *Mongolism*, or *Down's syndrome*, a defect in the DNA combines with improper diet during pregnancy to create a constitutional deformity. The original genetic defect is caused by an improper diet and way of life, and is therefore potentially preventable. In some cases, exposure to a very yin environmental stimulus, such as radiation, can weaken the quality of a woman's reproductive cells. However, whether or not an original defect develops into a severely retarded child can also be determined by what a mother eats during pregnancy as well as the child's diet following birth. Many cases of Mongolism, therefore, can be considered as disorders of both the *primary constitution*, which is determined by the quality of the parents' DNA, and of the *secondary constitution*, which is created by the mother's intake during pregnancy.

Among the many types of congenital retardation involving both primary and secondary constitution, four basic categories can be identified:

Type 1: Some retarded children have sharp, pointed teeth, very close-set eyes, and ears located high on the head. The ears have very little or no lobes and are often pointed at the top. These babies frequently make growling sounds. Occasionally their actions become wild and uncontrollable. This type of baby is produced when a woman consumes a tremendous quantity of meat throughout pregnancy, as often as two to three times per day.

Type 2: Many retarded children have a large, full face and square jaw. The eyes are usually far apart and widely opened. The sinuses are often clogged with deposits of fat and mucus. These children have a mild, gentle disposition, but their mental activity is often dull. They frequently make very long, gentle sounds and their skin is usually soft and milky white in color. Type 2 babies result from the overconsumption of milk and other dairy products during pregnancy.

Type 3: Another type of retarded baby has a small head and a very prominent nose. The mouth and lips often protrude and the eyes are larger than normal. These children move their heads with a rapid, jerky motion and have very agile necks. They also make sharp, clucking sounds. Type 3 babies arise from eating too much poultry and eggs during pregnancy.

Type 4: Some retarded children develop protruding teeth with many spaces between them. Their faces are generally smaller and more compact than normal and they are often mentally alert. The ears are usually small and thin, and these children frequently make rapid, high pitched noises. Type 4 babies result from the overintake of tropical fruit, fruit juice, nuts, and refined sugar.

These characteristics develop as a result of the types of food consumed during pregnancy. Many of these children can become nearly normal through the practice of macrobiotics, although recovery may take three to seven years. The speed of recovery depends upon how severe the deformity is and, in cases where the deformity was produced in pregnancy, at what stage during the pregnancy the deformity arose. In general, defects that are created during the early part of pregnancy or prior to pregnancy are more difficult to correct than those that arise later on. Although complete recovery may not be possible in every case, substantial improvements can often be achieved through the practice of macrobiotics.

Fetal Anomalies

Fetal anomalies result from extremes of yin and yang—usually in the form of dietary imbalances—over- or under-nutrition, drugs or medications that are toxic to the developing embryo, or external influences such as radiation. Abnormalities may influence structure or function. Functional abnormalities include conditions such as unusual protein metabolism, *hemophelia*, color-blindness, and *photophobia* (abnormal sensitivity to light). Structural abnormalities can be classified into the following general types, which result from apparently opposite causes that produce opposite manifestations:

1. *Developmental arrest*, in which only partial growth or development occurs (for example, dwarfism or *microcephaly*); or *developmental excess*, in which growth is exaggerated (for example, giantism, extra digits, or *hypertrophy of the clitoris*).

2. *Failure of fusion*, in which paired embryonic parts which normally fuse fail to do so, resulting in conditions such as *cleft palate* or double uterus; or *fusion*, in which parts normally paired are united, as in horse-shoe kidney.

3. *Splitting*, in which parts that are normally single are paired or split, such as a ureter; or *failure to subdivide*, as in fused digits.

4. *Persistence of embryonic ducts or openings which normally close;* or *stenosis*, an abnormal narrowing of a duct or opening (for example, *aortic* or *pyloric stenosis*).

5. *Failure of migration*, in which the normal shifting of an embryonic structure does not occur, as in *undescended testis*; or *migration of structures to abnormal positions*, as in the case of parathyroids occurring in the chest.

6. *Absence of an organ or a part* (for example, absence of an arm, a finger, or a leg); or *failure to atrophy*, in which an embryonic structure that normally atrophies persists.

7. *Misplacement*, as when organs normally found in the upper region occur in a lower position and vice-versa; or when organs normally found in the right side appear on the left, and vice-versa.

Congenital abnormalities result from defects in the primary constitution, which is determined by the quality of the genes transmitted through the egg and sperm, or in the secondary constitution which is determined by the quality of the blood supplied to the embryo, together with various external influences. The former category of defects is referred to as *inherited abnormalities* and the latter as *acquired abnormalities*.

In the process of development, each organ or structure passes through a critical period, at which time the growth rate accelerates and differentiation occurs. The organs and tissues are especially susceptible to various dietary or environmental influences at these times. Generally speaking, most abnormalities originate during the *embryonic period* (from the second to the eighth week, inclusive). It is during this time that all of the organ systems develop from their respective germ layers and the fundamental structure of each organ is established. Some of the critical periods for various parts of the body are presented below:

Weeks 1 and 2: Period in which the ovum divides, implantation occurs, and the bilaminar embryo develops.

1) A harmful substance or influence will damage all or most of the cells at this time, resulting in prenatal death, or the embryo will survive with few, if any, noticeable defects. However, the baby's fundamental constitution is being formed at this time, and the quality of foods and other influences plays a decisive role in the baby's future development.

Week 3: This is a highly sensitive time for the developing *heart* and *central nervous system*.

1) Highly sensitive for the *heart* from the middle of week 3 to week 6.

2) Highly sensitive for the *central nervous system* from early in week 3 through the beginning of week 6.

Week 4: The eyes, ears, arms, and legs begin to develop during this time.

1) Sensitive period for the *eyes* is the middle of week 4 to the middle of week

8.

2) Sensitive period for the *ears* is the middle of week 4 to the middle of week 9.

3) Sensitive period for the *arms* is the middle of week 4 to the end of week 7.

4) Sensitive period for the *legs* is the middle of week 4 to the end of week 7.

Week 6

1) The *teeth* are most sensitive between the end of week 6 until the end of week 8.

2) The *palate* is most sensitive between the end of week 6 until early in week 9.

Week 7

1) The *external genitalia* are most sensitive from the middle of week 7 until the end of week 9.

Periods of lesser sensitivity

1) *The central nervous system:* the beginning of the week 6 to term.
2) The *heart:* late in week 6 to the end of week 8.
3) The *arms:* during week 8.
4) The *eyes:* middle of week 8 to term.
5) The *legs:* during week 8.
6) The *teeth:* during weeks 9 and 10.
7) The *palate:* during week 9.
8) The *external genitalia:* the latter part of week 9 to term.
9) The *ear:* middle of week 9 to the end of week 16.

The factors that influence the embryo during these critical periods and throughout prenatal life are summarized below:

1. *Dietary factors:* The maternal diet influences the developing baby through the quality of blood supplied to the placenta. An unbalanced diet can produce malformation through mineral excesses, deficiencies, vitamin imbalances, or improper balance between the other nutritional factors. The overintake of alcohol, for example, has been implicated with prenatal and postnatal growth deficiency, mental retardation, microcephaly (an abnormally small head), joint abnormalities, and congenital heart disease. Hormones secreted by the mother's endocrine system also play a direct role in the development of the baby. The balance of hormones in the mother's bloodstream is largely determined by what she eats and drinks.

2. *Hormonal factors:* Aside from the influence of hormones secreted by the mother's endocrine glands, hormones such as androgens, synthetic progesterone, cortisone, and others which are taken therapeutically have been implicated in a variety of abnormalities. Thyroid drugs, for example, have been implicated in congenital *goiter*, while androgens have produced varying degrees of masculinization of female fetuses including labial fusion or clitoral hypertrophy. Diethylstilbesterol (DES) has been shown to produce long-term effects such as cancer mostly between the ages of sixteen and twenty-two and a variety of reproductive system disorders. The reproductive

abnormalities show up, of course, throughout adult life. DES has also been associated with abnormalities in male reproductive systems.

3. *Chemical factors:* A variety of drugs and medications has been implicated in fetal malformation. Antibiotics such as *Tetracycline* and *Streptomycin* are associated with distortion of bone growth, possible congenital cataract, infant deafness, and other abnormalities. Anticonvulsant drugs, including *Dilantin*, have been implicated with cardiac defects, cleft palate, intrauterine growth retardation, and other defects, while antitumor drugs have been implicated with a wide range of defects including those of the skeleton and central nervous system. Perhaps the most well known abnormalities resulting from the use of drugs are those which resulted from the use of thalidomide. Thalidomide use has resulted in malformation of the limbs, external ears, heart, and digestive tract. LSD and marijuana have also been associated with limb malformations and severe abnormalities of the central nervous system. Smoking, especially chemically treated tobacco, also has been indicated as a risk factor for a variety of abnormalities.

4. *Radiation:* Tissues in which cells are multiplying rapidly are especially susceptible to radioactivity. A sub-lethal dose of x-rays, radium, or atomic radiation produces a variety of anomalies in human fetuses. Therapeutic radiation, for example, has been implicated with microcephaly, skeletal malformations, and mutations in fetal germ cells.

5. *Disease and disease organisms:* The syphilis organism may cross the placental barrier and infect the embryo, resulting in a variety of abnormalities. Some of the other infectious agents associated with malformations include rubella (German measles), cytomegalovirus, toxoplasma gondii, herpes simplex virus, and varicella zoster virus.

Environmental pollutants can also produce malformations. Fish contaminated with mercury have caused fetal *Minamata* disease, with neurologic and behavioral disturbances including cerebral palsy, brain damage, mental retardation, and blindness.

Emotional and psychological influences also play an important role in prenatal development, as pointed out earlier, both through their direct electromagnetic effects and through their influence on the secretion of hormones in the mother's body.

Two recently developed medical tests now frequently used during pregnancy may also have a negative influence on the unborn baby.

Amniocentesis: Amniocentesis is now becoming a widespread method of testing for congenital abnormalities during pregnancy. In this procedure, the mother is given a local anesthetic and a long, thin needle is inserted through the abdominal and uterine walls into the amniotic sac and amniotic fluid is withdrawn with a syringe. When fetal cells in the fluid are subjected to chromosomal study, they reveal fetal deformities as well as the sex of the child. However, amniocentesis involves a number of risks including injury to the fetus or planceta (between one and two complications occur per 100 procedures), infection, bleeding, leaking of the amniotic fluid, premature rupture of the membranes, possible mixing of incompatible blood types, and hemorrhage following delivery. Some of these complications may lead to spontaneous abortion, and the rate of miscarriage is generally higher among mothers who have had this procedure.

Sonography or Ultrasound: In this procedure, an image is produced on a screen by bouncing sound waves through the abdomen. The fetus is located in a manner similar to that in which a submarine is located by radar. Ultrasound is used to detect certain congenital abnormalities, locate the placenta, diagnose an abnormal fetal position, measure the size of the head and estimate the age of the baby and the due date. It may be administered prior to amniocentesis. The effects of ultrasound on mother and baby have yet to be scientifically determined. However, this unnatural application may have unhealthy influences on neurological development, emotion, and behavior, as well as the quality of blood.

Birth Defects and Disorders of the Newborn

I have met many people whose experiences illustrate the importance of eating well both before and during pregnancy, and the power of food to help correct a variety of birth defects. In one instance, a popular, active, and healthy woman became pregnant after eating a very clean macrobiotic diet for about seven years. The father had only recently become macrobiotic, and, for about four or five years prior to starting the diet, had been a heavy and regular user of marijuana, LSD, and other drugs.

She became pregnant soon after she met him. Everyone was certain that she would have a very nice baby because she had been practicing macrobiotics so well and had become a very good cook. Nine months later, however, she gave birth to a seriously defective baby. He was born without a brain, a condition known as *anencephaly*, and died soon after birth.

To understand the cause of this tragedy, refer to Chapter 2 and our discussion of how each parent influences the development of the baby's major bodily systems. The digestive system is influenced primarily by the quality of the egg and the nervous system primarily by the quality of the sperm. In this case, the mother was very healthy and her influence was normal. But the father's DNA had been damaged by drugs. Consequently, half of the baby's DNA was fine while the other half, which influenced more the formation of the nervous system, was inadequate.

Another case involved a woman who had been seriously ill and had received an injection of strong medication. She became pregnant shortly afterward. Nine months later, she gave birth to twin boys: one was normal and healthy, the other was literally a monster.

The twins are now in their early twenties. When I met them, the deformed boy was totally unable to care for himself. His mother had to lift him to feed him. She had to take care of him twenty-four hours a day, seven days a week. There is a strong likelihood that the injection she had received prior to pregnancy had damaged one of her eggs. The damaged egg was later fertilized and developed into a severely deformed baby.

Following our meeting, she began feeding the child macrobiotically and applying various external treatments. I have seen him several times since then, and the results of his macrobiotic practice have been truly amazing. The boy has gotten continuously better; he can now utter a few words, chew his own food, and smile in response to others. He is gradually becoming more normal. Although he may not be able to completely reverse his condition, he has already experienced a substantial improvement in the quality of his life.

The number of American children reported born with physical abnormalities, mental retardation, or learning defects has doubled in the past 25 years, according to researchers at the Health Policy Program of the University of California. According to data from the National Health Interview survey, the number of birth defects rose from 70,000 in the late 1950s to 140,000 in 1983. In the late 1950s an estimated 2 percent of the babies in the United States were born with defects, compared with an estimated 4 percent in 1983.

Below are a number of common birth defects and newborn disorders, with a discussion of their dietary causes. In some cases, birth defects can be improved through the correct dietary practice. Of course, the ultimate goal of macrobiotics is the prevention of birth defects through proper diet and way of life, both before and during pregnancy.

Absence of Organs or Body Parts

Many birth defects involve missing organs, limbs, digits (fingers and toes) or other body parts. In some cases, the cause of the defect lies in the dietary and environmental factors which influence the parents prior to conception, or in other words, the quality of egg and sperm which unite at the moment of conception. In others, the defect is the result of the quality of foods and other environmental factors taken in by the mother, especially in the early period of pregnancy. Below are several of the more common defects involving missing body parts:

1. *Anencephaly or Microcephaly (absent or very small brain):* As the above case illustrates, anencephaly originates prior to conception with the quality of reproductive cells. The disorder is caused by extremely yin environmental or dietary factors, including the intake of drugs and medications, or the overconsumption of sugar, soft drinks, spices, tropical fruits, ice cream, and other frozen dairy products, and exposure to radiation or toxic chemicals. The quality of the father's sperm is largely responsible for this condition.

   Microcephaly, in which a baby is born with a poorly developed brain, results primarily from the quality of foods, beverages, and other factors consumed during pregnancy. Like anencephaly, it is caused largely by the overintake of extreme yin products.

2. *Absence of Umbilical Artery:* This defect is caused primarily by the overconsumption of extreme yin foods and beverages during the pregnancy.

3. *Absence of Lungs:* This defect originates prior to conception in the quality of the egg cell, or ovum. It arises from the mother's overconsumption of

Estimated Incidence of Specific Birth Defects in the United States, 1980

Central Nervous System
Spina bifida (open spine) and/or hydrocephalus
    (water on brain)   3,500

Heart and Circulatory System
Ventricular septal defect (hole between lower
    chambers of heart)   4,250
Atrial septal defect (hole between upper chambers
    of heart)   430
Valve stenosis and atresia (heart valve defects)   470
Patent ductus arteriosus (failure of opening between
    aorta and pulmonary artery to close at birth)   6,550

Respiratory System
Defects of larynx and/or trachea   800

Alimentary System
Cleft lip and/or cleft palate   4,650
Tracheo-esophageal fistula
    (opening between trachea and esophagus)   720

Genito-Urinary System
Undescended testicles   8,820
Hypospadias (abnormal position of male
    urethral opening)   9,480
Hydrocele (collection of fluid in covering of
    testicles)   9,940

Musculo-Skeletal System
Clubfoot (without central nervous system
    defect)   9,180
Hip dislocation   8,350

Skin, Hair, etc.
Defects of abdominal wall   2,160
Hemangioma of skin (birth mark made up of
    bundles of blood vessels)   7,780

Metabolic Disorders
Phenylketonuria (PKU)   430
Cystic fibrosis   250

Multi-System Syndromes
Rh hemolytic disease of newborn   5,360
Down syndrome   2,260
Toxoplasmosis   400

Source: Centers for Disease Control.
These estimates are based on hospital discharge notes covering about one-third of the births in the United States. Only those defects evident at birth are included.

From the March of Dimes Publication, "Facts 83."

extreme yin foods and beverages before conception.

4. *Absence of Kidneys:* This abnormality originates before conception in the quality of both egg and sperm. The dietary cause includes the overconsumption of extreme yin foods, beverages, or chemicals by both parents prior to conception.

5. *Reduction Deformity (underdeveloped or missing limbs):* This defect originates during the pregnancy, especially during the time when the limb buds begin to develop (see Chapter 2). Extreme yin foods, beverages, or drugs or medications are the primary contributing factors.

6. *Syndactyly (fused digits) or Polydactyly (extra digits): Fused digits* are caused by the quality of foods, beverages, and other factors taken in during the pregnancy. The overintake of extreme yin foods, beverages, and other items causes this defect to develop. *Extra digits* are also caused by the mother's intake during pregnancy, specifically the overconsumption of meat, eggs, poultry, fish, and other more yang items. *Webbed fingers*, another deformity of the hands, are also the result of the diet during pregnancy, and are caused by the overintake of liquids, sugar, fruit, fruit juices, spices, chemicals, and other more yin items, together with a lack of minerals and complex carbohydrates in the diet.

Biliary Atresia

Biliary atresia is a relatively uncommon birth defect in which the major bile ducts that carry bile from the liver to the small intestine are either malformed or missing entirely. It is caused primarily by the excessive consumption of fats and oils, especially saturated varieties, simple sugars, and extreme yin products such as tropical fruits, coffee, and drugs and medications during pregnancy. Biliary atresia causes jaundice, incomplete digestion of fatty foods leading to chronic diarrhea and malnutrition and, if the obstruction of the bile flow is complete with no possibility of repair, liver failure and death between the ages of one and three. The standard medical treatment for this condition is surgical repair of the malformed ducts.

Cerebral Palsy

Cerebral palsy occurs when the brain is damaged during pregnancy, at birth, or in early life. The impairment of brain function causes a variety of physical and mental defects. It currently affects about 750,000 people in the United States.

In more severe cases, a problem is evident from birth: newborns with this disorder are often irritable, vomit, and have difficulty nursing. Less severe cases may not be noticed until later when the child fails to develop properly, for example, he or she may not be able to sit up or walk when the appropriate time comes. About 25 percent of the children with cerebral palsy have convulsions. About one in three hundred babies in the United States is born with cerebral palsy.

Milder cases may manifest in the form of a slight weakness in the arms and legs, combined with mild spasticity, or unnatural muscle tension. Those more seriously affected are often severely crippled.

Cerebral palsy is classified into three general types, depending on the part of the brain most affected. More than one region of the brain is commonly involved, and the symptoms tend to manifest in the legs more frequently than the arms.

Children with cerebral palsy frequently suffer other disabilities. In one study, 16 percent had a variety of visual problems, 49 percent had speech defects, and 35 percent were found to have varying degrees of intellectual impairment. Specific learning disabilities occur in many cases, and as many as 70 percent of the children with cerebral palsy have some form of mental retardation, although retardation often appears worse than it actually is due to difficulties that patients have expressing themselves.

Children with cerebral palsy often have a history of problems such as jaundice, abnormal labor, birth trauma, and meningitis, all of which are thought to contribute to brain damage. Premature babies have a higher incidence of cerebral palsy than do full term infants. Researchers now suspect that impaired blood flow to the brain during labor and delivery, which can result in brain damage, may be a factor in many cases. However, the specific disorders or injuries associated with cerebral palsy are not present in all cases. In these instances, there is no apparent medical reason for the disorder.

There is presently no medical cure for cerebral palsy. Rehabilitation is directed mostly at minimizing symptoms and includes approaches such as speech training, muscle reeducation, and psychotherapy.

The dietary cause of cerebral palsy is the overconsumption of extreme yin items such as sugar, soft drinks, tropical fruits, milk and ice cream and the overintake of fluids in general. These items contribute to difficulties in labor, premature birth, meningitis, and other developments associated with brain damage. The standard macrobiotic diet—with a limited intake of fruit and fruit juices—can contribute toward improvement of this disorder, while the macrobiotic dietary practice prior to and during pregnancy can help reduce the risk of cerebral palsy.

Cleft Lip and Cleft Palate

The overintake of more yin foods and beverages, in combination with an insufficiency of minerals, vitamins and complex carbohydrates, often interferes with the complete fusion of the palate or of the region between the upper lip and nose. Cleft palate varies in severity from a small slit in the soft palate located at the back of the mouth at the opening of the throat, to a half-inch cleft extending from the soft palate across the roof of the mouth, or hard palate, to the upper gums. The gums and teeth may also be involved. Cleft-lip, or harelip, also varies in severity from a small cleft in the upper lip to a large gap stretching from the upper lip to the nose. A proper diet during pregnancy can help prevent this disorder.

Clubfoot

Clubfoot, a more yang abnormality, is caused by the overconsumption of animal proteins and minerals during pregnancy, often in combination with too many baked flour products, and a lack of fresh, lightly cooked vegetable dishes. In club-foot, the entire foot is bent downward and twisted inward. It may affect one foot or both. Even among vegetarians, this condition can arise when too many eggs or dairy products, especially cheeses, are consumed.

Crib Death

Every year, between sixteen and twenty thousand babies in the United States die from what is referred to as *sudden infant death syndrome*. There is no apparent reason for these deaths, which typically occur at night between the ages of five weeks and five months, with the greatest number occurring between two and four months. Sudden infant death rarely occurs before the age of three weeks or after six months.

The first three months after delivery comprise the initial period of adjustment between the baby's previous life in water and the present life on the surface of the earth. During this time, the baby must establish the ability to survive as an air-breathing organism. In order to take in and successfully use oxygen, which is a more yin element, a baby must have a more yang condition. Foods that weaken a baby's native constitutional vitality, including more yin items such as simple sugars, ice cream, and milk, diminish the ability to attract and absorb oxygen in the breathing functions as well as in the quality of red blood cells, and can contribute to the sudden collapse of breathing and metabolism that occurs in sudden infant death. This problem can arise when these foods are taken by the mother during pregnancy, while nursing, or when given directly to the baby. In some cases, milk or formula enters the respiratory passages. If the milk or formula has a very sticky quality, it may accumulate and block the intake of oxygen. Synthetic clothing and blankets, which interfere with the baby's intake of environmental energy forces, can also diminish breathing power.

Cystic Fibrosis

Cystic fibrosis is a chronic disorder affecting the mucus-producing glands, especially in the pancreas and air passages of the lungs. Thick, sticky mucus builds up in the air passages of children with cystic fibrosis. It clogs the small air tubes and produces coughing, labored breathing, and fatigue. Blockage of the air tubes leads to *emphysema*, the expansion and hardening of portions of the lung, and to *atelectasis*, the eventual collapse of lung segments. When untreated, the lungs become filled with mucus and pus, and breathing is severely hampered. The result is often permanent lung damage. Cystic fibrosis currently affects about 30,000 people in the United States.

In the pancreas, thick deposits of mucus clog the ducts that connect the pancreas with the main tube that empties into the small intestine. The flow of pancreatic juice, which contains enzymes that breakdown proteins, fats, and carbohydrates, is blocked and the pancreas becomes lumpy, scarred, shrinks to a small size, and is eventually destroyed. Digestion is greatly disturbed; the stools are fatty, bulky, and foul smelling, and contain food which is only partially digested.

The resulting insufficiency of nutrients creates symptoms such as potbelly, weight loss, and increased appetite.

In some affected newborns, the blockage of pancreatic enzymes causes incomplete digestion while the baby is still in the womb. As a result, sticky meconium blocks the intestine, often in several locations, resulting in a type of intestinal obstruction known as *meconium ileus*. This condition is normally treated surgically and occurs in about 15 percent of the infants with cystic fibrosis.

A small percentage of affected children develop liver inflammation and scarring, while children with the disorder are generally more likely to suffer from *nasal polyps* (overgrowths of the mucus membranes) and *prolapse of the rectum*. Persons with cystic fibrosis also have unusually high concentrations of salt in their perspiration, and the suspicion of cystic fibrosis is often confirmed by a test that measures the salt concentration of the sweat.

At present, there is no medical cure for cystic fibrosis. The primary treatments are aimed at restoring the function of the lungs and digestive system as much as possible and include feeding the child digestive enzymes, restricting the fat intake, physical therapy, such as chest pounding to shake loose stagnated mucus, and inhaling aerosol medications.

In general, the dietary cause of cystic fibrosis is the overconsumption of animal fats, especially those in dairy products, together with the overintake of simple sugars, including refined sugar, concentrated sweeteners, and fruit. Cystic fibrosis can be improved through proper dietary practice, especially when foods such as whole cereal grains and fiber-rich vegetables are consumed as a major part of the daily intake. The macrobiotic dietary guidelines may be practiced by the nursing mother or by the affected child if he or she is no longer breast-feeding. It is important that the intake of fats and oils be minimized, including those in vegetable oils, nuts, animal products, and dairy foods. Sugar, tropical fruits, and concentrated sweeteners tend to create mucus and fat in the body and are best avoided. The overconsumption of flour products is also not recommended.

Dislocation of the Hip

This condition occurs before birth and usually becomes evident several weeks or months after birth. It may occur on one or both sides and affects the connection of the head of the *femur*, or hip bone, into its socket in the pelvis. The hip joint develops early in the embryonic period. The socket develops as a result of being in close contact with the head of the femur. If close contact is not maintained, the socket will fail to grow and will remain underdeveloped and unable to accept the ball of the hip bone securely. The hip bone will then tend to slip further out of joint, and the condition becomes progressively worse. Some babies are born with completely dislocated hips, while others have partially dislocated hips that eventually become fully dislocated.

Congenital dislocation of the hip results from the intake of extreme yin foods and beverages during pregnancy, together with an insufficiency of minerals and complex carbohydrates. The condition is made worse when a mother continues to eat extreme yin foods and beverages while nursing or if the baby is fed artificially.

The standard macrobiotic diet, with frequent servings of mineral-rich sea vegetables and tough, fibrous greens, is recommended for the nursing mother. Fruit, fruit juice, concentrated sweeteners, and uncooked dishes are best minimized during the recovery period. It is important for this condition to be properly diagnosed and treated or the child could become severely crippled.

Fig. 37 Congenitally dislocated hip.

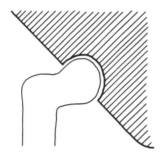 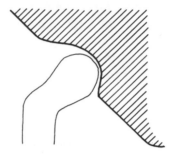

Normal hip socket and femur (head of the hip bone) in young infant.

Inadequately shaped socket and femur head of a congenitally deformed hip.

Heart Abnormalities

During the nine months of pregnancy, the developing embryonic heart is very sensitive to imbalances in the mother's diet and way of life. A wide variety of congenital abnormalities affect this organ as the result of improper diet and way of life. According to the Center for Disease Control in Atlanta, two of the more common congenital malformations—*ventricular septal defect (VSD)* and *patent ductus arteriosus (PDA)*—have increased substantially in incidence in recent years: the incidence of VSD doubled and that of PDA tripled between 1970 and 1976. These increases have continued into the 1980s; the rates of both conditions rose an additional 38 percent between 1976 and 1980.

Congenital heart defects can result when the maternal diet is deficient in minerals, complex carbohydrates, and other nutrients that produce a more contractive effect, in combination with the overconsumption of simple sugars, such as those in fruit, fruit juice, soft drinks, and concentrated sweeteners, and liquids, drugs, medications, and other more expansive items. The consumption of extreme yin items can cause the tissues that separate the various sections of the heart and normally close completely, to partially fuse and leave an opening. Incomplete fusion may occur in the tissues that divide the lower chambers of the heart *(ventricular septal defect)*, the upper chambers *(atrial septal defect)*, or those that divide the aorta and pulminary artery *(patent ductus arteriosus)*.

Other common defects include *valve stenosis* and *atresia*, in which the heart valves are abnormally narrowed or closed entirely, and *endocardial fibroelastosis*, in which the inner lining of the heart is abnormally thickened. Valve stenosis and atresia result from the overconsumption of meat, eggs, poultry, and other more yang animal foods, while endocardial fibroelastosis is caused by the overconsumption of fat, especially of animal origin.

The degree of impairment of heart function varies widely, depending on the type of defect. In many cases, congenital defects prevent the heart from pumping blood efficiently, and the result is chronic shortness of breath, coughing, pooling of blood and swelling of the liver, and accumulation of fluid, especially in the ankles. Another major complication occurs when a portion of the blood is prevented from passing through the lungs and exchanging carbon dioxide for oxygen. The blue color of this unoxygenated blood becomes visible through the baby's skin and is especially noticeable in the nail beds. Blue discoloration of the skin is known as *cyanosis*, and in very severe cases, the tips of the fingers become clubbed as a result of a lack of oxygen. Chronic fainting spells also occur.

The primary medical approach to congenital heart defects is corrective surgery. However, in some cases, the standard macrobiotic diet, when properly applied, can help restore the heart to a more normal function while strengthening the infant's condition as a whole. This is especially true in cases where the defect is the result of improper fusion of the heart tissues. Complex carbohydrates, especially those in whole cereal grains, aid in the establishment of a natural contracting process, as do foods rich in minerals, such as sea vegetables and hard, fibrous leafy greens. The proper use of seasonings and condiments is also very important. Foods such as fruits, raw foods, fats and oils, fluids and others which cause tissue expansion are best avoided or minimized during the recovery process, either by the nursing mother or child.

Hernia—Diaphragmatic

Diaphragmatic hernia is a rare congenital defect in which the diaphragm that divides the chest and abdominal cavities fails to develop properly. An opening persists, and the abdominal organs, including the stomach and intestines, frequently protrude into the chest cavity. Related complications include compression of the lungs and interference with breathing, or obstruction or strangulation of the digestive tract.

The underlying dietary cause of diaphragmatic hernia is the consumption of extreme yin foods, beverages, and medications during pregnancy, together with a deficiency of minerals and complex carbohydrates. Severe cases constitute a medical emergency, while milder cases may go undetected for several years. The standard macrobiotic diet, with the frequent inclusion of tough, fibrous vegetables and sea vegetables, is recommended for the nursing mother and for the child with this defect in order to minimize the expansion of the digestive organs which could lead to more serious complications. Extremely yin foods and beverages are best avoided or minimized, as is the intake of saturated fat. It is also best to keep the intake of vegetable oils to a minimum.

Hernia—Inguinal

In inguinal hernia, part of the intestine protrudes from the abdominal cavity and into the groin. At birth, a small portion of the *peritoneum*, or lining of the abdominal cavity, projects downward into the labia of the female and scrotum of the male. This peritoneal pouch eventually closes off and dissolves, but until it does so, the intestine may slip down into the pouch. In some cases, the sealing off of the peritoneal pouch is incomplete, leaving the possibility of hernia later in life.

Inguinal hernia is a relatively common condition, occurring in about five percent of children in the United States. Most hernias in childhood are discovered in the first year of life, and boys are affected almost ten times as frequently as girls. The most common symptom is a bulge in the groin which may come or go depending on whether the child is straining or relaxed. *A reducible hernia* is one in which the intestine slips in and out of the abdominal cavity, and *an incarcerated hernia* is one in which the intestine is stuck in the peritoneal pouch.

Fig. 38 Inguinal hernia.

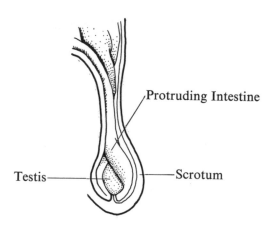

Inguinal hernia is caused by the consumption of sugar, concentrated sweeteners, fruit and fruit juice, soft drinks, milk, ice cream, spices, too many liquids, and other more expansive items. These items can influence the development of a hernia if they are taken by the mother during pregnancy or while nursing, or if they are given directly to the baby. They cause the intestines to expand beyond their normal limits and weaken and loosen the muscles of the inguinal canal. The standard treatment of hernia in infants is an operation known as *herniorrhaphy*, especially in cases of incarceration, since there is a possibility of the intestine becoming kinked and obstructed or of the blood vessels becoming compressed and leading to gangrene. However, surgery does not eliminate the cause of the problem nor change the weakened and overexpanded condition of the intestine and muscles of the inguinal canal. Their normally more contracted condition can only be established by avoiding the intake of more extreme foods and eating a moderately balanced diet. The standard macrobiotic diet is recommended as the basis for recovery, with the frequent inclusion of side dishes of tougher, more fibrous vegetables and side dishes which include *hijiki*, *arame*, or other sea vegetables.

Hydrocele

Hydrocele is the condition in which fluid accumulates around the testis. It occurs frequently when the peritoneal sac fails to seal off completely. Hydrocele is not painful and usually resolves itself. However, if it is large or continues for a year, it usually indicates that the peritoneal sac has not closed completely and that inguinal hernia may occur.

Hydrocele is a more yin condition resulting from the overintake of extreme yin foods and liquids. It can be corrected when the nursing mother avoids extremes and begins eating according to the standard macrobiotic diet. During the recovery period, it is important for the mother or the baby not to take in too many fluids and to reduce or avoid raw fruit, fruit juice, or salad and to use less water in cooking. The macrobiotic diet can help the peritoneal sac to close properly and prevent hernia from occurring by causing the baby's overexpanded organs and tissues to contract.

Hydrocephalus

Hydrocephalus, which used to be known as "water on the brain," results from an excess accumulation of spinal fluid in and around the brain. The brain tissue becomes thinner and more expanded, the bones of the skull spread apart, and the fontanel, or soft spot, becomes stretched. As a result, the head grows faster than normal and becomes enlarged.

A primary cause of hydrocephalus is an insufficient intake of minerals combined with an excessive intake of fluids during pregnancy including watery foods like fruit as well as beverages. This produces an imbalance between the baby's production of spinal fluid and the ability to reabsorb it. The intake of fats, oils, and simple sugars, which lead to mucus and fat accumulations in both mother and baby, can also contribute by causing obstructions to develop in the filtering sites on the meninges, or membranous sac, which surrounds the brain and spinal cord. The result is a backing up of excessive fluid.

Hydrocephalus can be mild or severe. Milder forms may cease spontaneously, while more severe cases can lead to stretching of the brain and to death. In some cases, the condition is present at birth and the baby's head is too large for normal delivery; while in others, the baby seems normal at birth but the head develops abnormally during the first year. The current treatment of hydrocephalus, in which excess fluid is surgically drained off, only relieves the symptoms of the condition without addressing the underlying dietary causes.

Hypospadias

In the most common form of hypospadias, the male urethral opening is abnormally located on the underside of the penis just below the normal site. In more severe cases, it is located further down on the shaft of the penis. In rare cases, the scrotum is divided into two and the opening lies between the sections. This disorder results from the overconsumption of extreme yin foods and beverages during pregnancy, especially sugar, soft drinks, ice cream, coffee and other stimulants, fruit, fruit juice, and alcohol.

Intussusception

Intussusception is an uncommon condition of infancy which usually occurs between the ages of four and eighteen months. It frequently occurs in fat and well-nourished boy babies. In this disorder, a portion of the small intestine telescopes into itself. The flow of blood through the vessels of the sucked-in section is cut off and swelling and obstruction of the intestine result. In some cases, gangrene develops, leading to *peritonitis* which is often fatal. The lining of the intestine becomes inflamed, and bloody mucus is discharged. A baby with this condition will experience sudden, severe abdominal cramps, which frequently come in short bursts, will vomit copiously, and pass stools which contain blood-tinged mucus, which are said to resemble currant jelly.

The cause of intussusception is the overconsumption of foods such as sugars, fruit, fruit juices, soft drinks, fats and oils, flour products, nuts, and excess fluids which weaken and expand the intestinal tissue. The standard macrobiotic diet, with the temporary avoidance of fruit, fruit juices, flour products, nuts, and oil can aid in the recovery process by strengthening the intestinal tissue. The current treatment by operation, although helpful in relieving the acute symptoms, does not rectify the underlying cause of the problem. Because this condition is so serious, however, emergency medical treatment is necessary. Afterward, dietary adjustments can be made to remove the cause and prevent a recurrence of this disorder.

Muscular Dystrophy

According to the Muscular Dystrophy Association, more than one million people in the United States have some type of neuromuscular disorder. One variety, muscular dystrophy, currently affects about 200,000 people. According to a spokesperson for the Association, these disorders have increased dramatically in incidence over the last 30 years.

In muscular dystrophy, the muscles of the body waste away and the patient becomes progressively crippled. Muscles under voluntary control tend to be affected most, especially those that control the legs. Muscular dystrophy develops in several ways; the most common type in children affects boys more than girls and appears as an increasing weakness in the hip and thigh muscles before the age of three. Affected children develop a waddling type of walk, have trouble climbing stairs, frequently fall down, and are unable to run. When they get older, they may lose the ability to climb stairs. After the age of puberty, most cannot walk without assistance and are confined to a wheelchair.

As the disease progresses, the patient is prone to develop pneumonia because of a limited ability to expand the muscles of the chest and cough up accumulated mucus. Some patients develop *scoliosis*, or curvature of the spine, due to weakness in the back muscles, and there is a greater tendency toward obesity due to inactivity.

Patients also develop *contractures,* or deformities in the joints due to abnormalities in muscle pull. One type of contracture occurs when the foot becomes loose and drops and causes the Achilles tendon to become tight and rigid. Contractures add to the difficulties that patients have in moving.

At present there is no medical cure for muscular dystrophy. Most therapies are aimed at increasing life expectancy through exercise and movement, and controlling the dietary intake to prevent obesity.

The dietary cause of muscular dystrophy is the overconsumption of extreme yin quality foods such as sugar, drugs, chemicals, fruits, fruit juices, soft drinks and others, together with the overintake of more yang quality food including meat, pork, eggs, and poultry. By avoiding or drastically reducing these foods, together with the inclusion of whole grains, vegetables, and other items in the standard macrobiotic approach, this condition can be improved considerably.

Obstruction of an Airway

Stridor, or *noisy breathing*, is common among infants today. It is the result of blockages that occur in the air passages—the nose, throat, larynx, or trachea. In some cases, the obstruction causes difficulty in breathing. A widespread cause of stridor in newborns is *laryngomalacia,* or congenital softening of the larynx. The larynx, or voice box, is normally firm and tight at the time of birth. However, when a woman consumes plenty of sugar, soft drinks, fruit and fruit juice, milk and other dairy products, highly acidic vegetables, and other extremely yin items during pregnancy and does not have an adequate intake of minerals and complex carbohydrates, the voice box may not become firm and compact toward the end of pregnancy but will instead remain soft and pliable.

The consumption of extreme yin items during pregnancy may cause the vocal cords to remain partially fused instead of becoming separate and distinct and may also cause the thyroid to enlarge and compress the vocal cords. Both conditions can produce stridor. A variety of tumors on the vocal cords and trachea, caused largely by the overconsumption of fats and oils, dairy foods, simple sugars, and drugs and medications, can also cause stridor.

PKU (Phenylketonuria)

Phenylketonuria is a metabolic disorder in which the body is unable to process one of the essential amino acids, *phenylaline*. In PKU, the enzyme *phenylaline hydrolase,* which is necessary for the processing of phenylaline, is deficient or defective. Phenylaline then accumulates in the blood and tissues and can damage the brain and cause mental retardation and seizures. It can also interfere with the child's overall growth and development. Children with a severe form of the disorder may vomit, eat poorly, and fail to thrive.

PKU is not a common condition. It affects about one out of ten thousand babies in North America. However, the practice of testing newborns for the disorder is widespread and is required by law in some states.

The primary treatment for PKU is dietary; the child is placed on a diet that provides only the required amount of this amino acid. Animal products, including eggs, meat, poultry, fish, cheese, milk, and other dairy products are high in phenylaline and are therefore not recommended for children with this condition. Foods such as whole cereal grains, vegetables, sea vegetables and other items included in the standard macrobiotic diet are generally lower in phenylaline and can therefore serve as the basis for the child's diet. Beans and their products, seeds, and nuts are generally higher in this amino acid and can be eaten less frequently and in smaller amounts.

If a baby with this disorder is unable to breast-feed, because the content of phenylaline is too high in the mother's milk, the cereal grain and other milk substitutes introduced in Chapter 6 can be used instead. Cow's milk and infant formula are generally too high in phenylaline for use by affected children. Synthetic milk in which the amount of phenylaline has been reduced is often given to babies with this condition. However, before artificial milk substitutes are given, the nursing mother can first reduce or avoid the intake of foods which are high in phenylaline and thereby alter the overall composition of her breast milk. If the amount of phenylaline in the breast milk cannot be reduced in this manner, the cereal grain and other natural milk substitutes can be introduced.

It is important for children with PKU to minimize or avoid the intake of animal foods throughout life. Women with PKU need to be careful of their dietary intake during pregnancy, since the overintake of foods high in phenylaline can result in the fetus being overexposed and can lead to retardation.

Polycystic Kidney Disease

An infant with this disorder develops enlarged kidneys which contain numerous cysts filled with clear or yellow fluid. Instead of the more dense tissue normally found in the kidneys, large fluid-filled spaces develop. The outflow of urine often becomes clogged or deficient as a result.

Cystic kidney disease often occurs with a similiar condition in other organs, especially the liver. In about 60 percent of those with polycystic kidney disease, the liver also develops fluid-filled cysts. One complication is pain caused by swelling of the liver capsule. This illness is most common in infancy and late adulthood.

The overconsumption of milk, cheese and other dairy products, flour products, sugar and foods treated with sugar, and foods which contain plenty of oil and fat contribute to the development of this condition. Accordingly, the avoidance of or drastic reduction in these foods, together with a shift toward whole grains and vegetables prepared according to macrobiotic dietary guidelines can contribute to improvement.

Pyloric Stenosis

Pyloric stenosis is a more yang condition in which the *pyloris*, or muscular valve between the stomach and duodenum, becomes thicker and blocks the flow of food and gastric juices. The obstruction may be partial or complete and causes the baby to vomit during a feeding or soon after. The condition is more common in

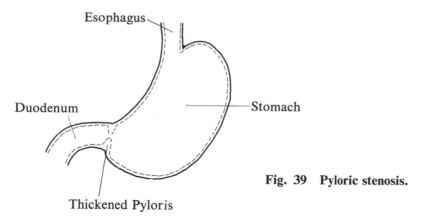

Esophagus

Duodenum

Stomach

Fig. 39 Pyloric stenosis.

Thickened Pyloris

boys and tends to recur in families. Vomiting is more forceful than the usual drooling or spitting up. Babies with this condition eventually lose weight, discharge fewer stools, and show signs of dehydration. The condition tends to worsen progressively with milder symptoms appearing before the baby becomes seriously malnourished. A baby with pyloric stenosis usually starts vomiting several weeks after delivery. The vomiting often begins as a slight spitting up and becomes progressively worse. The thickening of the pyloric muscle is known as a *pyloric tumor* and is usually about the size of a grape.

Pyloric stenosis is caused by the overconsumption of animal fats and proteins during pregnancy, including those in eggs, meat, poultry, fish, cheese and other dairy foods. The condition is accelerated when a mother continues to eat these foods while nursing or if the baby is fed cow's milk formula. The usual treatment of pyloric stenosis in the United States is an operation to remove the obstruction, while in other parts of the world, special feedings and antispasmodic drugs are recommended. However, unless the underlying dietary cause is corrected, these treatments bring only symptomatic relief.

Spina Bifida

In spina bifida (which means "two part spine"), the spinal vertebrae fail to fuse properly and do not close completely. The result is an opening in the vertebral structure. From one to six vertebrae are usually affected. When there is no associated defect of the spinal cord and nerves, the disorder does not produce symptoms and often remains undetected. This type is more common and is called *spina bifida occulta*. It results from the overintake of fluid, sugar, soft drinks, fruit and fruit juice, and other more yin items during pregnancy, together with an insufficient intake of minerals and complex carbohydrates.

In more extreme versions of the disorder, the meninges, or the membranous sac which encloses the brain and the spinal cord, protrudes through the surface of the skin. There are two general varieties of this disorder: a less extreme variety known as *meningocele*, in which the spinal cord or nerves are not present in the sac, and a more extreme variety, known as *myelomeningocele*, in which the cord and nerves are present in the sac. Meningocele results from a diet that is somewhat more extreme than that which causes spina bifida occulta, while myelomeningocele is caused by a diet that is far more extreme. In the latter condition, the part of the cord and nerves that protrudes into the sac is defective and the parts of the body which it controls do not function properly. The common treatment for both varieties is surgery and in some cases rehabilitation. However, when a mother whose child suffers from this disorder begins to eat macrobiotically, the quality of her milk can prevent further development of the condition and can serve for possible improvement.

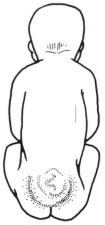

Newborn with spina bifida.

Fig. 40   Spina bifida.

Tracheoesophageal Fistula

In tracheoesophageal fistula, the esophagus is divided into upper and lower parts which do not connect with each other. The lower section extends upward from the stomach and merges with the lower end of the trachea. The upper segment of the esophagus extends downward from the mouth and ends in a pouch in the chest. A baby with this condition cannot eat or drink, while gastric juices may be regurgitated from the stomach into the trachea and lungs, leading to an infection. Aside from the inability to feed, symptoms include gagging, drooling, choking, poor color, and labored breathing. The present treatment for this relatively uncommon congenital defect is surgery.

Tracheoesophageal fistula is caused by the overconsumption of extreme yin foods and beverages, including sugar, soft drinks, drugs and medications, coffee and other stimulants, tomatoes, eggplant, and tropical fruits and juices. An example of a more yang deformity in the digestive tract is *rectal stenosis or atresia*, in which the rectum is abnormally narrowed or closed. This defect results primarily from the overconsumption of meat, eggs, poultry, fish, and other types of animal food.

Toxoplasmosis

Toxoplasmosis is an infection by a single-celled, animal parasite. The infection can be aquired by eating undercooked meat containing the organism or through contact with cat stools which contain the parasite.

When an adult is infected, there are usually few or no symptoms. It is estimated that a large proportion of adults in the United States have had the infection, but in most cases, no apparent illness has resulted. However, if a person is in a weakened condition, for example as a result of the repeated overintake of sugar, soft drinks, tropical fruits, milk, coffee, spices, and other extreme yin items, the infection is more likely to be severe. In some cases, symptoms such as mild fever, cough, sore throat, and swelling in the lymph glands can occur. Persons with cancer are more likely to experience severer forms of the disease, especially if they have received chemotherapy or radiation which weaken the body's resistance to infection. Severe toxoplasmosis can result in infection of the brain, lung, heart, liver, and other organs and can occur years after the original infection.

Toxoplasmosis can be of concern to the newborn if the infection is acquired during pregnancy. If a woman is infected before becoming pregnant, her baby will not be affected. When the organism is aquired during pregnancy, however, there is a chance that it will cross the placental barrier. If the unborn baby is thus infected, he or she may be born with a variety of deformities such as cataracts, enlargement of the liver or spleen, infection of the brain, and hydrocephalus. Permanent brain damage, blindness, or death may result. However, the majority of children who are infected in the womb develop a milder form of the disease in which no immediate symptoms are present.

Since uncooked meats are not included in the macrobiotic diet, toxoplasmosis which is acquired by this route is therefore entirely preventable. One precaution recommended by the medical profession is for pregnant women to avoid handling cats or anything that might be contaminated by their stool.

It is important to remember that the overconsumption of flour products, dairy and other fatty foods, sugar and sugar-treated foods, fruits and juices, soft drinks, and other extreme yin items can make the fetus more susceptible to infection.

If infection has been acquired, the severity of the illness can be minimized by basing one's diet around foods that strengthen the immune system and the body's ability to resist illness. These include whole cereal grains, sea vegetables, seasonings such as *miso, tamari* soy sauce, and *umeboshi*, tough fibrous greens such as *daikon*, carrot, and turnip tops, and various macrobiotic condiments. At the same time, it is recommended that sugar, tropical fruits, spices, soft drinks, animal fats, stimulant beverages, and drugs and medications, all of which weaken the immune system, be avoided.

Undescended Testis (Cryptorchism)

As pointed out in Chapter 2, the testes remain in the abdominal cavity until late in pregnancy and normally descend into the scrotum by the time of delivery. When one or both testes fail to descend, the condition is known as undescended testis, or *cryptorchism*. There are varying degrees of undescended testis; some remain high in the abdomen while others are further down. In some cases, a testis will enter the scrotum and be pulled back into the body cavity—a condition known as *retractile testis*.

Cryptorchism can be caused by the intake of eggs, meat, poultry, fish, and salt and other minerals during pregnancy, which causes the canal through which the testes normally descend to constrict and block their passage. Retractile testis is also caused by the overconsumption of more yang foods, although to a lesser degree than in undescended testis. If the testis remains in the body cavity through puberty, sperm will most likely fail to develop within it. If both testes remain in the body cavity through puberty, sterility frequently results. In some cases, undescended testis results from the overconsumption of extreme yin items such as sugar, fruit, fruit juices, too many fluids, milk and ice cream, together with the overintake of fatty, oily, and greasy foods, especially animal fats. These items can cause the testis to become too swollen and overexpanded to pass through the canal and down into the scrotum. Both varieties of undescended testis can be improved through dietary practice according to macrobiotic principles.

Wry Neck (Torticollis)

In torticollis, or wry neck, a baby develops the tendency to keep the head tilted forward and to one side. The abnormality usually becomes apparent within a short time after delivery. Foods such as sugar, fruit, fruit juice, soft drinks, and other more yin items taken during pregnancy weaken the muscle which controls the movement of the head and neck. When the muscle is in a weakened state, it is more easily bruised or torn during pregnancy or delivery. Then, if the mother consumes too much animal food and salt, the injured muscle can contract and pull the head out of position. Wry neck can be corrected with proper diet and exercises that strengthen and relax the overly-contracted muscle.

8 | Recipe Guide

Presented throughout this book are dietary and way of life recommendations for a variety of conditions affecting sexual and reproductive health, pregnancy and birth, and the newborn baby. A variety of special dishes and beverages are mentioned, which, when included as a part of the overall macrobiotic approach, have been found to be helpful in the recovery from disorders such as those included in this book.

In some cases, instructions for preparing the recommended dishes and beverages have been included in the text. Recipes that are not presented in the text are included below, in their order of appearance in the book. Dishes or beverages that are recommended in the text for more than one condition are presented below only once. Instructions for preparing home remedies such as the ginger compress, *tofu* plaster and others have been included in the text.

We have omitted recipes for most of the basic dishes used in macrobiotic cooking, as these are presented in the cookbooks and other titles listed at the back of the book. We recommend that you refer to these publications when planning meals, as the dishes presented here represent only a small sample of the many dishes used in macrobiotic cooking. It is also helpful to attend cooking classes and lectures presented at the Kushi Institute or at a macrobiotic or East West Center in your area, and to seek qualified advice when implementing the macrobiotic diet or any of the specific recommendations presented in this and other books which deal with macrobiotic healing.

Style Note for Recipes:

| 6"–8" | 6 to 8 inches | 2 Tbsp. | 2 Tablespoons |
| 3 oz. | 3 ounces | 1 tsp. | 1 teaspoon |

● **Chapter 1/Reproducing Ourselves. To help dissolve deposits of fat and mucus.**

Boiled Daikon, Daikon Greens and Kombu

> **2 strips *kombu*, 6"–8" long**
> **1 medium sized *daikon*, sliced into ½" rounds**
> **1–1½ cups chopped *daikon* greens**
> **water**
> ***tamari* soy sauce**

Place the *kombu* in a shallow dish and cover it with water. Soak for 3–4 minutes or until soft enough to slice. Slice the *kombu* into ⅓"–½" rectangles. Place the sliced *kombu* on the bottom of a pot. Slice the *daikon* into rounds and place it in layers on top of the sliced *kombu*. Add enough water to about half cover the *daikon.* Bring to a boil. Cover, reduce the flame to low and simmer until the *dai-kon* is translucent and very soft. This will take about 30–45 minutes.

Season with a little *tamari* soy sauce and simmer about 5–10 minutes longer. Place the chopped *daikon* greens on top of the sliced *daikon.* Cover and simmer several minutes longer until the greens are cooked. The greens should be bright green when done.

If there is an excessive amount of liquid remaining in the pot when the *daikon* is done, remove the *daikon, daikon* greens and *kombu.* Dilute a little *kuzu* and add it to the remaining *daikon* cooking water. Simmer until thick. Pour the thick sauce over the *daikon, daikon* greens and *kombu.*

Dried Daikon and Kombu

2 strips *kombu*, 6″–8″ long, soaked and very thinly sliced
3 oz. dried *daikon*, soaked about 5 minutes and sliced
***kombu* soaking water**
***tamari* soy sauce**

Place the *kombu* on the bottom of a pot. Place the *daikon* on top of the *kombu.* Add enough soaking water to almost cover the *daikon.* Cover and bring to a boil. Reduce the flame to low and simmer about 35–40 minutes. Season with a little *tamari* soy sauce and simmer until almost all the remaining liquid is gone. Mix and place in a serving bowl.

● **Chapter 2/A Healthy Pregnancy. To satisfy cravings during pregnancy.**

1.   Cravings for Animal Food

Broiled White-Meat Fish

4 oz. white-meat fish (flounder, fillet of sole, haddock or other white-meat fish)
¼ cup water
2 Tbsp. *tamari* soy sauce
1 tsp. freshly grated ginger

Wash the fish. Place water and *tamari* soy sauce in a bowl. Add the ginger and the fish. Marinate for about 15–20 minutes. Remove the fish and place on a baking sheet or dish which you can broil in. Broil the fish for about 5 minutes or until done. Remove and place on a serving dish. Garnish with a sprig of fresh parsley and serve with grated *daikon.*

Grated Daikon Garnish

2 Tbsp. freshly grated *daikon*
2–3 drops of *tamari* soy sauce

Grate the *daikon* on a flat grater. Place the *daikon* on a plate or in a small bowl.

Pour 2–3 drops of *tamari* soy sauce on top of the *daikon*. Serve with fish or with *tempura*.

Tempeh and Scallions

> 8 oz. *tempeh*, cubed
> 1 cup sliced scallions
> dark sesame oil
> water
> *tamari* soy sauce

Place a small amount of dark sesame oil in a skillet and heat the oil. Place the *tempeh* in the skillet and fry 1–2 minutes. Turn the *tempeh* over and fry the other side for about 1 minute. Add enough water to about half cover the *tempeh*. Cover and reduce the flame to medium-low. Simmer about 15–20 minutes. Season with a little *tamari* soy sauce. Simmer about 3–4 minutes longer. Add the scallions on top of the *tempeh*, cover and simmer 1–2 minutes. Mix and remove. Place in a serving dish and serve.

Seitan Kimpira

> ¼ cup burdock, sliced into matchsticks
> 1 cup carrots, sliced into matchsticks
> 1 cup *seitan*, cubed
> ¼ cup celery, sliced diagonally
> dark sesame oil
> 2 cups water
> 2–3 Tbsp. diluted *kuzu*
> *tamari* soy sauce

Place a small amount of dark sesame oil in a skillet and heat. Add the burdock. Sauté 1–2 minutes. Add the carrots, and celery. Sauté 1–2 minutes. Add the *seitan* and the water. Bring to a boil. Cover and reduce the flame to low. Simmer until the vegetables are done. Dilute the *kuzu* and add to the vegetables and *seitan*. Stir constantly to avoid lumping. Season with a little *tamari* soy sauce. Simmer until the sauce is thick and smooth. Remove and place in a serving bowl. Garnish with a few sliced scallions or chopped parsley.

Fu Soup

> 4–5 cups water
> 3 oz. *fu*, soaked 3–5 minutes and sliced
> 1 cup fresh green peas
> ½ cup diced onions
> 4 Tbsp. *kuzu*, diluted
> *tamari* soy sauce
> sliced scallions
> 1 strip *kombu*, soaked and cubed

Place the *kombu* and water in a pot. Bring to a boil. Cover and reduce the flame to low. Simmer 5 minutes. Add the onion, green peas and *fu*. Simmer about 15–20 minutes. Dilute the *kuzu* and add to the soup. Stir constantly. Cover and simmer about 5 minutes. Season with a little *tamari* soy sauce and simmer several minutes longer. Place in individual serving bowls and garnish each bowl with a few sliced scallions.

Boiled Tofu

> **4–5 slices fresh *tofu*, about ½″ thick each**
> **water**
> ***tamari* soy sauce**
> **grated ginger**
> **sliced scallions or chives**

Place the *tofu* in a pot. Add enough water to just cover. Place on a low flame and slowly bring to a boil. Simmer 1–2 minutes. Remove the *tofu* and place on a plate. Serve with a couple drops of *tamari* soy sauce, a pinch of freshly grated ginger and a few sliced scallions or chives on each slice.

Dried Tofu Miso Soup

> **4–5 cups water**
> **2 cups dried *tofu*, soaked in warm water and cubed**
> **1 cup onions, sliced in half moons**
> **½ cup *wakame*, soaked and sliced**
> **sliced scallions**

Place the water, onions, *wakame* and dried *daikon* in a pot. Bring to a boil. Cover and reduce the flame to medium-low. Simmer until the onions are soft and translucent. Reduce the flame to very low and add a small amount of barley *miso*. Simmer 2–3 minutes. Place in individual serving bowls and garnish with a few sliced scallions.

Nishime (A)

> **1 strip *kombu* 6″–8″ long, soaked and cubed**
> **½ cup carrots, chunks**
> **½ cup *daikon*, chunks**
> **1 cup butternut squash, chunks**
> **1 cup dried *tofu*, soaked and sliced into 1″ squares**
> **water**
> ***tamari* soy sauce**

Place the *kombu* in the bottom of a pot. Place the dried *tofu* on top of the *kombu*. Layer the *daikon* on top of the dried *tofu*, the carrots on top of the *daikon* and the squash on top of the carrots. Add enough water to about half cover the vegetables. Bring to a boil. Cover and reduce the flame to medium-low. Simmer for about 30–35 minutes. Add a small amount of *tamari* soy sauce and continue to simmer until almost all of the liquid is gone. Just before the liquid is gone, mix the vegetables to evenly coat them with the juice of the vegetables. Place in a serving dish.

Nishime (B)

    1 strip of *kombu*, soaked and cubed or sliced
    1 cup *daikon*, sliced into ½″ rounds
    1 cup fresh lotus root, sliced into ½″ rounds
    1 cup deep fried *tofu* cubes
    water
    ***tamari* soy sauce**

Place the *kombu* in the bottom of a pot. Set the *tofu* on top of the *kombu*. Layer the *daikon* on top of the *tofu*. Place the lotus root on top of the *daikon*. Add enough water to about half cover the vegetables. Bring to a boil. Cover and reduce the flame to medium low. Simmer about 30–35 minutes. Season with a little *tamari* soy sauce and simmer several minutes more until almost all of the remaining liquid is gone. Just before the liquid is gone mix the vegetables to evenly coat them with the vegetable cooking juice. Place in a serving dish and serve.

Miso Scallion Condiment

    2 bunches of scallions, sliced
    dark sesame oil
    3 tsp. puréed barley *miso*
    ¼ cup water

Wash the scallions and the roots. Slice the scallions and roots. Place a small amount of dark sesame oil in a skillet and heat. Add the scallion roots and scallions. Sauté several seconds. Arrange all the scallions and roots in a pile in the center of the skillet. Hollow out the center of the scallions and place the puréed *miso* in the hollow. Add water. Cover and simmer about 5 minutes or so. Do not mix the scallions and *miso* until they are done. The *miso* will filter down through the scallions. Mix and place in a serving dish. Eat about 1 Tbsp. at a meal.

    Other greens such as finely chopped carrot tops, dandelions, or chives can be prepared in the same manner as the above recipe to create different tasting condiments.

2.   Cravings for Sweets or Fruit

Amazake Pudding

    2 cups *amazake* drink
    2 Tbsp. *kuzu*, diluted in a little water
    1 tsp. raisins, garnish

Place the *amazake* in a sauce pan. Dilute the *kuzu* and add it to the *amazake*. Stir. Bring to a boil. Stir constantly to avoid burning and lumping. When thick and smooth remove and place in a shallow serving dish. Garnish with a few raisins in the center of the bowl. Serve hot or cool.

This dessert can be made with cherries or other fruits, puréed squash, etc. to create other seasonally appropriate puddings.

Stewed Fruit

> **3 cups water or apple juice**
> **1 cup pears, sliced**
> **1 cup apples, sliced**
> **½ cup raisins**
> **pinch of sea salt**
> **3–4 Tbsp. *kuzu*, diluted**

Peel fruit if waxed or sprayed and then slice. Place the raisins and water or juice in a pot. Add a pinch of sea salt. Bring to a boil. Cover and reduce the flame to medium-low. Simmer about 5–10 minutes. The longer you cook the raisins the sweeter the water becomes. Add the fruit slices, cover and simmer about 3–4 minutes. Turn the flame to low and add the diluted *kuzu*, stirring constantly to avoid lumping. Simmer until the *kuzu* forms a thick clear sauce. Serve as is or over cous cous cake or buckwheat pancakes.

Other fruit can be used in this recipe to create a variety of seasonally appropriate desserts. Some examples are peaches, cherries, strawberries, blueberries, dried apricots, etc.

Hot Amazake

> **1 cup *amazake* drink**
> **pinch of ginger (optional)**

Place the *amazake* in a saucepan and bring to a boil. Remove from the flame and add a pinch of freshly grated ginger. Drink hot.

Chestnut-Dried Apple Compote

> **1 cup dried chestnuts, washed**
> **½ cup raisins**
> **½ cup dried apples, soaked and sliced**
> **4 cups water**
> **pinch of sea salt**

Wash the chestnuts and place them in a dry skillet. Dry roast the chestnuts on a medium-low flame several minutes, stirring constantly to avoid burning and to evenly roast. Remove the chestnuts and place them in a bowl. Add water to just cover the chestnuts and soak them for about 10 minutes. Place the chestnuts and soaking water in a pressure cooker or a pot. Add the raisins, dried apples, and a pinch of sea salt. If pressure-cooking, cover and bring to pressure. When pressure is up reduce the flame to medium-low and cook for about 45 minutes. If boiling, place ingredients in a pot, cover and bring to a boil. Reduce the flame to medium-low and simmer until all the ingredients are soft.

Azuki, Chestnuts and Raisins

> 1 strip *kombu*, 6″–8″ long
> 1 cup *azuki* beans, washed and soaked 6–8 hours
> 1 cup dried chestnuts, washed, dry roasted and soaked for 10 minutes
> ½–¾ cup raisins
> water
> sea salt

Place the *kombu* on the bottom of a pot. Add the chestnuts, raisins, and *azuki* beans. Add water to cover the beans. Bring to a boil. Cover and reduce the flame to medium-low and simmer about 2 hours. When the beans are about 80 percent done season with a little sea salt. Simmer several minutes longer until all ingredients are soft.

To pressure-cook place ingredients in a pressure cooker in the same order as above. Cover and bring to pressure. When the pressure is up, reduce the flame to medium-low and cook for 45–50 minutes. Bring pressure down and remove the cover. Add a small amount of sea salt and simmer several minutes longer until all ingredients are soft. Place in a serving dish or serve over a piece of freshly toasted *mochi*.

Onion Butter

> 8 cups onions, sliced into halfmoons or diced
> water
> pinch of sea salt
> dark sesame oil (optional)

If you wish to use oil, brush a small amount of oil in a pot and heat. Add the onions and sauté several minutes until they are translucent. Add enough water to just cover the onions. Add a pinch of sea salt. Cover and reduce the flame to very low. Simmer on a low flame for several hours until all liquid is gone and the onions become very sweet and creamy in texture. Cool and place in a tightly sealed glass jar to store. Keep in a cool place. Serve on rice cakes or your favorite whole grain bread.

3.   Cravings for Sour Tastes

Tempeh and Sauerkraut

> 8 oz. *tempeh*, cubed or sliced

1 cup sauerkraut
½ cup sauerkraut juice or water

Place the *tempeh* in a skillet. Place the sauerkraut on top of the *tempeh*. Add the sauerkraut juice or water. Bring to a boil. Cover and reduce the flame to low. Simmer about 15–20 minutes. Remove and place in a serving dish. Garnish with chopped parsley.

Can *Seitan* be used in this recipe instead of *tempeh*.

Seitan can be used in this recipe instead of *tempeh*.

Red Radish Pickles

1 cup sliced red radishes
***umeboshi* vinegar**
water

Place the radish slices in a pickle press or bowl. Prepare a mixture of ½ water and ½ *umeboshi* vinegar. Pour mixture over the radishes. Press for 2–3 hours. Remove and serve.

If *umeboshi* vinegar is not available, place 3–4 *umeboshi* plums in 2 cups of water and bring to a boil. Reduce the flame and simmer several minutes. Remove from flame and allow to cool. Pour part of the cooled juice over the radishes and press same as above. Save remaining juice for future pickles or salad dressings.

Other vegetables can be used in place of radishes if sliced thin.

Umeboshi Dressing

2 *umeboshi* plums
2 tsp. grated onion
2 Tbsp. chopped parsley or sliced scallions
1 cup water

Place the meat of the *umeboshi* in a *suribachi*. Purée the *umeboshi*. Add the onion and purée again. Add water and mix well. Add the chopped parsley or sliced scallions. Pour over your favorite salad.

A little *tahiani* or sesame butter can be added to this recipe at the beginning to create a creamy dressing for noodles, salads, etc.

Whole Onions and Miso

4 whole onions
1 strip *kombu*, 6″–8″ long, soaked and sliced
barley *miso*
water
chopped parsley

Place the *kombu* on the bottom of the pot. Make 6–8 shallow slices in each of the onions so that you create a sectional effect. Do not slice all the way through the onions or they will fall apart while cooking. The slices will allow the onions to open up slightly while cooking to give a flowering effect. Place the whole onions in the pot on top of the *kombu*. Add water to about half cover the onions. Dilute about 1 Tbsp. of barley *miso* and place a small amount of it on top of each of the onions. Cover and bring to a boil. Reduce the flame to low and simmer until the onions are translucent and tender.

If there is too much liquid remaining after the onions are done, thicken it with a little diluted *kuzu* and serve as a thick sauce over the onions.

Remove the onions and place in a shallow bowl. Add a little of the water from cooking the onions. Garnish with chopped parsley.

Vegetable Soup

> 4–5 cups water
> 1 cup diced onions
> 1 cup diced carrots
> ½ cup diced celery
> ½ cup fresh sweet corn
> ¼ cup fresh green peas
> 1 strip *kombu*, soaked and diced
> 3–4 *umeboshi* plums (or you may use a small amount of *umeboshi* paste)

Place the *kombu*, *umeboshi* and water in a pot. Bring to a boil. Cover and reduce the flame to medium-low. Simmer about 7–10 minutes. Add the onions, carrots, celery, corn and peas. Cover and simmer until all the vegetables are soft. Serve hot with sliced scallions for garnish.

4. Dairy Cravings

Fried Tempeh

> 2 slices fresh ginger
> 8 oz. *tempeh*, sliced
> dark sesame oil
> *tamari* soy sauce
> water

Place a small amount of dark sesame oil in a skillet and heat. Add the *tempeh*. Fry on one side then turn over and fry on the other side. Add enough water to just cover the *tempeh*. Add the ginger slices. Season with a little *tamari* soy sauce and cover. Reduce the flame to low and simmer about 20 minutes. Remove the cover and cook off remaining liquid. Place in a serving bowl. Slice the ginger and serve as a condiment, or save and use in other dishes.

Tofu Dressing or Dip

> 1 cake *tofu*
> 3–4 *umeboshi* plums, remove pit
> 1 small grated onion

¼ cup chopped scallions, chives or parsley
water (only if you want thinner dip)

Place *umeboshi* in a *suribachi* and purée. Add the onion and grind. Add the *tofu* and purée until very smooth and creamy. Add water if you desire a thinner consistency but the volume of water should not be more than a half cup. Add chopped scallions, chives or parsley and mix. Place in a serving bowl and let sit for about 30 minutes before serving.

Tofu Cheese

1 cake of *tofu*, whole or quartered
barley *miso*

Place a thick layer of barley *miso* all around the cake of *tofu* so that the entire surface is covered. Place in a deep bowl or crock and let it sit for 1–2 days. The longer you allow it to ferment the saltier and cheesier the taste becomes. Remove from the *miso* when done and wash off any remaining *miso*. Slice and serve with your favorite crackers, rice cakes or bread. Refrigerate to store.

Hijiki with Tempeh and Vegetables

1 oz. *hijiki*, washed and soaked about 4–5 minutes
1 cup carrots, sliced in matchsticks
1 cup onions, sliced in halfmoons
8 oz. *tempeh*, cubed and deep fried (frying optional)
water
***tamari* soy sauce**

Wash the *hijiki* and soak it for 4–5 minutes. Slice the *hijiki*. Deep fry the *tempeh* cubes until golden brown in light sesame oil. Remove and drain the oil from the *tempeh*. Place the *tempeh* in a pot. Add the onions on top of the *tempeh*. Place the carrots on top of the onions. Next place the *hijiki* on top of the carrots. Add enough *hijiki* soaking water—or if the taste is too salty add plain water—to cover the *tempeh* only. Place a small amount of *tamari* soy sauce in the pot. Bring to a boil. Cover and reduce the flame to low. Simmer 45–50 minutes. Season with a little more *tamari* soy sauce and turn the flame to medium. Cook remaining liquid off. There will be a very small amount of liquid left when the *hijiki* is ready. Place in a serving bowl and serve.

If you wish to avoid using oil, do not deep fry. Simply place the *tempeh* cubes in the pot and add other ingredients in the same order as above. Cook same as above.

Arame can be used instead of *hijiki*. *Arame* does not have to be soaked. If soaked it looses much of its sweet flavor and its nutrients. Simply wash the *arame* very quickly and drain off all liquid. Let the *arame* sit several minutes before preparing. It will absorb the liquid on it from washing and expand.

Sautéed Cabbage and Carrots

> **1 cup cabbage, sliced**
> **½ cup carrots, sliced thinly on a diagonal or in matchsticks**
> **dark sesame oil**
> **pinch of sea salt**
> **water**
> **1 tsp. toasted black sesame seeds**

Place a small amount of dark sesame oil in a skillet and heat. Add the carrots and sauté 1–2 minutes. Add the cabbage and sauté 1–2 minutes. Add a pinch of sea salt and several drops of water. Cover and simmer on a low flame several minutes until the carrots and cabbage are done. The vegetables should be bright colored and slightly crisp when done. Place in a serving dish and garnish with a few toasted black sesame seeds. Serve.

There are many different vegetables and combinations of vegetables which can be sautéed in the same manner as above. Use whatever vegetables are in season and combine well to make a delicious tasting dish.

● **Chapter 4/Complications and Disorders**

1. Anemia

Miso Soup with Daikon and Wakame

> **4–5 cups water**
> **1 cup sliced *daikon***
> **¼–½ cup *wakame*, washed, soaked and sliced**
> **barley *miso*, puréed**
> **sliced scallions**

Place water, *daikon* and *wakame* in a pot. Bring to a boil. Cover and reduce the flame to medium-low. Simmer until the *daikon* is very soft. Reduce the flame to very low and add a small amount of puréed barley *miso* to make a mild tasting soup. Simmer 2–3 minutes longer. Place in individual serving bowls and garnish each bowl with a few sliced scallions. Serve hot.

Steamed Greens

> **2 cups sliced greens (kale, mustard greens, *daikon* greens, turnip greens, watercress, etc.)**
> **water**

Place a very small amount of water in a pot. Place a steamer in the pot. Place greens in the steamer and cover. Bring to a boil. Steam until done. Different greens take different cooking times so adjust the time accordingly.

If you do not have a steamer, simply place about ½ cup of water in a pot and bring to a boil. Add the greens and cover. Cook until done. The greens should be bright green and slightly crisp when done. (Watercress takes less than 1 minute to cook whereas kale, which is harder, takes maybe 2–3 minutes to cook.)

Azuki Beans, Squash and Kombu

> 1 strip *kombu*, 6″–8″ long
> 1 cup *azuki* beans, soaked 6–8 hours
> 1 cup winter squash, cubed (carrots may be used as a substitute for squash. Make
>   sure to leave the skin on the squash if it is unwaxed.)
> water
> sea salt

Place the *kombu* on the bottom of a pot. Place the squash on top of the *kombu*. Next place the *azuki* beans on top of the squash. Add water to just cover the squash. Bring to a boil. Cover and reduce the flame to medium-low. Simmer until the beans are about 80 percent done which will take about 2 hours. If additional water is needed while cooking, add only enough to cover the squash and not the beans. When 80 percent done, season with a little sea salt and continue to cook until the beans are completely soft. Place in a serving dish and serve.

   Soaked wheat berries, fresh or dried lotus root, soaked, or soaked lotus seeds can be cooked with *azuki* beans in the same manner as above. In this case add water to just cover the beans.

Boiled Salad with Dulse

> 1 cup broccoli, flowerettes
> 1 cup cauliflower, flowerettes
> ½ cup carrots, sliced in chunks
> ½ cup Chinese cabbage, sliced
> ¼ cup *daikon*, quartered and sliced about ¼″ thick
> ½ cup dulse, washed, soaked and sliced
> water

Place about ½ inch of water in a pot and bring to a boil. Add the Chinese cabbage and boil about 1 minute. Remove and drain. Place the cabbage in a bowl. Next add the broccoli. Boil 2–3 minutes. Remove, drain and place in a bowl. Next add the carrots and cook until soft. Remove and drain. Place the carrots in the bowl with the cabbage and broccoli. Place the cauliflower in the water and boil until done. It should be slightly crisp. Remove, drain and add to the bowl with the other vegetables. Last add the *daikon* and cook until done. Remove, drain and add to the other vegetables. Mix the vegetables. Wash the dulse quickly and soak it for 3–4 minutes. Slice and add the dulse to the vegetables. Mix, place in a serving dish and serve plain or with your favorite salad dressing.

2.   Backaches

Shiitake Mushroom Tea

1 *shiitake* mushroom
1 cup water
tamari soy sauce

Place water and *shiitake* mushroom in a saucepan and bring it to a boil. Reduce the flame to medium-low and simmer several minutes. Add a couple of drops of *tamari* soy sauce and simmer another minute. Remove from the flame and place in a cup. Drink hot.

3.   Constipation

Azuki Beans and Wheat Berries

1 strip *kombu*, 6″–8″ long
1 cup *azuki* beans soaked 6–8 hours
¼ cup wheat berries, soaked 6–8 hours or more
water
sea salt

Place *kombu* on the bottom of a pot. Add wheat berries. Place *azuki* beans on top of the wheat berries. Add enough cold water to just cover the *azuki* beans. Bring to a boil. Reduce the flame to low and cover. Simmer about 1½–2 hours or until the beans are about 80 percent done. Add a small amount of sea salt to season and continue to simmer until the beans and wheat berries are completely done. Remove and place in a serving bowl.

Brown Rice and Wheat Berries

1 cup brown rice
¼ cup wheat berries, soaked 6–8 hours
pinch of sea salt per cup of grain
1¼–1½ cups of water per cup of grain

Place the wheat berries and rice in a pressure cooker. Mix. Add water. Place the cooker on a low flame, without sea salt or a cover. After the 20 minute soaking period on a low flame is over, add sea salt and place the cover on the pressure cooker. Bring to pressure. Place a flame deflector under the cooker and reduce the flame to medium-low. Cook for 50 minutes. Remove from the flame and allow pressure to come down. Remove rice and place in a wooden bowl. Serve.

4.   Cramps

Tamari-Bancha

1 cup hot *bancha* tea
1 tsp. *tamari* soy sauce

Place *tamari* soy sauce in a cup and pour hot *bancha* tea over it. Stir and drink while hot.

5. Swelling

Boiled Daikon

> 1 medium *daikon*, sliced into ½″ rounds
> 1 strip *kombu*, soaked and sliced (10″–12″ long)
> water
> *tamari* soy sauce

Place the *kombu* in a pot and place the *daikon* on top of the *kombu*. Add enough water to half cover the *daikon*. Bring to a boil. Cover and reduce the flame to medium-low. Simmer until the *daikon* is translucent and the *kombu* and *daikon* are very soft. Season with a little *tamari* soy sauce and simmer 2–3 minutes longer. Remove and serve.

6. Heartburn

Ume-Sho-Bancha

> ½–1 *umeboshi* plum, remove the pit and pull into two or three pieces
> ½–1 tsp. *tamari* soy sauce
> 1 cup hot *bancha* tea

Place the *umeboshi* plum and *tamari* soy sauce in a tea cup. Pour hot *bancha* tea over it and stir well. Drink while hot.

7. Herpes Simplex Infections

Waterless Sautéed Vegetables

> ½ cup burdock, sliced into matchsticks or shaved
> 1 cup carrots, sliced into matchsticks
> water
> *tamari* soy sauce or sea salt

Place a small amount of water (just enough to lightly cover the bottom) in a skillet. Bring to a boil. Add the burdock and sauté about 1 minute. Add the carrots. Cover. Reduce the flame to low and simmer until the carrots and burdock are almost done. They should be slightly crisp. Season with a small amount of *tamari* soy sauce or a pinch of sea salt. Remove the cover and sauté, moving the vegetables around constantly with chopsticks to cook them evenly, until all liquid is gone. Remove and place in a serving dish.

   Just about any type of vegetable can be cooked in this manner. Instead of cooking off all the liquid, you may add a small amount of diluted *kuzu* and make a thick sauce for the vegetables. *Tofu*, dried *tofu*, or *seitan* and *tempeh* may also be added to create delicious oilless vegetables.

8. Miscarriage

Koi-Koku (Carp Soup)

> **1 carp, freshly caught**
> **burdock, shaved or cut into matchsticks (volume of burdock should be about 2–3 times**
> **more than the volume of carp.)**
> **dark sesame oil**
> *bancha* **tea twigs and leaves (used from making tea. Do not use fresh** *bancha* **twigs**
> **as they will cause the soup to become very bitter tasting.) volume of tea twigs is**
> **about ½–1 cup**
> **water**
> **grated ginger**
> *mugi miso*, **puréed**
> **cheesecloth**

Buy a carp and ask to have the gallbladder and yellow bone removed at the fish
market, being careful not to break the gallbladder. Leave the head, tail, fins, bones
and scales on the fish. Have the insides removed and discarded. If the carp is a
female, and has eggs inside, have the market leave the eggs for you to cook in the
soup. Have the carp cut into several chunks about 3 inches or so wide, as it is very
difficult to cut at home without the proper knives.

Shave the burdock. Place a small amount of dark sesame oil in a pot or pressure cooker and heat it up. Add the burdock and sauté several minutes, stirring
constantly to avoid burning and to evenly sauté.

Tie the used *bancha* twigs and leaves in a piece of cheesecloth, forming a sack,
so that the leaves and twigs can not fall out while cooking in the soup. Place the
twig sack in the pot or pressure cooker on top of the burdock.

Place the carp chunks on top of the twig sack and the burdock. Add enough
water to cover the carp. Bring to a boil if not pressure-cooking. Cover and reduce
the flame to medium-low. Simmer for about 5–6 hours. If pressure-cooking, cook
for 2–2½ hours.

When the bones are soft remove the tea sack and discard. Purée a small amount
of *miso* with a little water or soup broth. Add enough *miso* to make a mild tasting,
not salty, soup. Simmer another hour or so. Just before serving add a little freshly
grated ginger.

If you want very soft, well cooked carp, place the carp under the burdock while
cooking. Instead of making the soup with water, light *bancha* tea can be used. This
will make the carp bones much softer. Make sure that the *bancha* tea you use is
not too strong, or it may cause the soup to have a bitter taste. The best type of
miso to use, if available, is three-year-old barley (*mugi*) *miso*. Female carp are preferable to male carp, if available, because they are more yin.

To store, place in a tightly sealed glass jar and refrigerate. *Koi-Koku* will keep
for about 1 week if refrigerated.

Garnish with a few scallion slices, or chives when serving.

● **Chapter 5/Birth and Recovery**

Homemade Mochi

> **2 cups sweet brown rice**
> **1–1¼ cups water to each cup of grain**
> **pinch of sea salt per cup of grain**

Wash sweet rice gently but quickly. Place in pressure cooker and smooth the surface so that the grains present a flat, even surface. Pour the water down the side of the pot so as not to disturb the grains. Add salt. Place cover on pressure cooker and turn flame to high. When the pressure guage begins to hiss loudly or jiggle, remove pot from flame and place a metal flame deflector on the burner. Place the pressure cooker on the flame deflector.

Reduce the flame to low and cook for 45–50 minutes. When the rice is done, remove from flame and allow pressure to come down. Remove rice from cooker with a bamboo rice paddle and place in a large, heavy wooden bowl.

Then, pound the rice vigorously with a large wooden pestle (similar to the *surikogi* which is used with a *suribachi*, but in this case, somewhat larger and heavier), until all the grains are broken and the rice becomes like a thick, sticky paste. (This may take an hour or more of pounding, so be sure to have your husband or some friends do it for you while you are resting.) The pestle can occasionally be dipped in water and a few drops of water can be sprinkled on the rice to prevent sticking.

After the *mochi* has been sufficiently pounded, wet your hands and form the thick paste into small cakes and place them on a cookie sheet that has been dusted with rice flour or oiled lightly with sesame oil to prevent sticking. You may also mold the pounded sweet rice into oblong loaves about 10 inches long, 4 inches wide and ½–1 inch thick. Dust the *mochi* with rice flour. It may be eaten as is, baked until it puffs up, or allowed to dry by leaving it exposed to the air and eaten at some later time. You may also refrigerate it to prevent mold from forming. If mold does form, simply cut it off and eat the remaining part. *Mochi* is also delicious when pan-fried in a dry skillet over a low flame. Cover the skillet and periodically turn the *mochi* over to prevent burning. Cook until each piece puffs up. *Mochi* is delicious when eaten plain or seasoned with several drops of *tamari* soy sauce and wrapped in strips of toasted *nori*. *Mochi* may also be added to *miso* soup as in the following recipe.

Miso Soup with Mochi

> **4–5 cups water**
> **1 cup *daikon*, cut into ½″ wide × ¼″ thick rectangles**
> **½ cup *wakame*, soaked and sliced**
> **4–5 pieces *mochi*, pan toasted in a dry skillet**
> **barley *miso*, puréed**
> **sliced scallions**

Place the water, *daikon* and *wakame* in a pot. Bring to a boil. Cover and reduce the flame to medium-low. Simmer until the *daikon* is very soft and translucent.

Slice the *mochi* into pieces about 2″ × 3″. Place the *mochi* in a dry skillet (preferably cast iron or heavy stainless steel) and cover. Reduce the flame to low and toast the *mochi* until golden on one side. Turn the *mochi* over and toast the other side until golden brown and the *mochi* puffs up. Remove the *mochi*. Place the soup in individual serving bowls. Add one piece of *mochi* to each bowl of soup. Garnish with sliced scallions and serve while hot.

Toasted Mochi and Grated Daikon

> **2 pieces of *mochi***
> **1–2 Tbsp. grated *daikon***
> **¼ sheet *nori*, toasted and cut into thin strips**
> ***tamari* soy sauce**

Roast the *nori* and cut it into thin strips. Place it in a small dish. Grate the *daikon* and place it in another small serving dish. Place 1–2 drops of *tamari* soy sauce on top of the grated *daikon*.

Place the *mochi* in a heavy skillet, on a low flame. Cover and toast until golden brown on one side. Turn the *mochi* over and toast the other side until golden brown and the *mochi* puffs up. Place the *mochi* on a plate. If desired, pour 1 or 2 drops of *tamari* soy sauce on each piece of toasted *mochi* before eating. If your condition is too yang you may omit the *tamari* soy sauce on the *mochi* and eat it plain.

Eat the *mochi* with the grated *daikon*, which will aid in the digestion of the *mochi*, and the toasted *nori* strips.

Seitan Stew

> **4–5 cups water**
> **2 cups cooked *seitan*, sliced into bite-sized chunks**
> **1 cup onions, quartered**
> **1 cup carrots, chunks**
> **½ cup celery, sliced thickly on a diagonal**
> **1 strip *kombu*, soaked and sliced (8″–10″ long)**
> **3 *shiitake* mushrooms, soaked, stems removed and quartered**
> **¼ cup barley, washed and soaked 6–8 hours**

Place the *kombu* and *shiitake* in the bottom of a pot. Add the onions next. Then add the celery and carrots. Place the barley on top of the carrots and the *seitan* on top of the barley. Add water. Bring to a boil. Cover and reduce the flame to medium-low. Simmer until the barley and vegetables are very soft. You may pressure-cook for 45–50 minutes instead of boiling if you wish. You may season with a little more *tamari* soy sauce, but the stew is best if it has a mild salty taste.

Garnish with sliced scallions, chopped chives, or chopped parsley and serve.

Other types of grains and vegetables may be used to make different tasting stews. Also the stew can be thickened with the *seitan* starch water left from rinsing the *seitan* or with *kuzu* if desired.

● **Chapter 6/The Newborn Baby.** *Common Problems*

1. The Overuse of Salt

Dried Daikon, Shiitake and Kombu

> **3 oz. dried *daikon*, soaked 3–4 minutes, and sliced**
> **2 strips *kombu* 8″–10″ long, soaked and very thinly sliced**
> **4–5 *shiitake* mushrooms, soaked, stems removed and thinly sliced**
> ***daikon* soaking water**
> ***tamari* soy sauce**

Place the *kombu* on the bottom of a pot. Add the sliced dried *daikon* and *shiitake* mushrooms. Add enough soaking water to cover the *daikon*. Bring to a boil. Cover, reduce the flame to low and simmer about 45 minutes or until the *kombu* is very soft. Season very lightly with *tamari* soy sace and continue to cook for several minutes more until almost all liquid is gone. Place in a serving bowl and serve.

2. Constipation

Sweet Kuzu

> **1 cup water**
> **1 tsp. *kuzu*, diluted**
> **1 tsp. barley malt or yinnie rice syrup**

Place the sweetener and water in a saucepan and bring it to a boil. Reduce the flame to low and add the diluted *kuzu*. Stir constantly to avoid lumping. Simmer until the *kuzu* becomes thick, creamy and translucent. Drink while hot.

3. Fever

Roasted Brown Rice Tea

> **2 Tbsp. brown rice, washed**
> **1 quart water**

Place the rice in a light-weight skillet and heat. Roast the rice until it is golden brown and releases a nutty fragrance. Stir constantly to avoid burning. Remove the rice and place it in a saucepan with the water. Bring to a boil. Reduce the flame to medium-low and simmer several minutes. Drink while hot.

Roasted Barley Tea

> **2 Tbsp. unhulled barley or hulled barley**
> **1 quart water**

Prepare same as above. If you are using unhulled barley, toast it until it is dark brown but not burnt.

9 | Pregnancy and Birth Experiences

Pamela Snyder, Baltimore, Maryland

Over the past ten years, I have had the opportunity to attend many births. After the home birth of my first child, I became very interested in natural birth, especially home births, and I started to attend the deliveries of all my friends' babies. At that time there were many births in our community, as many of us were newly married and starting our families. After a few years of being a birth attendant, I met a lay midwife who was willing to give classes in lay midwifery. I took these classes for over a year and during this time attended both home and hospital births, macrobiotic and nonmacrobiotic. As a result of these experiences, I noticed some differences between the pregnancies and births of women who were macrobiotic and those who were not.

Generally, I would say that most of the macrobiotic births were uncomplicated. However, difficulties did arise on occasion. One of the problems was slow labors —labors that would start but not progress. Contractions were usually frequent but mild and ineffective. Another of the difficulties was labors that started out well, with good contractions and progression, but that suddenly stopped.

At these times I tried a variety of things. In the first case, I would ask the mother to become a little more active, by walking and doing mild exercise. Sometimes I would give her strong hot *bancha*-ginger tea in the hopes of improving her circulation and getting things going. Also, I would do mild *shiatsu* massage on certain pressure points. Usually this proved to be very effective.

In the second case, it was important to pinpoint the cause of the slow-down of a labor that was initially doing well, especially if the bag of waters had already broken. Usually, I would try the points mentioned above. If after a few hours, no progress was made, I would try *moxibustion** on the points previously massaged and also give the woman something yin to drink—yinnie *kuzu*, apple juice, or beer—which proved highly effective. I would also rub, in a kneading fashion, the *fundus* (upper uterus) and this stimulated contractions. Sometimes it was necessary to rub the uterus at two or three minute intervals for a period of hours, with the woman's body eventually doing the contractions on its own. Sometimes the source of the problem was exhaustion. In this case, a warm bath and sleep would do the trick. If a woman had a lot of fear, this would also stop labor. At times I tried guided imagery. I would have her shut her eyes, talk to the child, encouraging its arrival. I would try to get her to visualize the birth in hopes this would build her confidence in herself and in her baby's well-being.

With nonmacrobiotic women, I found their labors to be longer and more pain-

* Stimulation using the active vibration of fire to release stagnation along the body's energy pathway (meridians). Dried mugwort is placed on various acupuncture points and lighted to tonify the organs and bodily processes.

ful. Sometimes I would be at a birth for three days. Because of longer labors, it was often harder for them to stay on top of the contractions, and many times they would ask for drugs. Most of these women were not very receptive to alternate ways of dealing with their problems in labor.

Another noticeable difference between these labors was the appearance of the child after birth. With nonmacrobiotic women there was considerably more vernix (the oily coating on a newborn's skin), blood, and birth fluids covering the babies. Also, these women bled a lot more. This is very ironic considering that macrobiotic women were sometimes below the required iron levels according to doctor/midwife charts.

Macrobiotic women tend to become dehydrated more quickly during birth, so it is important for them to drink throughout labor. This dehydration can lead to an overly yang condition that often goes undetected and can be a cause of interrupted labor patterns. During labor, women lose a lot of body fluid, so a little *bancha* tea or spring water is most helpful. However, we generally do not recommend giving a woman more yin herbal teas, fruit juices, teas sweetened with honey, maple syrup, or iced or chilled beverages.

Most of my experiences were with macrobiotic women at home. They were all wonderful, growing experiences for me, and I am truly grateful to each and every one of them, macrobiotic or not, for allowing me to participate.

Wendy Esko, Brookline, Massachusetts

My name is Wendy Esko and I am thirty-three years old. My husband, Edward, and I have four children, all boys.

Our first child, Eric, was born at home on October 15, 1974. This pregnancy was probably one of my easiest. I experienced no morning sickness at all. My weight gain was 17 pounds. I was very active during this pregnancy, working at the East West Foundation, in Boston. I had been eating macrobiotically for about three-and-a-half years and was doing secretarial and bookkeeping work. I was also attending Michio Kushi's evening lectures, which were given three to five days per week and often all day on weekends. My main physical exercise was in the form of walking. During this pregnancy I found that my main cravings were for high-protein foods such as beans, *seitan*, *fu*, *tofu*, and fish. During this pregnancy and all of my others, I had routine prenatal checkups with my obstetrician, a traditional doctor who has delivered hundreds of babies at home. I feel this is very important to ensure that all is proceeding well with the pregnancy. My doctor also had a midwife, who was macrobiotic, working with him. I felt extremely happy about this, and I am sure having her present helped me to be more relaxed. My labor began at 8:00 A.M. and Eric was born at 10:58 A.M., which is a total of 2 hours and 58 minutes.

The pain that I experienced with Eric and with my other children was not the same type of pain that one experiences when you hit your finger with a hammer or bruise yourself. I felt that it was more like intense menstrual cramps. One thing that I found very helpful during labor was to keep my eyes open and concentrate on some object in the room. I must have read about 100 book titles on our bookshelf! By keeping my eyes open I found it much easier to concentrate and also to relax. Whenever I closed my eyes, I found that I became too tense, and my energy was more inward. The cramping sensation became more intense with my eyes closed. This labor was somewhat different from the others in that I had no lower back cramps or abdominal cramps. Instead I had cramping sensations in my thighs. Very simple, light *shiatsu* massage on my thighs by the midwife helped to relieve this. When Eric was born he immediately began to cry, but as he was handed to me he stopped. He was very alert, looking around the room and at me.

I became pregnant with Mark in August of 1976, and he was born May 28, 1977. This pregnancy was a little more difficult in some ways than the first. I found that I often became too yang or contracted, and it was a little more difficult for me to maintain a balance. Several things which I think influenced this were: taking too much salt and *miso*, not getting outside enough and walking (winter time was a little difficult for me to get out especially since I was also working and teaching in my home), taking too many flour products, and smoking. I really recommend not smoking during pregnancy. Mark was the smallest of our children and has had some lung troubles which I believe are due to my smoking. Mark was born in a hospital because he was breech, and my doctor did not have a midwife or nurse to assist him in a home delivery. I am not sure but it is possible that having smoked the entire pregnancy may have been a contributing factor in his being breech. I was constantly thirsty, which was probably from smoking and eating too many flour products. Consequently, I drank a lot of tea and soup, which may have expanded my uterus too much, making it easier for Mark to move around instead of keeping his head down. My labor began at about 11:00 P.M. and my doctor came over. He examined me and told me that the baby was breech. I was shocked and somewhat frightened by this. My labor completely stopped because of my emotional state. I kept reflecting on what I had eaten or done to cause this situation. I went to the hospital with the doctor and a macrobiotic woman friend of mine. I was very upset by this time and found it difficult to relax. After pacing the floor in the hospital for several hours and reading many magazines and newspapers, I decided that if I was going to have the baby via natural childbirth and without any complications I had to stop blaming myself and become more positive. I began to think of my baby instead of myself and how much I wanted him to be born without any problems. My doctor was very patient and helped by reminding me that he was going to deliver the baby naturally if at all possible. Finally, I became relaxed enough to fall asleep. I awoke at 8:00 A.M. and my labor began almost immediately. My water broke at about 10:47 and Mark was born naturally, feetfirst, at 10:56 A.M. Again, a 2 hour and 56 minute labor. I left the hospital that afternoon and went home with another beautiful baby boy. Mark was an extremely good baby. He was so quiet that I hardly knew he was around. He would eat for about 5 to 10 minutes and sleep for 4 to 5 hours. He slept all night from the day he was born.

I became pregnant with Daniel in May of 1979, and he was born February 5, 1980. Although I think that this pregnancy was my most difficult, the birth was very easy. We had been living in Japan for about 10 months when I became pregnant. We left Japan just a couple of weeks after I became pregnant. I thought that I might be pregnant but did not say anything to Edward about it, as we had a 25-hour flight back to Boston and I was sure he would have worried too much about me traveling. I became extremely tired after the plane trip back. I became very yang, even sunlight made me feel sick. I was also craving all the foods we were used to eating in Japan and nothing seemed to satisfy my cravings when we got back. It took me about 3 months to finally adjust to the different tastes of the foods here and to really feel comfortable and balanced. I was slightly anemic during this pregnancy because of my imbalanced condition. Several things which helped me to correct this were a sprig of raw parsley every day in my soup or on my rice, roasted sea vegetable powders, leafy greens and *nori*.

The last few months of my pregnancy I felt very good. As with the other pregnancies, I continued my routine prenatal checkups with the doctor who had delivered our first two children. At this time he had another midwife working with him so a home delivery was done. My labor began at about 11:00 P.M. I called my doctor and midwife. As soon as the doctor arrived my labor stopped. It started up again around 12:30 A.M. and Daniel was born at 3:10 A.M. The labor went smoothly as I was very relaxed. It was very quiet in the house with the children asleep, but I forgot about keeping my eyes open during the contractions and they were very intense. As soon as the doctor cut the umbilical cord, Daniel began to cry, but then he started to make the most beautiful sounds—almost like he was singing. Even the doctor and midwife were surprised by the sounds he was making.

I became pregnant with our fourth child, Thomas, in September 1981, and he was born June 18, 1982. This pregnancy and the birth, I think, were the easiest of all our children. I did experience some morning sickness but it was again because my stomach was too tight. Simple adjustments in my diet and going for morning walks in the fresh air took away all traces of morning sickness. I read so many books when I was pregnant with Thomas; often reading until very late at night and then not getting enough rest. I think this also contributed to my stomach problems. With this pregnancy I ate the most balanced of all. My cravings were very simple. I had no cravings for fish as before but instead craved things such as green peas, corn on the cob, sauerkraut, and *natto*. Thomas is as peaceful and contented as I was during my pregnancy, and he is very happy all the time. Again, I continued my routine prenatal checkups with my pediatrician and also saw a midwife who was working with him. On June 17th we moved into a new house, which was somewhat unsettling as I was about to deliver any day. On June 18th I woke up very early and began to clean and put things away in our new home so that everything would be orderly when the baby arrived. I was doing my laundry when the contractions started at 3:00 P.M. They were very strong. I called my doctor and the midwife and a macrobiotic woman friend of mine who is studying to be a midwife. The doctor arrived around 3:30 P.M. and the midwife around 3:50 P.M. Thomas was born at 4:00 P.M. which would be 1 hour total labor. I remained active during labor as much as I could, which is probably why it went so fast. Thomas was born at home without any complications.

Throughout all of my pregnancies one thing that I constantly felt was that everything would be fine and that our children would be born healthy and strong.

I think having a positive and happy outlook is very important. Having a vision of how things should turn out can be compared to a seamstress having a pattern, a cook having a menu or ideas of how the meal will turn out, an architect having a blueprint, or a conductor having a musical score. To these people it is probably unthinkable to begin work without these definite ideas or plans. This vision became so clear to me during my last pregnancy with Thomas. Twice during the last two or three weeks of my pregnancy I actually had the same dream. I saw the birth taking place always with the same ending. The labor would be extremely short, and both times I saw his beautiful little face looking up at me and all was fine. Well, that was exactly the way the birth happened.

I practiced embryonic education (*Tai Kyo*), as described in an earlier section, with each of my pregnancies—eating good food, getting exercise, and keeping active with working, writing, cooking, cleaning, and just being a mother and wife. I did not watch violent movies, which I think is important not only when you are pregnant but also as long as you are of childbearing age. If you are exposed to overstimulating or violent scenes and situations, these experiences could affect your unborn child. I prefer not to expose myself or my children to these influences at all. I also took walks and observed and appreciated nature very much. I was so thankful to be alive and have happy healthy children, husband, and family. If you practice the form of embryonic education which is explained in this book, all will go very well for you, your baby, and your family.

It is important to give our children the best possible start in life, and I have found through personal experience that this approach does work. Of course, we must also be flexible and not rigid during pregnancy. If you have cravings, first try to find a good quality substitute. If this does not work, try having a very small amount of what you crave, avoiding meat, eggs, and sugar. There are many other substitutes for these foods which will satisfy you.

Again, keep in mind that what you eat becomes your blood, which nourishes your unborn child. I hope that we can all create happy, healthy, and peaceful children who will contribute greatly to the health, peace and happiness of all humanity and the world.

Carol Smith, San Francisco, California

My name is Carol Smith and I am thirty-two years old. I've been living a macrobiotic lifestyle now for seven years. During this time many things have changed for me. My own health has gradually improved. I'm no longer afflicted with vaginal infections, cystitis, irregular menstrual periods, kidney infections, or a preulcerated stomach. My emotional health has improved remarkably. Most of the time, I feel calm, peaceful, happy, and ready to handle any situation. I'm amazed when I look back on myself as a college student and even earlier in my life. I actually considered myself healthy and all of the problems I had as just something everyone had to put up with. Macrobiotics has changed my whole outlook on life. One attitude which I used to have was that I wasn't going to have children until I was too old to do anything else. Now I'm the mother of three beautiful children.

The first of these children was born a year before I became macrobiotic. During my pregnancy, I ate a lacto-vegetarian diet with some fish and poultry. I was constantly bothered with digestive and emotional problems. Although these are common problems in most pregnancies, I found them to be much less severe with my next two macrobiotic pregnancies. In particular, during my third pregnancy, I felt very emotionally stable and had normal digestive processes. I found many other differences between my earlier and later pregnancies, labors, and postnatal adjustments.

The amount of energy I've had for daily tasks during pregnancy has increased with each pregnancy in spite of the fact that my third pregnancy began four months after my second baby was born. The condition of my birth canal and bone structure became much stronger and more flexible. When I was carrying my first child, my doctor remarked that if it was a large child then I would have trouble because of not having much room inside. After becoming macrobiotic, with the next two pregnancies the doctors remarked that I didn't have any fat inside to obstruct childbirth and had plenty of room for any size baby. Luckily for me, since my third child weighed almost eight pounds. I was very flexible too.

Another difference between my earlier and later pregnancies concerned anemia. During my first pregnancy, I was anemic and took many iron pills. With the next two pregnancies, I took no supplements but ate a lot of greens and sea vegetables. In spite of the last two pregnancies being very close together, I didn't have problems with anemia. I believe this was due to a macrobiotic diet which strengthened my intestines and blood. My diet with the last two pregnancies consisted basically of whole grains, vegetables, sea vegetables, beans, and some fish. When I craved something that I didn't normally eat, I would first try to satisfy the craving by thinking of what I might be lacking either nutritionally or because of body imbalances. If that didn't work, I would fix something sensorially appealing in the way that the food I was craving appealed to me. As a last resort, I would have the smallest amount possible of the food that I craved. The effects of different foods are so profound on the fetus. As my babies were born, I could easily see a direct relationship between their weaknesses, strengths, and my eating habits during the pregnancy and before conception.

With my first child I didn't eat macrobiotically but lacto-vegetarian with a little fish. I also took in a lot of extreme sweets which were mostly made with honey but also some with sugar. This child has always had a very weak condition in many ways. His weaknesses, although better now, seem to be mostly in his nervous system and emotional balance. During my second pregnancy, I had taken in too much salt before becoming pregnant and I really wanted to eat raw fruit. I overconsumed and consequently my daughter has just now recovered from weaknesses in her legs, arms, and hips. By the time of my third pregnancy I was more stable in my eating and emotions, and a little wiser overall. My third baby, who is now ten months old, is very strong and happy. While pregnant with him, I ate most of my fruit cooked, some fish, and a basic diet composed of grains, vegetables, sea vegetables, and beans.

It is also interesting to me that my third child was my easiest labor and delivery. My first two labors were extremely long with unusual presentations—the first child was posterior until the very end of labor and the second child was a frank breech presentation (rear end first). My labor with the first child was very painful and of medium length (fifteen hours of hard labor). However, although my second child was breech, I noticed a big difference in my ability to relax during labor and the intensity of the labor pains, in spite of having twenty-two hours of hard labor. After all of my labors, I've felt strong again fairly quickly. However, I think that the amount of rest you get afterward, as well as the foods you eat, are extremely important. With the third child, I found my recovery period to be easier emotionally and physically even though there were two other children to take care of.

The diet that I found to work best after birth is one composed of strong but relaxing foods. I ate a basic diet of grains, beans, sea vegetables, and vegetables —as during pregnancy—with additions of *koi-koku* (carp soup), more *mochi* (pounded sweet rice), and lots of lightly cooked vegetables. I have found that for the most part it is best to avoid fruit and flour for a while after birth and then to have only small amounts. I also avoided eating a lot of oil. If I felt myself not being able to relax then I would have more lightly cooked vegetables, a little less grain, and some non-fruit dessert like yinnie-*kuzu*.

The problems that I've always had to deal with after birth are cracked nipples and breast infections. By following the above mentioned diet, I found the adjustment to nursing to be much easier. Also helpful for these problems are chlorophyll plasters to draw out infections and unblock milk ducts; sesame oil and sunshine for cracked nipples; and most important, proper rest.

As my babies grew older, I let the coming of teeth, interest in food, and hunger in spite of nursing dictate when I began solid foods. When I began weaning them, I first introduced grains cooked with just a pinch of sea vegetables. Shortly after this, I found it necessary to introduce vegetables into their diet. The grains alone didn't seem to be satisfying or relaxing enough for them. They were much happier having a balance of grains and vegetables. From here my children's diet gradually widened to include fruits, beans, and other foods. I've never fed my children much salt. In fact, not any salt at all until they were around five-years-old, with the exception of *miso* and sea vegetables. My children ate a basic macrobiotic diet of grains, vegetables, sea vegetables, beans, fruits, and occasional fish. I have given them more or less the above foods depending on their condition at the time. I found with my little girl that, due to her weakness from my fruit consumption while she was in the womb, it was necessary to feed her more strong foods, whereas my youngest is so strong that he needs more food to help him relax. So I give him lightly cooked vegetables often.

My oldest child is now of school age and that has caused some interesting changes in his diet. When he eats at home, his diet is standard macrobiotic. However, owing to peer pressure at school, I send a lunch of good quality macrobiotic foods that are prepared to look like the lunches of all the other children. This might consist of a sandwich, corn chips, juice, and a sweet snack. Now instead of thinking his lunches strange, the other children all want to eat them. My life with my children, which began with conception and which will go on forever, has been my best education. I think I now understand a little of what Michio meant when he said that men must work very hard in their lives to experience spiritual growth while all that women have to do is to have babies. I'm grateful for the growth that my children are bringing to me, and now it is my turn to help them with their development. I only hope that as the years pass I can be as effective a teacher for them as they have been for me.

Judith Waxman, Brookline, Massachusetts

My name is Judith Waxman. I was born in Nikossia, Cyprus, and raised in Israel. Currently, our family resides in the Boston area. I have been living by the macrobiotic way approximately 14 to 15 years.

Once, years before marriage, I saw a child and mother. The mother hit her child, and he cried unhappily, bitterly. But it was to her he clung for comfort and solace. Such tender beings children are. So soft, at first, yielding to be moulded into any character. I thought: Poor, grown children, many adults, hardened in the distortions of unhappiness. I always wanted children. They are humanity's treasure, preserving the fragile dream of human existence and creativity.

Through her children a woman can uncover a source of limitless and selfless love that can grow to encompass many others. Through raising children the mother can develop a natural, subtle sense of authority and an understanding of people. I, personally, did not realize the extent of my own unhappiness until after the first child's arrival, when a more lasting contentment replaced feelings of dissatisfaction. When I knew that I was pregnant for the first time, I felt a sense of awe. This was the greatest thing, of utmost importance. I thought this was so great a thing, that I would not dare handle it with the stupidity of my mind. I would not impose my own notions and concepts that must inevitably be imperfect.

Fortunately, my appetite was exaggerated to an almost unreasonable degree. Whole grains were desired (although rice, for quite a while, was unappealing) along with the full range of macrobiotic foods, but cravings for fruit were uncontrollably great. During that pregnancy, on several occasions, I ate refined commercial sweets and drank coffee. June came and labor. Long, long hours of labor. The baby came in a posterior position. A screaming boy with long earlobes. That was Hiram. This was nearly nine years ago in Philadelphia. At that time, our own understanding of the care of new mothers was vague, and our friends, who were then new to macrobiotics, had an even vaguer idea. Both baby and I were too yang, and I remained feeling weak for quite a while. Hiram was picked up the very instant he began screaming, and he began screaming, always, the very instant he was put down. As his first teeth began showing I tried feeding him grain milk but in vain. He refused. As more and more teeth came in, he refused and refused. When he was nearly a year old he was still refusing. We went to my parents' house, and when I thought that he was getting hungry, I would disappear. When he got very, very hungry, without me, he accepted the grain milk from my mother and became used to eating. At the age of one year, he was weaned. First he ate strained grain liquids that were gradually thickened, and mashed vegetables, Eventually he could eat soft whole grains, whole soft vegetables, a little weak *miso* soup, and some noodles. He received a little fruit. Later I realized that I caused him to become somewhat too yang.

Soon after Hiram was weaned the second child was conceived. That was a happy realization. During this pregnancy my appetite was great. I wanted to eat everything: rice, vegetables, sea vegetables, *miso* soup, fish, fruit, and some non-macrobiotic foods. This baby too was in a posterior position but turned during birth. At midnight some amniotic fluid began leaking. Labor began. As with Hiram I was again at Booth Maternity Hospital (where natural childbearing is respected). But labor stopped completely. As the hours went, the midwives became worried. Finally the doctor came and told us that if labor did not continue, she would have to induce labor, for fear of infection (since the water, somewhat, seemed to have broken.) We discovered the existence of an herb used by Indians—birthroot. A friend quickly brewed some and brought it to me. It worked exactly as the textbook said it should. Joseph was born. This time baby and I had the best care. A Japanese friend looked after us. She would not permit anyone to see me (except for husband and parents). She would scold me if I did anything, move out of bed or even read. Daily she would come to tidy the room, wash the floor, open the windows. She would bathe the baby, taking care not to rub off the protective film that coats the skin after birth. Each day she would bring hot water and a washcloth, sponge bathe the whole body lightly, and bring a clean gown. The hair would be unbraided and rebraided neatly, without brushing (so as not to stimulate the head and thereby cause upward movement of *ki* and blood). The bed would be remade. All this for two complete weeks.

All these small and simple attentions made a great difference in making the two weeks pleasant and more easily tolerable. After this care, there was a feeling of newness and brightness. A stronger and steadier condition. The baby was much calmer than the first baby.

The baby exhibited the same appetite that I had while carrying him. He ate everything eagerly. He loved plain grain milk and vegetables when the time came for them, etc. But this time, grain sweeteners such as barley malt or yinnie syrup entered the baby's diet. This baby never could have constant and immediate attention, since his older brother was too demanding and also since our lifestyle became more demanding. He very quickly learned to cry only when hungry or wet, or if something was really wrong with him. He grew to be content with whatever he had and was also very patient.

We were very happy again when the next baby was conceived. This was now after years of macrobiotic living. My appetite now was much more simple and there was no need for extremes.

Labor began during an East West Foundation meeting in Philadelphia. While timing contractions it was still possible to participate in the meeting. All ladies present noticed and understood. But my husband didn't have a clue. After the meeting I asked him to drive me to the hospital. He looked both puzzled and annoyed. The girls were laughing and impatient, calling to him to get moving. Finally and reluctantly he understood. No sooner did we arrive than the baby began making its way into the world and soon easily entered it. This one was our daughter Naomi. With proper care and rest we were both comfortable and strong.

The food was carefully prepared, appropriate for the occasion. Again *koi-koku* was made from a whole, fresh carp and burdock. However, this time we found it too yang and so I ate only one bowl and after that had it in small quantities diluted in light *miso* soup. There was *azuki* bean rice with vegetable *tempura* for good milk, *mochi* in soup, plenty of fresh greens, sea vegetables, root vegetables, etc. Plain *kanten* with *tamari* soy sauce and a ginger and scallion dip seems helpful in easing the mother's bowel movements right after delivery.

Fruits were avoided, but when there was need, *bancha* tea with a small amount of barley malt was helpful or very light *kuzu* drink with just a hint of sweetness.

Before continuing, I would like to pause and consider the importance of proper rest and care after childbearing. Mothers who rise from bed soon after having given birth often find that they have an amazing surge of energy. In fact, it is so great that they lose control of it and themselves, run about frantically, and are unable to cease. Their bodies, on the other hand, are frail from the great exertion of giving birth and adjusting to the process of nursing. It is as though they are flooded by a surge of energy too great for the now somewhat fragile frame. This leads to a weakening of one's condition, a high pitched nervousness, and can lead even to the loss of milk. Even while resting in bed, if one begins to talk and goes on, she becomes overly excited and cannot rest again, cannot sleep, etc. Even thoughts can run away into a frantic pace, unless deliberately calmed. It seems that there is a great power, at that time, deep within the body. It will stay there and heal, if it remains untapped and undisturbed, and will restore the body to a sound and strong condition, with the help of proper food. Then the baby receives a better quality of milk and is also healthier and happier. Women who do not follow the macrobiotic way are encouraged by their doctors to move and exercise right after delivery, for danger of blood clots. Macrobiotic women, all over the world, have proven different, as their conditions are different.

These two weeks of rest are well worth taking advantage of, as they are likely to be a mother's only opportunity for thorough rest in a long time to follow.

At this time our children are eight, six, and four years old. At home they eat a lot of rice but love noodles best. They will eat *miso* soup only if it is light and sweet. They like only lightly cooked vegetables, especially when boiled with *kombu*. Beans they love excessively at times, but avoid completely at other times. *Natto*, *tempeh*, *tofu*, *seitan*—they will eat whenever in front of them.

Sometimes a child will refuse everything but one food. Whether it is only rice or only vegetables, if the child is allowed to follow his own appetite, he will soon seek to balance himself. Sometimes however a child may refuse all vegetables, etc. from having become too yang. Then the mother needs to be ingenious and invent ways and tricks to make him eat something to change his direction. Once the child begins to eat more yin food, he will follow eagerly of his own accord.

Unintentionally and unknowingly we may make mistakes. With young children especially, we must keep our eyes open. They are wholly dependent on what we give to them, and their ability to balance by their own choices depends on the range of foods and the variety we make available to them. However, children often make themselves unbalanced if they are too free to choose since their judgment is often sensory.

In every way, our children make us grow wiser.

Tonia Gagne, Brookline, Massachusetts

In the early 1970's, nineteen-year-old Tonia Gagne was diagnosed as having endo-metriosis, a disease that results from an implantation of tissue within the walls of the uterus and around the ovaries and intestines. She had just had a baby, which she gave up for adoption, and soon after began to have a profuse vaginal dis-charge and agonizing cramps. Following two months in the hospital, she had her left ovary and Fallopian tube surgically removed. Doctors put her on hormonal therapy and prescribed Enovid-10. As a result of taking this pill three times a day for nine months, her hair began to fall out and her mental state, already fragile, deteriorated.

In 1973 Tonia went to live at the Zen Center in San Francisco, and meditation helped center her life. A friend introduced her to macrobiotics and the principles of ecological cooking. Nevertheless, Tonia, whose ancestry was partly Puerto Rican, was still attracted to some of the tropical food on which she grew up. "One of the things I loved was fried bananas," she said, looking back on this time in her life. "When I was told that if I wanted to practice macrobiotics correctly, I would have to give up fried bananas, I said, 'Oh no, not that.' " She included some brown rice, miso soup, and vegetables in her diet but continued to eat dairy food, sugar, and fried bananas. She went off Enovid-10, but her health continued to worsen.

In April 1976, Tonia returned to New England, and doctors at South Boston Community Center told her that the endometriosis had come back. Medical tests showed that she also had uterine cysts, and her right ovary had swollen to the size of a tennis ball. The doctors told her they would have to operate and she would never be able to have children again.

Tonia decided against the operation and moved into a macrobiotic study house where trained cooks prepared a special diet for her condition. Within three months on balanced food and no fried bananas, the cyst had disappeared. Over the next year her health improved, but the vaginal discharge persisted, and she still suffered from occasional cramps. In August 1977, Tonia and her new husband came to see me at the East West Foundation's summer program in Amherst.

"I sat down with Michio and he looked at my left hand and my left foot," she noted afterward. "He looked into my eyes and examined my face and then he said to me, 'You have no left ovary, right? Also, right ovary not so good, right? Also, tumor in your descending colon.' Then he looked at me and said, 'Maybe you have cancer.' "

I took out a piece of paper and drew a diagram describing the exact proportions of food she should be eating. I told her to eat 60 percent whole-cereal grains, the rest cooked vegetables, miso soup, various condiments, and to avoid all animal products, especially dairy food and meat. I told her to eliminate all oil, flour products, and fruits from her diet until her condition improved and to take regular hip baths in daikon leaves and to apply a plaster of taro potato over her repro-ductive organs to loosen the accumulation of fat and mucus.

"Within two weeks after I started that diet," Tonia reported, "the pain subsided. I had a feeling of elation. My energy came back and a lot of worry was gone."

During the next two years, Tonia had to eat very strictly. Even the slightest deviation, such as an occasional peanutbutter cookie or a carob brownie, would bring back the pain, cramps, and other symptoms of endometriosis. Gradually, however, she began to enjoy macrobiotic cooking and adjusted to living in a temperate climate without eating bananas and other tropical foods. About seven months after she began to practice the diet correctly, she became pregnant. Six weeks after giving birth to her son, Taran, she underwent a full examination by her physician. Medical tests showed no sign of endometriosis.

"Now I find myself much happier and more fulfilled," Tonia concluded several years after fully restoring her health. "Macrobiotics isn't any kind of religion or belief system. I had thought that macrobiotics would take the fun out of my life, but instead, I have learned to have more fun. I've learned balance. My life (and sense of enjoyment) is much simpler and much more fulfilling than I have ever before felt."

In January 1981, Tonia gave birth to a second child by natural childbirth at her home and experienced no complications. For a woman who was told she would never have children again, Tonia has become a living example of faith in the healing powers of nature. A balanced diet is the birthright of us all.

Sources: "Endometriosis and Tumor in the Colon," *The Cancer Prevention Diet* (Brookline, Mass.: East West Foundation, 1981, pp. 90–91), Tom Monte, "Journey to Motherhood: Tonia's Triumph Over Illness and Infertility," *East West Journal*, March 1982, pp. 44–48, and Michio Kushi and Alex Jack, *The Cancer Prevention Diet* (New York: St. Martin's Press, 1983, pp. 184–186).

Carolyne Cesari, Brookline, Massachusetts

A few years ago on a rainy Monday in upstate New York Carolyne Cesari heard her doctor say, "Carolyne, your condition could be fatal unless you have a hysterectomy. I've scheduled the operation for Thursday." In less than four days, 24-year-old Carolyne was slated to join the annual three-quarter million American women who have their wombs (and often their ovaries and Fallopian tubes as well) surgically removed.

Exploratory surgery a week earlier had revealed a massive abscess which had not only damaged her uterus but parts of her intestines as well. The surgery followed weeks of pain and inflammation caused by an IUD. Now, as she was still experiencing pain, the physician insisted on the necessity of a hysterectomy.

"I refused to sign a waiver during the exploratory surgery which would have given the doctors permission to take out whatever they wanted." Carolyne recalled while breast-feeding Charles, her handsome little boy born less than two years after the scheduled hysterectomy. "I really wanted to have children and had to find an alternative to the operation."

Carolyne was already accustomed to looking for alternatives to conventional medical treatment. From the age of seventeen, she had suffered from rheumatoid arthritis, a painful and debilitating disease, from which both her mother and grandmother also suffered.

"The pain was so bad I'd wake up in the mornings crying," Carolyne told me. "I couldn't even stand the weight of the bedsheets on my knees." She often required codeine or morphine to get through the day, as well as twice-weekly injections to control the pain and swelling in her legs. The medication made her stomach bleed, and left her dizzy and in a mental fog. Once Carolyne had to be hospitalized because she contracted hepatitis from a needle used during a blood test to measure the effects of her medication.

One particular visit to her doctor, however, proved far more positive than any she had known. In the waiting room she happened upon a medical journal advocating a dietary approach to rheumatoid arthritis. The author advised eliminating red meat, coffee, sugar, and chocolate in order to control the disease. Encouraged by her physician, Carolyne embarked on what at the time seemed like a bold experiment—she stopped eating beef.

"The bedsheets stopped bothering me almost immediately. Within a month 50 percent of the pain had gone away." Encouraged, she gave up all meat, coffee, and sugar. The last item to go was her favorite, chocolate. Within three months, she was totally free of pain.

The new vegetarian steadily improved until several years later when she had an IUD inserted. Her complaints of discomfort were dismissed by her physician as simply abdominal pain; he even refused to remove the offending IUD. Later, the contraceptive device was removed, but damage and infection had already set in. A trusted gray-haired gynecologist, whom she had known for years, examined her and insisted on exploratory surgery. He wanted permission to remove whatever was necessary once he was inside. Carolyne refused.

"In my 35 years of operating, I've never seen a woman's insides look so bad," he told her the day after the operation. "If the pain returns, we'll have no choice but to perform a hysterectomy." He was leaving for a vacation and directed Carolyne to see his associate should any emergency situation develop.

Out of the hospital, Carolyne was in pain again. She avoided the associate and found another physician whom she hoped would offer a less final second opinion. His verdict, however, was the same. Surgery would have to be performed.

Carolyne protested that she wanted to have children. "It is very unlikely that you could, you are scarred so badly," the gynecologist told her, perhaps attempting to minimize her sense of loss at the impending operation.

The next morning, following a friend's advice, Carolyne flew to Boston for a macrobiotic consultation. She met Edward Esko, a macrobiotic counselor, who recommended that she eat a diet of pressure-cooked whole grains, three different types of beans, lightly steamed vegetables, and a sea vegetable condiment. She had to strictly avoid fish, flour products, oil, and nuts as well as dairy foods. In addition to the dietary recommendations, Esko told her to make a compress from taro potato, and apply it to the area of her surgery.

That night Carolyne peeled the hairy skin from the taro and mashed the sticky potato into a poultice. She pressed it across her pelvic area, and carefully covered it with a gauze bandage. She then fell into an exhausted sleep, until a strange smell interrupted her slumber. "I reached over to the night table and smelled the unused portion of the taro. It was clean and still had a slightly perfumed scent. I then opened the gauze and took the plaster off. It had turned black, was filled with pus, and had a decaying smell."

Her condition began to improve dramatically. She returned home, free of fears of surgery, but uncertain about the basics of macrobiotic cooking. Her roommates, however, supported Carolyne in her early efforts at cooking.

She began taking classes from Kay Dara in nearby Syracuse and both her cooking and health continued to improve. She also met Bob Cesari, a jazz musician and longtime student of macrobiotics. They fell in love, were married, and Carolyne then became pregnant.

Carolyne, Bob, and Charles now live in Boston and during most of her pregnancy Carolyne worked and studied at the Kushi Institute. Her midwife recalls that delivering Charles was exceedingly easy. The Cesaris are a healthy-looking family, full of joyful energy. Charles's birth and Carolyne's narrow escape from surgery stand in sharp contrast to the fate of most American women scheduled for hysterectomy, and serve as a reminder that alternatives to "the knife" do exist.

Source: "Escape from Hysterectomy, by Carolyne Cesari and Steve Minkin, *East West Journal*, October, 1983, pp. 47–48.

❀|Classes and Pregnancy Counseling

Further information on the macrobiotic approach to pregnancy, childbirth and childcare can be obtained from **The East West Foundation**, a non-profit institution established in 1972. The East West Foundation, and its seven major affiliates or regional offices around the country, offer ongoing classes for the general public in macrobiotic cooking, pregnancy and prenatal care, natural birth, and care of the newborn. They also provide pregnancy and dietary counseling services with trained consultants and referrals to pediatricians, nurse-midwives, and other professional health care associates. There are also **Macrobiotics International** and **East West Centers** in Canada, Mexico, Latin America, Europe, the Middle East, Africa, Asia, and Australia. The whole foods and naturally processed items described in this book are available at thousands of natural foods and health food stores, as well as a growing number of supermarkets. The macrobiotic speciality items are also available by mail order from various distributors and retailers.

Contact the Boston office for further information on any of the above services or whole foods outlets in your area.

BOSTON HEADQUARTERS:
Macrobiotics International and
The East West Foundation
17 Station St.
Brookline, MA 02147
(617) 731–0564

Baltimore
4803 Yellowwood Rd.
Baltimore, MD 21209
(301) 367–6655

California
708 N. Orange Grove Ave.
Hollywood, CA 90046
(213) 651–5491

Colorado
1931 Mapleton Ave.
Boulder, CO 80302
(303) 449–6754

Connecticut
184 East Main St.
Middletown, CT 06457
(203) 344–0090

Illinois
1574 Asbury Ave.
Evanston, IL 60201
(312) 328–6632

Philadelphia
606 S. Ninth St.
Philadelphia, PA 19147
(215) 922–4567

Washington, D.C.
Box 40012
Washington, DC 20016
(301) 897–8352

For those who wish to study further, the Kushi Institute, an educational institution founded in Boston in 1979 with affiliates in London, Amsterdam, and Antwerp, offers full- and part-time instruction for individuals who wish to become macrobiotic teachers and counselors. **The Kushi Institute** publishes a *Macrobiotic Teachers and Counselors Directory*, listing graduates who are qualified to offer guidance in the macrobiotic approach to health. The Cook Instructor Service is an extension of the Kushi Institute and is comprised of specially qualified graduates of the Institute's advanced cooking program. These men and women are available to assist individuals and families in learning the basics of macrobiotic food preparation and home care in their own home.

> **Kushi Institute and Cook Instructor Service**
> Box 1100
> Brookline, MA 02147
> (617) 731–0564

Ongoing developments are reported in the Kushi Foundation's periodicals, including the *East West Journal* (*EWJ*), a monthly magazine begun in 1971 and now with an international readership of 200,000. The *EWJ* features regular articles on the macrobiotic approach to health and nutrition, as well as ecology, science, psychology, the arts, and pregnancy, natural birth, and childcare.

> ***East West Journal***
> 17 Station St.
> Brookline, MA 02147
> (617) 232–1000

✵|Bibliography

Books

Aihara, Cornellia, *The Do of Cooking*, Chico, Calif.: George Ohsawa Macrobiotic Foundation, 1972.

——, *Macrobiotic Childcare*, Oroville, Calif.: George Ohsawa Macrobiotic Foundation, 1971.

Child Health Encyclopedia, Boston: The Boston Children's Medical Center, 1975.

Dick-Read Grantly, M. D., *Childbirth Without Fear*, New York: Harper and Row, 1944.

Dietary Goals for the United States, Washington, D. C.: Select Committee on Nutrition and Human Needs, U.S. Senate, 1977.

Diet, Nutrition, and Cancer, Washington, D. C.: National Academy of Sciences, 1982.

Dufty, William, *Sugar Blues*, New York: Warner, 1975.

Esko, Edward and Wendy, *Macrobiotic Cooking for Everyone*, Tokyo: Japan Publications, 1980.

Esko, Wendy, *Introducing Macrobiotic Cooking*, Tokyo: Japan Publications, 1978.

Feinberg, Alice, *Macrobiotic Pregnancy*, Oroville, Calif.: George Ohsawa Macrobiotic Foundation, 1973.

Fukuoka, Masanobu, *The One-Straw Revolution*, Emmaus, Pa.: Rodale Press, 1978.

Gilbert, Margaret Shea, *Biography of the Unborn*, New York: Hajner Press, 1962.

Healthy People: The Surgeon General's Report on Health Promotion and Disease Prevention, Washington, D. C.: Government Printing Office, 1979.

Hippocrates, *Hippocratic Writings*, edited by G. E. R. Lloyd, translated by J. Chadwick and W. N. Mann, New York: Penguin Books, 1978.

I Ching or *Book of Changes*, translated by Richard Wilhelm and Cary F. Baynes, Princeton: Bollingen Foundation, 1950.

Jacobson, Michael, *The Changing American Diet*, Washington, D. C.: Center for Science in the Public Interest, 1978.

Kohler, Jean and Mary Alice, *Healing Miracles from Macrobiotics*, West Nyack, N. Y.: Parker, 1979.

Kushi, Aveline, *How to Cook with Miso*, Tokyo: Japan Publications, 1978.

Kushi, Aveline and Wendy Esko, *The Changing Seasons Macrobiotic Cookbook*, Wayne, N. J.: Avery Publishing Group, 1983.

Kushi, Aveline with Alex Jack, *The Joy of Macrobiotic Cooking*, New York: Warner, 1984.

Kushi, Michio, *The Book of Do-In: Exercise for Physical and Spiritual Development*, Tokyo: Japan Publications, 1979.

——, *The Book of Macrobiotics*, Tokyo: Japan Publications, 1977.

————, *Cancer and Heart Disease: The Macrobiotic Approach to Degenerative Disorders*, Tokyo: Japan Publications, 1982.

————, *The Era of Humanity*, Brookline, Mass.: East West Journal, 1980.

————, *How to See Your Health: The Book of Oriental Diagnosis*, Tokyo: Japan Publications, 1980.

————, *Natural Healing Through Macrobiotics*, Tokyo: Japan Publications, 1978.

————, *Your Face Never Lies*, Wayne, N. J.: Avery Publishing Group, 1983.

Kushi, Michio and Alex Jack, *The Cancer Prevention Diet*, New York: St. Martin's Press, 1983.

————, *Diet for a Strong Heart*, New York: St. Martin's Press, 1984.

Kushi, Michio and the East West Foundation, *The Macrobiotic Approach to Cancer*, Wayne, N. J.: Avery Publishing Group, 1982.

Mendelsohn, Robert S., M. D., *Confessions of a Medical Heretic*, Chicago: Contemporary Books, 1979.

————, *Male Practice*, Chicago: Contemporary Books, 1980.

Ohsawa, George, *Cancer and the Philosophy of the Far East*, Oroville, Calif.: George Ohsawa Macrobiotic Foundation, 1971 edition.

————, *You Are All Sanpaku*, edited by William Dufty, New York: University Books, 1965.

————, *Zen Macrobiotics*, Los Angeles: Ohsawa Foundation, 1965.

Pregnancy, Birth and the Newborn Baby, Boston: The Boston Children's Medical Center, 1972.

Price, Weston, A., D. D. S., *Nutrition and Physical Degeneration*, Santa Monica, Calif.: Price-Pottenger Nutritional Foundation, 1945.

Pryor, Karen, *Nursing Your Baby*, New York: Harper and Row, 1973.

Sattilaro, Anthony, M. D. with Tom Monte, *Recalled by Life: The Story of My Recovery from Cancer*, Boston: Houghton-Mifﬂn, 1982.

Yamamoto, Shizuko, *Barefoot Shiatsu*, Tokyo: Japan Publications, 1979.

The Yellow Emperor's Classic of Internal Medicine, translated by Ilza Veith, Berkeley: University of California Press, 1949.

Periodicals

East West Journal, Brookline, Mass.

Macromuse, Washington, D. C.

Nutrition Action, Washington, D. C.

"The People's Doctor" by Robert S. Mendelsohn, M. D. and Marian Tompson, Evanston, Ill.

❋| About the Authors and Editors

Michio Kushi was born in Kokawa, Wakayama Prefecture, Japan in 1926. His early years were devoted to the study of international law at the University of Tokyo, and an active interest in world peace through world federal government in the period following the Second World War. In the course of pursuing these interests, he encountered Yukikazu Sakurazawa (known in the West as George Ohsawa), who had revised and reintroduced the principles of Oriental medicine and philosophy under the name "macrobiotics." Inspired by Mr. Ohsawa's teaching, Mr. Kushi began his lifelong study of the application of traditional understanding to solving the problems of the modern world.

Mr. Kushi came to the United States more than thirty years ago to pursue graduate studies at Columbia University. Since that time he has lectured on Oriental medicine, philosophy, culture and macrobiotics throughout North and South America, Europe and the Far East; he has also given numerous seminars on macrobiotics and Oriental medicine for medical professionals and personal counseling for individuals and families. While establishing himself as the world's foremost authority on the macrobiotic approach, he has guided thousands of people to restore their physical, psychological and spiritual health and well-being as a fundamental means of achieving world peace. He has also presented an address to a special White House meeting and two addresses to the delegates of the United Nations on the applications of macrobiotic principles to world problems.

Mr. Kushi is founder and president of the East West Foundation, a federally-approved, nonprofit, cultural and educational organization, established in Boston in 1972 to help develop and spread all aspects of the macrobiotic way of life through seminars, publications, research, and other means. He is also the founder of Erewhon, Inc. the leading distributor of natural and macrobiotic foods in North America, and of the monthly *East West Journal* and the quarterly *Order of the Universe* periodicals. In 1978 Mr. and Mrs. Kushi founded the Kushi Institute of Boston, an educational institution for the training of macrobiotic teachers and practitioners, with affiliates in London, Antwerp, and Amsterdam; and at the same time, as a further means toward addressing world problems, established the annual Macrobiotic Congresses of North America and Western Europe. A nonprofit organization, the Kushi Foundation, was established in 1981 to assist with the coordination of educational and research activities.

Mr. Kushi's published works presently include *Natural Healing through Macrobiotics*, *The Book of Macrobiotics*, *The Book of Dō-In*, *How to See Your Health*, *Oriental Diagnosis*, *Visions of a New World: The Era of Humanity*, and *The Cancer Prevention Diet*. Mr. Kushi presently resides in Brookline, Massachusetts, with his wife Aveline, children and grandchildren.

Aveline Kushi was born in 1923 in Yokata, Shimane Prefecture, Japan. She taught elementary school, junior high, and kindergarten after graduating from Teacher's College in 1944. Aveline began her lifelong study of macrobiotics in 1950 under the guidance of George Ohsawa and came to the United States the following year. She married Michio Kushi in 1952 and began to teach macrobiotic and natural food cooking in New York soon afterward.

Michio and Aveline moved to Boston in 1965 and together sponsored a variety of enterprises and educational institutions, including Erewhon, one of the leading distributors of natural and macrobiotic foods in the world, several macrobiotic and natural food restaurants, including Open Sesame, the *East West Journal* monthly, the East West Foundation, the Kushi Institute, and the Kushi Foundation. Aveline's classes in macrobiotic cooking, pregnancy, childbirth and childcare, and other subjects have attracted students from all over the world, and since 1974, she has presented international seminars with her husband in England, France, Denmark, Holland, Belgium, Germany, Italy, Spain, Portugal, Austria, Switzerland, Ireland, Costa Rica, Brazil, Hong-Kong, and her native Japan.

Aveline is the mother of five children—Lilian, Norio, Haruo, Yoshio, and Hisao—and the grandmother of three. She lives in Brookline, Massachusetts, and teaches regularly in addition to traveling, writing, and other activities. She is the author of *How to Cook with Miso* and the *Changing Seasons Macrobiotic Cookbook*, and is presently writing a comprehensive cookbook to be published in 1984.

Edward and Wendy Esko have authored or edited numerous books and publications on the macrobiotic approach, including *Introducing Macrobiotic Cooking, Macrobiotic Cooking for Everyone*, the *Changing Seasons Macrobiotic Cookbook*, and *Natural Healing through Macrobiotics*. They live with their four children in Brookline, Massachusetts and teach at the Kushi Institute, as well as throughout the United States and internationally.

✳ | Index